DISABILITY RIGHTS AND WRONGS REVISITED

In the past forty years, the field of disability studies has emerged from the political activism of disabled people. In this challenging review of the field, leading disability academic and activist Tom Shakespeare argues that disability research needs a firmer conceptual and empirical footing.

This new edition is updated throughout, reflecting Shakespeare's most recent thinking, drawing on current research, and responding to controversies surrounding the first edition and the *World Report on Disability*, as well as incorporating new chapters on cultural disability studies, personal assistance, sexuality, and violence. Using a critical realist approach, *Disability Rights and Wrongs Revisited* promotes a pluralist, engaged and nuanced approach to disability. Key topics discussed include:

- dichotomies – going beyond dangerous polarizations such as medical model versus social model to achieve a complex, multi-factorial account of disability
- identity – the drawbacks of the disability movement's emphasis on identity politics
- bioethics – choices at the beginning and end of life and in the field of genetic and stem cell therapies
- relationships – feminist and virtue ethics approaches to questions of intimacy, assistance and friendship.

This stimulating and accessible book challenges disability studies orthodoxy, promoting a new conceptualization of disability and fresh research agenda. It is an invaluable resource for researchers and students in disability studies and sociology, as well as professionals, policy makers and activists.

Tom Shakespeare is a Senior Lecturer in Medical Sociology at the University of East Anglia, UK. He was until recently a member of the Disability and Rehabilitation team at WHO, where he was an author and editor of the *World Report on Disability*. He has previously held academic posts at the Universities of Sunderland, Leeds and Newcastle.

'*Disability Rights and Wrongs Revisited* is an enormously important book for anyone who wants to understand what disability studies has already achieved, what it has failed to achieve, and what it should aspire to achieve in the future. Tom Shakespeare's writing is irreverent, clear, and wise.'

Dr Erik Parens, Senior Research Scholar, The Hastings Center, USA

'In this thoughtful and insightful book, Tom Shakespeare, a leading scholar, brings together current arguments and emerging concerns to review where disability studies now stands, how the field arrived at this point, and where it might – and should – go in future. Applying a disability perspective to some of the key ethical issues of our time – from prenatal diagnosis to personal relationships, violence to end of life choices, Dr Shakespeare raises as many intriguing questions as he answers. The result is an engaging and important contribution to the literature that should be required reading for anyone interested in disability studies, in ethics and in human rights.'

Professor Nora Ellen Groce, Director, Leonard Cheshire Disability & Inclusive Development Centre, University College London, UK

'The first edition of *Disability Rights and Wrongs* rapidly became a must-read text for any scholar interested in disability. This updated and substantially reworked edition is sure to be as influential and as important. By critically engaging with much of the recent literature in disability studies it consolidates and develops the arguments found in the first edition. The book argues that if we are to understand fully what disability is and what it means we have to adopt a broad approach. It also foregrounds the importance of social relationships and the book challenges us to understand the social, cultural and biomedical aspects of disability.'

Professor Nick Watson, Strathclyde Centre for Disability Research, University of Glasgow, UK.

DISABILITY RIGHTS AND WRONGS REVISITED

Second edition

Tom Shakespeare

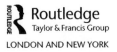

Routledge
Taylor & Francis Group

LONDON AND NEW YORK

First edition published 2006
by Routledge
This edition published 2014
by Routledge
2 Park Square, Milton Park, Abingdon, Oxon, OX14 4RN

and by Routledge
711 Third Avenue, New York, NY 10017

Routledge is an imprint of the Taylor & Francis Group, an informa business

British Library Cataloguing in Publication Data
A catalogue record for this book is available from the British Library

Library of Congress Cataloging-in-Publication Data
Shakespeare, Tom, 1966-
Disability rights and wrongs revisited / Tom Shakespeare.
pages cm.
Updated edition of the author's Disability rights and wrongs.
1. Disability studies. 2. Sociology of disability. 3. People with disabilities. I. Title.
HV1568.2.S53 2013
305.9'08--dc23
2013013948

ISBN13: 978-0-415-52760-6 (hbk)
ISBN13: 978-0-415-52761-3 (pbk)
ISBN13: 978-1-315-88745-6 (ebk)

Typeset in Bembo
by Taylor and Francis Books

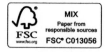

MIX
Paper from
responsible sources
FSC
www.fsc.org   FSC® C013056

Printed and bound in Great Britain by
TJ International Ltd, Padstow, Cornwall

Dedicated to Ivy and Robert

CONTENTS

ACKNOWLEDGEMENTS

As well as those people thanked in the first edition of the book, I would like to acknowledge the support and advice of Halvor Hanisch, Chris Mikton, Alana Officer, Sashka Posarac, Rannveig Traustadóttir, Simo Vehmas, and Nick Watson and apologise to any colleagues who may feel bruised by their academic encounters with me.

1

INTRODUCTION

This book is my attempt to offer a chart, a better way for disability studies. While I value the achievements that have been won through the close alliance of disability politics and disability research, I think that disability studies has failed to balance the demands of radical social change and intellectual rigour. Translation of ideas and ideologies from activism to academia has not been accompanied by a sufficient process of self-criticism, testing and empirical verification. The British materialist tradition in disability studies that has successfully inspired generations of activists has not translated into an adequate body of good empirical research, perhaps partly because of the reliance on an overly narrow and reductionist conception of disability. Meanwhile, it is my view that the cultural version of disability studies, which also espouses political commitment, has become fatally contaminated by post-structuralist and post-modernist theory, and thus failed to provide helpful analysis or evidence.

It is vital to state that in rejecting the 'strong' social model of disability, I am not rejecting the human rights approach to disability (UN, 2006). Many activists and writers appear to believe that the materialist social model is the only appropriate or effective analysis or definition of disability. There seems to have been an assumption that without the 'strong' social model, there can be no political progress and no social movement of disabled people. If I believed that this was the case, it would be very much more difficult for me to suggest that the social model should be revised.

In the first edition of this book, I demonstrated that the 'strong' social model is not the only progressive account of disability, and explained how there is a family of social approaches to disability, of which the British social model is just one example: others include the North American minority group approach, the social constructionist approach, the Nordic relational model. All of these approaches reject an individualist understanding of disability, and to different extents locate the disabled person in a broader context. To varying degrees, each of these approaches shares a basic political commitment to improving the lives of disabled people, by promoting social inclusion and removing the barriers that oppress disabled people.

In the first edition, I also demonstrated how the term 'medical model' is often used as a slur word (Kelly and Field, 1994: 35), concealing the many examples of empirical research within medical sociology and social policy which have made space for environmental and social factors in the construction of disability (Goffman, 1968a, 1968b; Safilios-Rothschild, 1970; Albrecht, 1976; Blaxter, 1976; Carver and Rodda, 1978; Laura, 1980; Locker, 1983; Marinelli and Dell Orto, 1984; Stone, 1984; Hedlund, 2000; see also the discussion in Noreau and Boschen 2010). Even the WHO's International Classification of Impairments, Disability and Health (ICIDH) was originally an attempt to shift emphasis away from the medical diagnosis towards the social consequences of impairment (Bury, 2000).

The first edition of this book was my attempt to offer a way beyond the impasse of 'social creationist' disability studies. While I valued the achievements that have been won through the close alliance of disability politics and disability research, I suggested that the weaknesses of the British approach outweighed the benefits. In this edition of the book, I also look at a 'social constructionist' approach, which emerges from the academic work of disabled and non-disabled scholars. Rather than the Marxist theory which underpins the work of Mike Oliver, Colin Barnes and others in the British social model tradition – which in this new edition I am labelling materialist disability studies – the Critical Disability Studies approach is more likely to draw on post-structuralist and post-modernist philosophers such as Michel Foucault, Judith Butler, and Gilles Deleuze and Félix Guettari. This approach to disability often takes a step back from the political commitments of the social model tradition, to explore cultural representations and the role of discourse. Scholars sometimes appear more concerned with deconstructing the category of disability or intellectual disability than in changing the social conditions of disabled people or people with learning difficulties. Responding to the theoretical deficits which I, among others, identified (Shakespeare, 1999b), these scholars have been active in building disability studies as a discipline within academia, particularly in the

North American humanities field. I will argue that Cultural Disability Studies is over-theoretical and does not offer much in the way of practical help in understanding the lives of disabled people, let alone changing them for the better. While there are some interesting examples of empirical social research coming out of this tradition, particularly in Europe, I question whether this approach can advance policy and practice in disability. When it comes to theory, my motto is taken from William of Ockham: 'Do not multiply entities unnecessarily', or alternatively, as Einstein once said, 'Make everything as simple as possible, but not simpler.'

The disability rights movement has gone through different phases, since its origins in the 1970s. For the first decade, it was primarily an oppositional force, criticising the status quo, and calling for barrier removal and social inclusion. In the second decade, the formation of the Independent Living Fund in 1988, the shift to community care in the early 1990s, and the passing of the Community Care (Direct Payments) Act 1996 not only enabled more disabled people to live in their communities, it also led the disability movement to respond by becoming a major service provider in many localities, as far afield as Avon and Norfolk. Meanwhile, the Disability Discrimination Acts of 1995 and 2005 meant that public buildings and transport services became far more accessible. Now with the global financial crisis and the advent of a deficit-reducing Conservative–Liberal Democrat government, austerity has led to cutbacks in both welfare benefits and services, which have often appeared deliberately to be targeted at disabled people (Strathclyde Centre for Disability Research and Glasgow Media Unit 2012, www.wearespartacus.org.uk 2012). The few thousand activists in the core disability movement have not appeared greatly to renew or revise their analysis or ideology during this period, although there have been generational changes as key individuals have retired or died. The 'strong' social model that I criticised in the first edition of this book still seems to hold sway. Indeed, the crude dichotomies of the British social model have also strongly influenced international thinking on disability, as expressed, for example, in the UN Convention on the Rights of Persons with Disabilities (UN, 2006).

Over the same period, I and others have been writing and talking about the need for a new approach to understanding disability, which enables research and practice to progress, forms new alliances, and advances an agenda of disability equality. This work has been controversial. However, I suspect that there is support and agreement and interest in new approaches from many quarters, and therefore I have tried to consolidate my ideas and work in different fields in the current volume. The resulting book brings together two decades' worth of thinking and talking about disability, bioethics and care. It represents my attempt to establish a balanced, rational and coherent analysis of disability, based on a critical realist approach that will be of value to practitioners, researchers, and disabled people themselves. I have particularly tried to ensure that issues concerning people with learning difficulties are not ignored (Chappell, 1998).

The book draws on my experiences of being a disabled person, and the son, father, husband and friend of disabled people. It has been influenced by my personal experience of disabled people's organisations and other voluntary organisations. The book draws on qualitative research I have conducted over the past decade, as well as the wealth of research on disability within disability studies and medical sociology. In first writing, and subsequently revising this book, I have tried to ground my discussions in the available empirical research evidence at all times. Too often, disability studies is not grounded in an adequate understanding of what I call 'actually existing disability', which means comprehending both the diversity of illness and impairment experiences and contexts, and the breadth of everyday life. Discussions with philosophers and professionals have also been very valuable to me in shaping my ideas. The resulting book therefore reflects an interdisciplinary perspective, drawing on sociology, social policy, social work, philosophy, psychology and development studies. I have tried to be scholarly, but also to orient the discussion towards politics and policy, with a view to supporting progressive social changes that benefit disabled people and their families. The target audience includes disabled people and those who work with them, as well as academics and policy-makers. I have tried to write clearly and accessibly, with a view to helping non-academics think deeper about questions that matter in their lives, as well as contributing to a reinvigorated and empirically-based disability studies.

Outline of the book

Part I, 'Foundations', tries to establish some firm foundations for understanding disability. I think it is reasonable to suggest that there are currently at least four approaches to disability on offer within the social sciences. First, there is the sociology of chronic illness. Helpfully, Carol Thomas (1999, 2007, 2012) has explored this tradition in some depth. Although I do not fully accept her critique of medical sociology, I do not want to repeat her good work, and I do not have space to discuss this literature here. Second, there is the social model-inspired British materialist tradition, exemplified by the work of Michael Oliver and Colin Barnes and Carol Thomas. Third, there are the various approaches that emphasise discourse and the role of culture, which I have labelled 'cultural disability studies'. These include the dominant North American disability studies authors, recent arrivals such as Rob McRuer and Fiona Kumari Campbell, and also authors who propose the term 'Critical Disability Studies' for their approach, such as Dan Goodley, Helen Meekosha and Russell Shuttleworth. These authors 'trouble' the category of disability, and emphasise the role of discourse rather more than the impact of material forces. Reviewers suggested that I devote attention to them in the second edition, and I have complied with this request, with a reluctance that should become evident by the end of the chapter. Fourth, I want to aggregate an even more diverse set of approaches that rely on a realist or critical realist ontology and seek to establish a relational understanding of disability. Many of the researchers within the Nordic countries adopt this perspective, and I am happy to locate myself in this emerging tradition which seeks to provide adequate empirical evidence on how disability arises as a complex interaction of factors. To offer a crude headline, people are disabled by society *and* by their bodies and minds. Finally, Part I ends with Chapter 5 exploring the complex issues in disability identity, questioning whether the disability rights movement can represent the diversity of disabled people, and suggesting that identity politics may cause more problems than it solves.

I realise in retrospect that Part II, 'Applications', reveals the sociological and philosophical issues which most interest me. My predominant focus is the relationships between people and their experiences in the most personal areas of life. The intellectual approach is multi-disciplinary, bringing together social, psychological and ethical concepts and evidence. I am interested in roles and responsibilities, feeling and emotions, and duties and values. These come together when we need to understand issues such as prenatal diagnosis, end-of-life support and assistance, families, friendship, love and sex, and even violence. It is not that I think that education and housing and transport are unimportant, far from it. But I do confess to finding them less interesting, on a personal level. For me, it is the relational aspects of life that are of the greatest fascination.

My academic journey

Like all researchers, my personal background and experience of disability have influenced my work in disability studies, and in the first edition of this book, I felt it was appropriate to include a brief description of my own journey, describing how I was born with achondroplasia, and how my father and children shared this restricted growth condition.

After 2006, my life changed in two ways. First, I went to work at the World Health Organization, the technical agency for health within the United Nations system. The major part of my responsibilities was to contribute to the writing and production of the first *World Report on Disability* (WHO, 2011), published in association with the World Bank, and to promote barrier removal and mainstreaming throughout WHO. For the first time, I had to learn about disability on a global scale: not only was our team prioritising research from low- and middle-income countries, but also I was to travel widely in our efforts to launch the *World Report* and promote disability inclusion. Moreover, such a report has to be based solely on facts: no opinion, no 'advocacy', but simply the scientific evidence, which meant refereed articles, reports of human rights bodies, and reliable statistics. The consultation, editorial, refereeing and editing process which the team undertook to produce a reliable report was the most rigorous intellectual exercise I have ever experienced, and I have huge respect for the WHO's Alana Officer, who oversaw the efforts of our small team and who, together with Aleksandra Posarac from World Bank, achieved such success with the *World Report*. I think that the *World Report on Disability* will contribute very significantly to the impact of the UN Convention on the Rights of Persons with Disabilities (UN, 2006). I was delighted, at the age of 45, to have such a huge learning experience, and I returned to academia in 2013 with a new global interest and a strengthened commitment to the best available scientific evidence, which I hope is reflected in the improvements to this volume.

Less welcome was becoming paralysed in 2008. My incomplete spinal cord injury (L2) was a complication of achondroplasia, and developed over a few days after a summer of pain from a prolapsed disc. I underwent spinal surgery, and spent ten weeks in rehabilitation, learning how to use a wheelchair, manage bowel and bladder, and maximise my functioning. Physiotherapy continued as an outpatient for two years, during which time I was lucky enough to regain the ability to weight-bear and walk with difficulty. However, I am still currently dependent on a wheelchair for most of the day. Acquiring an impairment in addition to my congenital impairment was very difficult. I had experienced pain and limitation throughout my adult life, but now I was dependent and restricted. I experienced my increased disability as resulting more from my own lack of functioning than as a result of inaccessible environments, although of course I have experienced my share of those. This change in my life expanded my understanding of disability greatly. For example, for the first time I now understood the significance and value of rehabilitation, which has been a very neglected topic in disability studies. However, this experience reinforced rather than challenged my rejection of the 'strong' social model. I remain convinced that the relational account of disability that I provided in the first edition of this book is the best way of understanding the complex and multi-dimensional experience of disablement. Now I have returned to academic life, I hope to apply my learning to develop engaged and useful research about disability both in Britain but also in the majority world.

PART I
FOUNDATIONS

2

MATERIALIST APPROACHES TO DISABILITY

> Few new truths have ever won their way against the resistance of established ideas save by being overstated.
>
> (Isaiah Berlin, *Vico and Herder* (1976))

Introduction

The social model of disability has been called 'the big idea' of the disability movement (Hasler, 1993). To many, it appears to be the fundamental political principle that both first initiated and now sustains the disability rights challenge to mainstream society. Both in Britain but also increasingly on the global disability rights stage, the term 'social model' has become synonymous with progressive approaches to disability, while 'medical model' sums up everything which is backward-looking and reactionary.

Neither in this chapter, nor in my wider disability research, do I reject the idea that disability is powerfully shaped by social forces. In the first edition of this book I wrote of the 'family of social contextual approaches', of which the British social model is a leading example. The role of factors such as the environmental, social and economic policies, cultural representations, individual attitudes in disabling people with health conditions cannot be denied. In North America, Australia and other countries, activists and scholars talk of the social model, but generally as a looser social-contextual concept, often entwined with a minority group approach (Hahn, 1988, 1985; Davis, 1995). However, in this chapter I want to focus on the British version of the social model, sometimes also called the 'strong social model'.

The British social model itself is a very simple and brief statement that turns the traditional definition of disability on its head. As the Union of Physically Impaired Against Segregation (UPIAS) activists argued: 'In our view, it is society which disables physically impaired people. Disability is something imposed on top of our impairments, by the way we are unnecessarily isolated and excluded from full participation in society' (UPIAS, 1976: 3).

The benefits of all social approaches are that they shift attention away from individuals and their physical or mental deficits to the ways in which society includes or excludes them. Mike Oliver (1990) coined the term 'social creationist' to describe the British social model approach, distinguishing it from both the biological determinism of the 'medical model' and the less materialist approaches associated with social constructionism (discussed in Chapter 3). Like social constructionism, the materialist approach signals that the experience of disabled people is dependent on social context, and differs in different cultures and at different times. Rather than disability being inescapable, it becomes a product of social arrangements, and can thus be reduced, or possibly even eliminated. However, unlike the social constructionist approach, social creationism roots the problem firmly in material social forces and physical environments, not just ideas, cultures and discourses.

The redefinition of disability in the British social model parallels the feminist movement's redefinition of women's experience in the early 1970s. Anne Oakley (1972) and others had distinguished between *sex* – the biological difference between male and female – and *gender*, the socio-cultural distinction between men and women, or masculine and feminine. The former was biological and universal, the latter was social, and specific to particular times and places. Thus, it could be claimed that sex corresponds to impairment, and gender corresponds to disability. The disability movement was following a well-established path of de-naturalising forms of social oppression, demonstrating that what was thought throughout history to be natural was actually a product of specific social relations and ways of thinking.

The British social model was crucial to the disability movement for two reasons. First, it identified a political strategy: barrier removal. If people with impairments are disabled by society, then the priority is to dismantle these disabling barriers, in order to promote the inclusion of people with impairments. Rather than pursuing a strategy of cure or rehabilitation, it is better to pursue a strategy of social transformation. In particular, if disability could be proven to be the result of discrimination (Barnes, 1991), then campaigners for anti-discrimination legislation saw civil rights – on the model of the Americans with Disabilities Act, and the British Equal Opportunities and Race Relations laws – as the ultimate solution.

The second impact of the social model was on disabled people themselves. Replacing a traditional deficit approach with a social oppression understanding was and remains very liberating for disabled individuals. Suddenly, people were able to understand that it was society that was at fault, not them. They did not need to change; society needed to change. They did not have to feel sorry for themselves; rather, they could be angry. Just as with feminist 'consciousness-raising' in the 1970s, or with lesbians and gays 'coming out', so disability activists began to think of themselves in a totally new way. They became empowered to mobilise for equal citizenship. Rather than a demeaning reliance on charity, disabled activists could now demand their rights.

In the world of academia, the British social model opened up new lines of enquiry. Whereas the medical sociology of disability had traditionally investigated issues such as individual adjustment to impairment, and explored the consequences of impairment for identity (Thomas, 2007), the social model inspired researchers in the new field of disability studies to turn their attention to topics such as discrimination (Barnes, 1991), the relationship between disability and industrial capitalism (Finkelstein, 1980; Gleeson, 1999), or the varying cultural representations of people with impairment. The social model enabled the focus to be widened from studying individuals to exposing broader social and cultural processes. Disability studies self-consciously emulated the precedents of Marxism, feminism, lesbian and gay studies and post-colonial studies, all intellectual movements that had asked new questions and generated new insights and evidence on the basis of an overt political affiliation with social movements of liberation.

This brief sketch signals how real and how widespread the benefits of the disability rights movement have been in Britain. Changes such as the Disability Discrimination Acts of 1995 and 2005, the Equality Act 2010, the removal of barriers to access, and the development of independent living and direct payments, have all begun to transform British society. Given that, in Britain, disability rights and disability studies have up to this point been inseparable from the social model concept, then certainly any scholar has to give credit to the mobilising power and strategic impact of the British social model redefinition of disability. Activists created the social model, which inspired new generations of activists, who fought for the structural changes that the social model mandated.

It is impossible to know whether the British disability movement would have moved so far, or so fast, in the absence of the social creationist approach. Disability rights movements in other countries seem to have progressed just as quickly, and in some cases rather further, in the absence of the strong version of the social model (Charlton, 1998). This suggests that while a social approach to disability may be indispensable, it does not have to take the particular form of the British social model. Indeed, the strength and simplicity of the strong social model of disability has created as many problems as it has solved.

By looking back at the origins of the British social model, it is possible to trace how an important and unarguable insight – that many of the problems which disabled people face are generated by social arrangements, rather than by their own physical limitations – evolved into a rigid ideology claiming that disability was everything to do with social barriers, and nothing to do with individual impairment. Examining the history carefully shows how in Britain, one particular form of the social-contextual approach to disability – the social model – triumphed over other, less extreme, versions of disability politics.

The Union of Physically Impaired Against Segregation (UPIAS) was one of a number of disabled people's organisations that emerged in the 1970s. The Disablement Income Group (DIG) had formed in 1966, to advocate for improved social security benefits for disabled people. However, DIG developed neither a critique of residential institutions, nor a broad-based campaign for disabled people to have control over their own lives. Frustration with DIG drove both the formation of the Marxist-inspired UPIAS, as well as that of the Disability Alliance, a more reformist group, that offered an alternative solution to the social problems of disabled people.

UPIAS originated when Paul Hunt, a resident of the Le Court Cheshire home, wrote a letter to the *Guardian* newspaper which was published on 20 September 1972, calling for the formation of a consumer group to represent those living in institutions. Hunt had spent his childhood, and much of his adult life, in residential institutions. He had actively researched independent living, inclusive education and welfare benefits, through contacts with the USA and Nordic countries. In 1966, he had edited *Stigma*, a collection of essays by disabled people reflecting on the prejudice and exclusion they experienced. Another key player in UPIAS was Vic Finkelstein, a spinal cord-injured psychologist. In 1968, Finkelstein, subjected to a banning order by the South African apartheid regime for his civil rights activism, came to Britain as a refugee. He was able to make the connection between the liberation struggles of Black South Africans and the situation of disabled people. Paul Hunt, Vic Finkelstein and a small number of other politicised activists created UPIAS (Finkelstein, 2001). For the first couple of years, the network seems to have concentrated on discussion and debate, in the attempt to develop a political ideology of disability.

According to their resulting policy statement (adopted December 1974), the aim of UPIAS was to replace segregated facilities with opportunities for people with impairments to participate fully in society, to live independently, to undertake productive work and to have full control over their own lives. The policy statement defined disabled people as an oppressed group and highlighted barriers: 'We find ourselves isolated and excluded by such things as flights of steps, inadequate public and personal transport, unsuitable housing, rigid work routines in factories and offices, and a lack of up-to-date aids and equipment' (UPIAS, 1976, Aims, paragraph 1).

However, the policy statement did not contain a definition of disability as social barriers or as oppression. The terms 'physically impaired people' and 'disabled people' were used interchangeably and there was a reference to 'physical disability', a usage incompatible with the strong social model. The UPIAS statement called for alliances with other groups – such as the 'mentally handicapped' and 'mentally ill' – and with non-disabled allies. However, only people with physical impairments were eligible to become full members of UPIAS: there was clearly a fear of the new grouping being taken over by non-disabled people.

The first surviving statement of what was to become the British social model of disability appeared in the publication, *Fundamental Principles of Disability* (UPIAS, 1976), which reported on discussions in November 1975 between UPIAS and the Disability Alliance. Founded in 1974, the Disability Alliance was a cross-impairment grouping which sought to promote a comprehensive income scheme. Chaired by the academic Peter Townsend, it sought to bring together a coalition of disability groups and disabled individuals, together with non-disabled academics and experts. The Alliance agreed with UPIAS that disability was a social problem, but argued that financial problems were fundamental to the isolation and segregation of disabled people. In response, UPIAS demanded a more comprehensive approach, not just a continuation of the previous DIG focus on incomes. Unlike the Alliance, which was a coalition of existing disability groups, UPIAS explicitly set out to create a mass grassroots organisation of disabled people.

The 'Fundamental Principles' which formed the starting point of the discussions between the two organisations were written by Paul Hunt, and at the outset defined disability as follows:

> Disability is a situation, caused by social conditions, which requires for its elimination, (a) that no one aspect such as incomes, mobility or institutions is treated in isolation, (b) that disabled people should, with the advice and help of others, assume control over

their lives, and (c) that professionals, experts and others who seek to help must be committed to promoting such control by disabled people.

(UPIAS, 1976)

The Disability Alliance felt able to subscribe to this view. During the discussion itself, recorded on the third page of the document, UPIAS elaborated their position on disability:

> In our view, it is society which disables physically impaired people. Disability is something imposed on top of our impairments, by the way we are unnecessarily isolated and excluded from full participation in society. Disabled people are therefore an oppressed group in society.

This is a more precise development of Paul Hunt's fundamental principle, which explicitly distinguishes impairment from disability in a way that the 1974 Policy Statement did not. The statement continues as follows:

> To understand this it is necessary to grasp the distinction between the physical impairment and the social situation, called 'disability', of people with such impairment. Thus we define impairment as lacking all or part of a limb, or having a defective limb, organism or mechanism of the body and disability as the disadvantage or restriction of activity caused by a contemporary social organisation which takes little or no account of people who have physical impairments and thus excludes them from participation in the mainstream of social activities.
>
> *(quoted in Oliver, 1996: 22)*

This further formalises the impairment/disability distinction. UPIAS thinking seems to have been evolving quickly: it appears that between the first Policy Statement and the Fundamental Principles document, their position had strengthened. Even within the Fundamental Principles document, it is possible to see the social model definition of disability as social exclusion becoming more specific and definitive. When the sociologist Michael Oliver became involved with social model theory in the early 1980s, the impairment/disability distinction and the social creationism approach were further reinforced at the core of the disability rights ideology. My claim in this reading of the origins of the UK disability movement is that the source of the recent sterile debates about the social model of disability lies in the increasingly ideological definition of disability which developed from the initial insights of Paul Hunt and his colleagues about the social factors in disabled people's experience.

A good idea became ossified and exaggerated into a set of crude dichotomies that were ultimately misleading.

In retrospect, UPIAS has been celebrated as the inspiration for the British disability movement, and as the pioneers of the social model. It was certainly the intellectual and political heart of the movement. But distance and mythology risk obscuring its limitations. UPIAS never grew into a mass movement. It was dominated by wheelchair users, perhaps because many had previously been able-bodied, and had been involved with other political movements (Finkelstein, 2001: 4). Some activists remember it as being sexist (Campbell and Oliver, 1996: 52), and as dominated by a typically masculine form of politics, which was hard, ideological and combative (ibid.: 67). It seems to have operated a Leninist democratic centralism, meaning that after discussion and agreement, dissent from the party line was not tolerated: individuals who disagreed either left the network, or were expelled.

The political dangers of the social model of disability

Perhaps only the most powerful counter-claim could have effectively dislodged the deep-seated idea that disabled people are defined by their incapacity. So from one extreme – the cultural assumption that disability is equated with dependency, invalidity and tragedy – the disability movement swung to another – the political demand that disability be defined entirely in terms of social oppression, social relations and social barriers. From seeing disability as entirely caused by biological deficits, the radical analysis shifted to seeing disability as nothing whatsoever to do with individual bodies or brains. This unprecedented attempt to turn traditional views of disability upside down appears, several decades later, to be one of the most brave and transformative move in the history of political thought, because it goes against deep-seated intuitions. However, the social model had logical consequences that were problematic both at the political and the conceptual level.

These difficulties include the following. First, if disabled people share a common experience of oppression, regardless of impairment – just as Black people share a common experience of racism, regardless of ethnic origins – then to organise or analyse on the basis of impairments becomes redundant. Both impairment-specific organisations – whether traditional charities, or more modern self-help groups (see, for example, Hurst, 1995) – and impairment-specific responses become problematic. Michael Oliver has been quite clear that 'the social model is incompatible with taking an impairment-specific approach to disabled people' (Oliver, 2004: 30). In the 2012 edition of *The Politics of Disablement*,

Oliver and Barnes again reiterate: 'Furthermore, impairment-specific labels may have relevance when accessing appropriate medical and support needs, but otherwise they are usually imposed rather than chosen and therefore socially and politically divisive' (Oliver and Barnes, 2012: 21).

The only exception Oliver concedes is the need for specific services for Deaf people. It should be noted that Finkelstein (2001) differs from Oliver on this point.

Second, if disability is about social arrangements, not physical or mental impairments, then attempts to mitigate or cure medical problems may be regarded with intense suspicion. They will appear to be irrelevant or misguided responses to the true problem of disability, and distractions from the work of barrier removal and civil rights (Oliver and Barnes, 2012: 19). Thus, the role of rehabilitation is summarily dismissed in the recent *The New Politics of Disablement*:

> Clearly the concept of rehabilitation is laden with normative assumptions clustered around an able-bodied/mind ideal. And, despite its limitations in terms of returning people with acquired impairments such as spinal cord injury, for example, to their former status, it has little or no relevance or meaning for people born with congenital conditions such as blindness or deafness other than to enforce their sense of inadequacy and difference.
>
> *(ibid.: 42)*

Third, if disability is not to be understood in terms of individual experiences, but as the product of structural exclusion, then the numbers of disabled people no longer become relevant. The imperative for social change and disability provision is to remove environmental and social barriers, rather than to meet the special needs of impaired individuals. So there has been a generalised suspicion of surveys of the disability population, or of particular impairment groups (Oliver, 1990; Abberley, 1992).

These positions provide evidence of how social model thinking became rigid and ideologically narrow in the 1980s and 1990s. There appears to be no intrinsic reason why a single-impairment organisation might not be progressive and helpful, given that people with different impairments experience specific issues and problems, both medical and social. Nor is it logical to think that a focus on social barriers necessitates a neglect of medical intervention. To accept – or even to prioritise – wider structural change does not necessitate the abandonment of medical research or clinical interventions. For example, evidence about the role of parents in rehabilitation after cochlear implantation of their deaf children contradicts the specific claim about the irrelevance of rehabilitation to deaf people (Mauldin, 2012). Finally, understanding the number of disabled people in society would seem to be important for many different areas of social policy in the real world of budgetary constraints and service planning. For example, an inclusive school system would need to provide special needs assistants for disabled pupils, and therefore it would be important to understand how many people might need those services. Fully including Deaf people would require provision of sign language interpreters, and therefore it would be necessary to know how many Deaf people are present in a particular locality in order to provide enough interpreters (Harris and Bamford, 2001). Setting parameters for the disability category necessitates a potentially arbitrary definition of the population being counted, and in that sense, an unavoidable circularity results: the numbers found are an artefact of the definition used (Abberley, 1992). Yet the contingent nature of the disability category does not mean that there is no purpose or value of such surveys, only that each survey can only be understood in terms of the purposes for which it was intended and the definition of a disabled person on which it relies (Bickenbach *et al.*, 1999).

These cases are examples of the way that the 'strong' social model of disability became a kind of litmus test, by which disability activists assessed interventions. If an initiative or organisations appears to contradict the social model, it was rejected as inappropriate, misguided, or even oppressive. The simplest form of this 'disability correctness' arises from basic terminology: the social model mandates the term 'disabled people', because people with impairment are disabled by society, not by their bodies. The phrases 'people with disabilities' or worse, 'people with physical disabilities' become unacceptable because they imply that 'disabilities' are individual deficits. Those who refer to 'people with disabilities' are thus adopting the 'medical model' and must be re-educated or repudiated.

In the UK, many who use the phrase 'people with disabilities' do so because they are striving to be respectful and supportive of disability rights and social inclusion. Rather than defining someone in terms of their impairments, they choose 'people first' terminology to express the common humanity which disabled people share. In other words, while terminology is important, it is not important as underlying values. 'People-first' language is the dominant terminology in the global disability rights field, hence the 'UN Convention on the Rights of Persons with Disabilities' (UN, 2006), and is the politically progressive choice in America, Australia and other English-speaking countries. Quibbling over 'disabled people' versus 'people with disabilities' is a diversion from making common cause to promote the inclusion and rights of disabled people.

The unchanging social model

There are several reasons why the social model has now become an obstacle to the further development of the disability movement and disability studies. These reasons are not external to the social model, but intrinsic to its success. The strengths of the social model are also its weaknesses. First, the social model began as the definitions that underpinned a set of practical political positions, from where it became simplified into a series of memorable slogans such as 'disabled by society, not by our bodies'. Developed by ordinary activists, whom Oliver (1990) celebrates as 'organic intellectuals', it was designed as a political intervention, not a social theory. Politics requires simple and emotionally powerful phrases. The social model was ideally suited to this purpose: it could be explained very quickly, and its implications were obvious and life-transforming.

Second, the social model was developed and promoted in the context of identity politics. For disabled people, the social model was important not just because it highlighted what needed to be changed – the barriers and prejudices and discriminations which they faced daily in their lives – but also because it provided the basis for a stronger sense of identity. Rather feeling ashamed of impairment, activists could deny that impairment was relevant to their situation. In other words, activists had a strong psychological and emotional attachment to the social model analysis, which became incorporated into their sense of self.

Third, the social model was first devised in the 1970s. It was developed in academic form in the publications of Vic Finkelstein (1980) and Michael Oliver (1990) and further promoted through the work of Colin Barnes (1991), Carol Thomas (1999, 2007) and other disability studies scholars. Yet it has barely evolved over the past thirty years. Over and again, the dominant voices of disability studies and the disability movement have reiterated that the fundamental principles of the social model are correct and indispensable (Finkelstein, 2001; Oliver, 2004; Thomas, 2007; Oliver and Barnes, 2012). Other social movement ideologies, such as feminism, have developed over time, have contained multiple different interpretations and emphases, have responded to criticism and have changed to respond to the changing circumstances, while retaining underlying values and commitments. Not so the British social model tradition, which must be one of the only areas of academia that still proudly maintains allegiance to Marxist orthodoxy: 'it was the coming of capitalism that created disability as an individual problem and that it was not until the latter half of the twentieth century that this came to be challenged, largely by politicized disabled people' (Oliver and Barnes, 2012: 3).

The one significant development within the materialist approach has been the contribution of Carol Thomas, a rather more subtle thinker than Oliver or Barnes. She theorised the term 'disablism', defined as: 'a form of social oppression involving the social imposition of restrictions of activity on people with impairments and the socially engendered undermining of their psycho-emotional well-being' (Thomas, 2007: 73). She and other feminist-inspired researchers, such as Donna Reeve, have focused on this psycho-emotional disablism, exploring how interactions between disabled and non-disabled people can be experienced as oppressive (Reeve, 2012). While welcome, it should be noted that this does not fundamentally undermine or revise the social creationist approach, with its focus on barriers and oppression as the basis of disability. There is a greater willingness to discuss impairments, for example, when Thomas (1999) gives some space to what she calls 'impairment effects', and when Reeve (2012) discusses the ways in which inaccessible environments or difficulties claiming welfare benefits can make impairments worse. Yet the role of impairments in contributing to social disadvantage is largely ignored.

The goal of the disability movement has always been to promote disability equality and the inclusion of disabled people in society. There is certainly no need for these goals to change. However, the social creationist approach was only ever a means to this end. If the contradictions and confusions of the strong social model have become overwhelming, the approach should be revised or replaced. There are three central reasons that suggest that this is the case.

The impairment/disability distinction

The distinction between impairment and disability lies at the heart of the social model. It is this distinction that separates British disability rights and disability studies from the wider family of social contextual approaches to disability. Impairment is defined in individual and biological terms. Disability is defined as a social creation. Disability is what makes impairment a problem. For social modellists, social barriers and social oppression constitute disability, and this is the area where research, analysis, campaigning and change must occur.

At first glance, many impairment/disability distinctions appear straightforward. If architects include steps in a building, it clearly disadvantages wheelchair users. Sensory impairments can be remedied by social arrangements such as sign language interpreters, or information in alternative formats. Yet looking closer, the distinction between biological/individual impairment and social/structural disability is conceptually and empirically very difficult to sustain. For example, learning difficulties may be associated with stigma and discrimination, but the individual deficits and the social responses shade into each other, and it is hard to extricate the contribution of each factor (Stalker, 2012). Impairments, even sensory impairments, can cause discomfort (Corker and French, 1999: 6). Pain itself is generated through the interplay of physiological, psychological and socio-cultural factors and thus the individual experience can never be separated from the social context (Wall, 1999).

There are several straightforward reasons why impairment and disability cannot be easily extricated, or to put it another way, why the social and the biological are always entwined. First, disabling barriers come into play when one has an impairment in the first place. If you can walk, steps generally are not a problem. If you can see well, you are not disadvantaged by information only being provided in print. Impairments may not be a sufficient cause of the difficulties which disabled people face, but they are a necessary one. If there is no link between impairment and disability, then disability becomes a much broader and more vague term that describes any form of socially imposed restriction.

Second, impairments are often caused by social arrangements (Abberley, 1987). For example, a considerable proportion of the global burden of impairment is generated by poverty, malnutrition, war and other collectively or individually imposed social processes. Paul Abberley used this argument to try and deal with the problem of impairment, by suggesting that impairment itself could be conceptualised as socially created. Yet because not all impairment is caused by social arrangements, the argument does not work to bolster the strong social model. Moreover, impairments are often exacerbated by social arrangements. Environmental and social barriers make impairments worse, both through action and omission. In the first case, having to negotiate physical obstacles, or use badly designed seats or toilets or transport, puts people at risk, and may cause pain or injury. In the second case, individuals might experience pain or other symptoms that could be alleviated by drugs or therapies, which are unavailable due to particular prescribing regulations, or to lack of income, or rationing. In each of these cases, are the problems to be defined as socially imposed restriction of activity or impairment effects (Thomas, 1999)? If social provision was improved, the restriction might disappear, or at least be minimised. But if it were not for the impairment, there would not be any restriction in the first place. The problem arises out of the combination of impairment effects and social restrictions.

Third, what degree of physical or intellectual limitation counts as impairment is often a social judgement. Many health conditions are on a continuum, for example, think of visual impairment, or mild intellectual disability, which is defined as two standard deviations below average intelligence (as measured by IQ tests). Here, the numbers of impaired people depend on the definition of what counts as an impairment, or rather, what counts as average – or normal – vision or intelligence. The visibility and salience of impairment depend on the expectations and arrangements in a particular society, for example, dyslexia may not become a problem until society demands literacy of its citizens, or conversely deafness may be less disadvantaging if everyone in a remote community knows sign language (Groce, 1985).

What these examples show is that impairment is bound up with social factors, while disability is almost always intertwined with impairment effects. Impairment is only ever experienced in a social context. When is a restriction of activity not a social restriction of activity? If disability is defined as social, while impairment is defined as biological, there is a risk of leaving impairment as an essentialist category. Impairment is not a pre-social or pre-cultural biological substrate (Thomas, 1999: 124), as Tremain (2002) and Areheart (2011) have argued in papers that critique the untenable ontologies of the impairment–disability and sex–gender distinctions. According to these post-structuralist or post-modernist thinkers, the words we use and the discourses we deploy to represent impairment are socially and culturally determined and so there is no such thing as impairment as a natural category, an argument to which I will return in the next chapter.

In practical terms, the inextricable interconnection of impairment and disability is demonstrated by the difficulty in understanding, in particular examples, where the distinction between the two aspects of disabled people's experience lies. While theoretically or politically it may appear simple to distinguish impairment from disability, qualitative research has found it very difficult to operationalise the social model because it is hard to separate impairment from disability in the everyday lives of disabled people, for example, people with learning difficulties (Stalker, 2012).

As mentioned above, Carol Thomas (1999, 2007, 2012) and Donna Reeve (2003, 2012) have been pioneers in exploring 'socially engendered undermining of psycho-emotional well-being'. For them, this is about extending the social model to show how it is inter-personal encounters and social relations that cause problems, not just physical or economic barriers. This is a helpful development. But of course, illness and impairment also undermine psycho-emotional well-being, and this aspect is neglected in their work. Having a spinal cord injury or being diagnosed with a degenerative condition can cause depression, anxiety and problems with self-esteem. Thus, a person with an impairment may at the same time experience socially engendered psycho-emotional problems, and impairment-engendered psycho-emotional problems. In practice, how easy would it be to distinguish between those two causes of mental distress? For example, consider a person with multiple sclerosis. She might be experiencing psycho-emotional effects for a number of reasons:

1 She may be in pain or suffering other physical symptoms and limitations.
2 She may experience depression as one of the symptoms of the neurological condition itself.
3 She may be experiencing negative reactions from her family, friends and employers, which cause her anger and distress.
4 She may be existentially distressed at the prospect of a disease which will limit her life. This distress may be made worse by the negative cultural representations of MS.
5 She may be experiencing social barriers which make her daily life more of a struggle, for example, inaccessible environments or difficulties negotiating welfare benefits.
6 She may have other reasons for distress that are not directly connected with either impairment, or the social reaction to it, for example, her cat may have died, or her partner may have left her.

As this individual presents her feelings, how easy is it to distinguish the effects of impairment from the effects of disablement (whether defined as barriers or oppression)? What sense would it make to distinguish these different factors in the complexity of an individual psyche? How does 'distress at the prospect of a limiting disease' shade into 'distress at the prospect of a limiting disease which is represented culturally as a fate worse than death'? Could the contribution of the different factors be separated or quantified? It seems likely that the different factors would be inextricably linked, compounding each other in a complex dialectic.

As soon as disability studies researchers turn to empirical research, it becomes difficult to sustain the impairment/disability distinction or advance a rigid social model perspective. For example, Mark Sherry's doctoral project was based on qualitative interviews with people who experienced acquired brain injury (2002). Following a social model approach, Sherry attempted to distinguish between the effects of the injury and the role of barriers or oppression. Yet he was left with a residuum of experiences which could not be classified as either 'impairment' or 'disability' and which he discussed in a chapter called, after Lyotard, 'Differend Perspectives'. Sherry concluded that impairment and disability experiences and identities were best conceptualised as a fluid continuum, not a polar dichotomy.

Another empirical example was the study by Lock *et al.* (2005) that took a social model approach to exploring the experience of stroke survivors, finding: 'Predictably, the social model focus on social barriers and social oppression proved to some extent incompatible with the exploration of stroke survivors' experiences' (ibid.: 34).

Their initial focus group data found that respondents experienced impairment effects, such as memory and cognition, speech and language, vision, fatigue and walking difficulties, all of which made employment more difficult (ibid.: 43). But of course, they also experienced various disabling barriers: 'Stroke survivors and partners in the focus groups saw their impairments as barriers to work. However, impairments were generally seen as just one element within a complex constellation of actors that act and interact to influence work reintegration' (ibid.: 43).

Another example is offered by Helen Lester and Jonathan Tritter's research with people with serious mental illness: while the authors endorse a social model perspective, their data shows that respondents found it impossible to ignore their impairment and the impact of what they call 'embodied irrationality'. However, social situations and professional attitudes exacerbated symptoms – what the authors called 'the elision of embodied irrationality and disability' (Lester and Tritter, 2005: 662). My interpretation of all these research studies is that they show the inter-penetration of impairment and disability, rather than simply endorsing the social model perspective. In fact, I would argue that any qualitative research with disabled people will inevitably reveal the difficulty of dis-tinguishing impairment and disability (e.g. Watson, 2002, 2003; Grech, 2009; Söder, 2009; Hwang and Charnley, 2010). The data in these studies is much better explained via the critical realist approach which I will outline in Chapter 4.

In responding to criticisms of the materialist social model, Mike Oliver has sought to deal with the problem of impairment by arguing that a social model of impairment is needed alongside the social model of disability (1996: 42). More recently, he and Barnes state: 'The dis-tinction between impairment and disability is a pragmatic one that does not deny that some impairments limit people's ability to function inde-pendently [and] a simplified representation of a complex social reality' (Oliver and Barnes, 2012: 23).

While Oliver's recognition of the importance of impairment and the limitations of the social model is welcome, it would be neither straightfor-ward nor desirable to create a social model of impairment separately from the social model of disability, precisely because impairment and disability are not dichotomous. It is difficult to determine where impairment ends and disability starts. But such vagueness need not be debilitating. As I will argue later, disability is a complex interaction of biological, psychological, cultural and socio-political factors, which cannot be extricated except with imprecision.

The importance of impairment

> It is not individual limitations, of whatever kind, which are the cause of the problem, but society's failure to provide appropriate services and adequately ensure the needs of disabled people are fully taken into account in its social organisation.
>
> *(Oliver, 1996: 32)*

The social model defines disability in terms of oppression and barriers, and breaks the link between disability and impairment. This has led to the common criticism that social model approaches have neglected the role of impairment. For example, Jenny Morris, in her book, *Pride Against Prejudice* (1991), discussed features of disability which had been neglected by the dominant, UPIAS-inspired ideology of the British disability movement: culture, gender, personal identity. Most importantly, she acknowledged that impairment itself created pain and difficulties that were not solely attributable to disabling factors in society:

> While environmental barriers and social attitudes are a crucial part of our experience of disability – and do indeed disable us – to suggest that this is all there is to it is to deny the personal experiences of physical and intellectual restrictions, of illness, of the fear of dying.
>
> *(ibid.: 10)*

Throughout her book, Morris uses disability interchangeably to stand for both social barriers and individual restriction. Following this lead, in 1992, Liz Crow published a paper in *Coalition*, the journal of the Greater Manchester Coalition of Disabled People (subsequently published as Crow, 1996), in which she criticised the social model for failing to encompass the personal experience of pain and limitation which is often a part of impairment. While she expressed commitment to the social model itself, she called for it to be developed in order to find a place for the experience of impairment: 'Instead of tackling the contradictions and complexities of our experiences head on, we have chosen in our campaigns to present impairment as irrelevant, neutral and, sometimes, positive, but never, ever as the quandary it really is' (ibid.: 208). Crow did not suggest that impairment was an explanation for disadvantage, but that it was an important aspect of disabled people's lives:

As individuals, most of us simply cannot pretend with any conviction that our impairments are irrelevant because they influence every aspect of our lives. We must find a way to integrate them into our whole experience and identity for the sake of our physical and emotional well-being, and, subsequently, for our capacity to work against Disability.

(Crow, 1992: 7)

In the 1993 Open University course book, *Disabling Barriers, Enabling Environments*, Sally French also wrote an important and careful article about the persistence of impairment problems: 'I believe that some of the most profound problems experienced by people with certain impairments are difficult, if not impossible, to solve by social manipulation' (French, 1993: 17). As a person with visual impairment, she gave the example of being unable to recognise people, and failure to read non-verbal cues in interaction, explaining how these aspects of being a visually impaired person caused problems interacting with neighbours and with her students. According to French, no amount of barrier removal or social change could entirely remedy or remove the problem of visual impairment. French also explored the reasons for resistance to these alternative perspectives:

It is no doubt the case that activists who have worked tirelessly within the disability movement for many years have found it necessary to present disability in a straightforward, uncomplicated manner in order to convince a very sceptical world that disability can be reduced or eliminated by changing society, rather than by attempting to change disabled people themselves.

(ibid.: 24)

Most recently, Carol Thomas (1999), from within the materialist social model tradition, has developed an approach to disability which makes space for the exploration of personal experience, of the psycho-emotional dimensions of disability, and for the impact of what she calls 'impairment effects'. She uses the latter concept 'to acknowledge that impairments do have direct and restricting impacts on people's social lives' (Thomas, 2004b: 42).

All these writers have argued from within a social model perspective, calling for reform or development of the model, rather than its abandonment. Nevertheless, many of these critical voices have encountered strong opposition from within the British disability movement and disability studies. Advocates and materialist academics frequently use scare-quotes and phrases such as 'labelled with learning difficulties', 'viewed by others as having some form of impairment' (BCODP, n.d.; Oliver, 2004) or 'perceived impairment' (Oliver and Barnes, 2012). Mental health campaigners use the terminology 'survivors of the mental health system':

> The construct of 'mental illness' is part of a modernist project which devalues the diversity of human experience and perceptions and is preoccupied with analysis, eradication, physicality and mechanical and chemical constraint, rather than understanding, empathy, support and an holistic approach to body and self.
>
> *(Beresford and Wallcraft, 1997: 71)*

While attention to labelling and discourse is important, there is a danger of ignoring the problematic reality of biological limitation. Linguistic distancing serves as a subtle form of denial. In Chapter 3, I will discuss further how the social constructionist approach moves disability studies away from the material realities of life with a different form of embodiment.

Aside from questions of logic and data, there are a number of wider reasons why it might be important for disability studies to engage with impairment:

1 Disability studies should pay attention to the views and perspectives of disabled people, rather than accepting medical claims about the nature and meaning of impairment. Many respondents say that impairment is an important part of their experience.
2 Disability studies should be concerned with medical responses to impairment. Is treatment effective? Are there side effects? Is research funded effectively? Does the NHS prioritise disabled people's impairment needs?
3 Disability studies should be concerned with the prevention of impairment. If there is an interest in the quality of life of disabled people, then this includes minimising the impact of impairment and impairment complications.
4 Disabling barriers both cause and exacerbate impairment. For example, poverty and social exclusion make impairment worse and create additional impairments, particularly risk of mental illness.
5 Impairment explains some of the disadvantages that disabled people face. As UPIAS pioneers were aware, disabling barriers are an additional burden on top of the disadvantages that physical, sensory or cognitive limitations cause. Understanding and, wherever possible, compensating for, intrinsic limitations should be a priority.

Rachel Hurst (2000) makes a familiar comparison of disability to gender, claiming that just as it would be inappropriate to analyse details of women's biology in political debates, so there is no need to analyse individual characteristics of disabled people: 'to concentrate on the personal characteristics of the disabled individual and the functional limitations arising from impairment is, itself, disablism' (ibid.: 1084). It is common to hear such analogies being made between the experiences of disabled people and those of women, minority ethnic communities and lesbians and gays (e.g. Gordon and Rosenblum, 2001). For example, Carol Thomas sees the concept 'disablism' as on a par with concepts such as sexism, racism and homophobia. The term 'disablism' was also deployed by the disability charity, Scope, in the last decade. Perhaps alarmed at being the target of the Direct Action Network and other disabled rights campaigners, Scope adopted a more radical position, with the 'Time to get Equal' campaign. They defined 'disablism' as 'discriminatory, oppressive or abusive behaviour arising from the belief that disabled people are inferior to others'. There is an implicit borrowing here from the celebrated definition of institutionalised racism in the Macpherson Report after the death of the black teenager, Stephen Lawrence: 'processes, attitudes and behaviour which amount to discrimination through unwitting prejudice, ignorance, thoughtlessness and racist stereotyping'.

But is the analogy between different movements and oppressions meaningful? As social movements, women's liberation, gay rights, disability rights and anti-racism are similar in many ways. Each involves identity politics, each challenges the biologisation of difference, each has involved an alliance of academia and activism. There are parallels between the theorisation of disability, and the theorisation of race, gender and sexuality, as the many citations of other oppressions within disability studies literature demonstrate. Yet the oppression that disabled people face is different and in many ways more complex than sexism, racism and homophobia. Women and men may be physiologically and psychologically different, but it is no longer possible to argue that women are made less capable by their biology: 'Gender, like caste, is a matter of social ascription which bears no necessary relation to the individual's own attributes and inherent abilities' (Oakley, 1972: 204).

Similarly, only racists would see the biological differences between ethnic communities as the explanation for their social differences. Nor is it clear why being lesbian or gay would put any individual at a disadvantage, in the absence of prejudice and discrimination. But even in the absence of social barriers or oppression, it would still be problematic to have an impairment, because many impairments are limiting or difficult, not neutral.

Comparatively few restrictions experienced by people with impairment are 'wholly social in origin'. If someone discriminated against disabled people purely because they had an impairment, and imposed exclusions which were solely on this basis, and nothing to do with their abilities, then this would be a wholly social restriction. Examples clearly exist of this form of discrimination: nightclubs which exclude disabled people because they cater only to attractive young people; the notorious 'ugly laws' in early twentieth-century Chicago and elsewhere which prohibited disfigured people from public spaces (Schweik, 2009). Here, disability discrimination parallels racism, sexism and other social exclusions exactly. But in most cases, disabled people are experiencing both the intrinsic limitation of impairment, and the externally imposed social discrimination, as we demonstrated in our research with people who have restricted growth who experience both pain and mobility restriction, but also public mockery and employment discrimination (Shakespeare *et al.*, 2009). When Mike Oliver and Colin Barnes state, in the new edition of *The Politics of Disablement*, that 'This social model breaks the causal link between impairment and disability. The reality of impairment is not denied but is not the cause of disabled people's economic and social disadvantage' (Oliver and Barnes, 2012: 22), I consider that they are wrong: impairment is *one of the causes* of economic and social disadvantage, for example, when it prevents some people with impairments from working, or when it means that people with conditions such as restricted growth have to work part-time or retire early (Thompson *et al.*, 2010). Clinical research in Canada that tested the International Classification of Functioning, Disability and Health model (WHO, 2001) found that impairments do contribute to participation restrictions, and that after joint replacement surgery as a response to arthritis, older people experienced fewer activity limitations and therefore more participation, for example, paid employment (Davis *et al.*, 2012). Looking further afield, Shaun Grech discusses the failures of the strong social model to account for the disadvantage of disabled people in countries like Guatemala. Not only are basic health needs a priority, but also 'In majority world contexts impairment remains a pivotal concern because poor livelihoods (and ultimately survival) are often dependent on hard physical labour (e.g. agriculture), making a healthy body an imperative' (Grech, 2009: 776). When disabled people are equated with other historically oppressed groups in a simplistic way, it leads to conclusions that are unwarranted. For example, in her introduction to an important North American collection about disability research, Marcia Rioux argues that once disability is seen as a citizenship issue, traditional research has to change:

Studying the genetic make-up of people from non-white racial groups is sceptically viewed. Research into genetic engineering that could be used to prevent female children is sceptically viewed … Disability ought not to provide a rationale for research that is unacceptable for other groups in society.

(1994: 6)

The implication of the comparison is that genetics is as irrelevant to disabled people as it is to women and non-white ethnic minorities. But this is surely wrong. Unlike the comparator groups, disabled people often experience major disadvantages as a result of their genetic endowment, whereas members of other historically oppressed communities experience either minimal or non-existent biological disadvantages. For a few disabled people, their genetic condition is the most salient aspect of their entire existence.

To take another example, if women or black people or disabled people have higher rates of unemployment than men or white people, then the explanations might include direct barriers – discrimination by employers (e.g. Wilson-Kovacs *et al.*, 2008; Shier *et al.*, 2009) – and indirect barriers caused by people lacking appropriate qualifications, training or confidence. However, does this entirely account for labour market statistics (e.g. Smith and Twomey, 2002) which show that 48 per cent of disabled people of working age are in work, compared to 81 per cent of non-disabled people? Is the disadvantage caused solely by external barriers, or additionally by the particular problems associated with impairment? The 20 per cent of disabled people whose impairments do not limit the kind or amount of work they are capable of undertaking do not seem to face as much discrimination. In fact, they are substantially less likely to be unemployed than non-disabled people. The people who are least likely to be working are those with mental illness, of whom only 18 per cent are in work, and those with learning difficulties, of whom only 21 per cent are in work. Some of this can be explained by discrimination, or by the failure of employers to adapt working arrangements to include people with mental illness or learning difficulties. But some of it is because many people with learning difficulties are very limited in the work they can do, and many people with mental health problems find it difficult to cope with regular, stressful work.

Similarly, the workers with restricted growth in our own study faced discrimination, but they also worked part-time and retired early, because of the effects of their impairments (Shakespeare *et al.*, 2009). Data across Europe suggests that 'it is not discrimination, but the way in which part-time jobs can accommodate health concerns, which primarily explains the high rate of part-time work among people with disabilities.' (Pagan, 2012: 101). In the United States, Schur (2002) found that 29.8 per cent of disabled people worked part-time, as compared to 13 per cent of non-disabled people.

Another example is a study of workers with cystic fibrosis (Edwards and Boxall, 2010). The majority of respondents were successful in finding jobs, despite their medical conditions which meant they needed time off for hospital visits, breaks for treatment, and flexibility in work hours. Considerable reasonable adjustment and understanding were required from employers. Even so, it was not possible for all the respondents to continue working, as in the case of this respondent:

> Fitting in up to three hours a day of physiotherapy and other treatments required to maintain her health, at the same time as holding down a job, became too much for Sally, even after a reduction in working hours.
>
> *(ibid.: 447)*

Yet the authors of the paper seem reluctant to accept that cystic fibrosis is a serious illness (Edwards and Boxall, 2010: 249), and continue to try to theorise their data from a social model perspective, claiming that people with CF are as able as their non-disabled peers (ibid.: 250).

The inference I take from these examples is that impairment often has explanatory relevance in ways that the colour of someone's skin, or their sex, or their sexual orientation usually does not. If social model approaches cannot account for the role of impairment, then they will fail to explain the complexities of disabled people's social situation. Moreover, disability rights academics and activists risk creating stories about disability which many disabled people will not recognise as describing their own experience. As disabled feminists have argued, impairment is an important part of the disability experience. Impairment affects individuals in different ways, particularly when it is acquired as the result of trauma or illness. Charmaz suggests: 'Chronic illness assaults the body and threatens the integrity of self. Having a serious chronic illness shakes earlier taken-for-granted assumptions about possessing a smoothly functioning body' (1995: 657). Some people are comparatively unaffected by impairment, or else the main consequences of impairment arise from other people's attitudes. For others, impairment limits thir experiences and opportunities, or shapes their sense of self. In some cases, impairment causes progressive degeneration and premature death. These features of impairment cause distress to many disabled people, and any adequate account of disability has to give space to the difficulties which many impairments cause. As Simon Williams has argued: 'Endorsement of disability solely as social oppression is really only an option, and an erroneous one at that, for those spared the ravages of chronic illness' (1999: 812). While Carol Thomas acknowledges the impact of what she calls 'impairment effects', she claims they are of transient significance: 'These impairment effects are, of course, crucially important in people's lives – but they generally become of secondary or irregular significance to disabled people as time moves on' (Thomas, 2012: 211).

This claim seems questionable. If you have a degenerative condition, impairment effects will not disappear, they will likely worsen, as the cystic fibrosis study cited earlier shows. Even with a so-called static condition, the body does not suddenly become insignificant – in my experience of spinal cord injury, neuropathic pain continues to be debilitating, and occasional bladder infections or pressure sores regularly cause discomfort or anxiety. In low-income countries, these complications of spinal cord injury are major causes of premature mortality.

Of course, impairment may also lead to opportunities, for example, to experience the world in a different way, as with those who claim the label of 'neurodiversity' (Wheeler, 2011), or to enjoy the richness of Deaf cultures based on sign language (Corker, 1998), or to develop one sense or aptitude because others are unavailable. Moreover everyone, even the supposedly able-bodied, experiences limitations: it is not just the wheelchair user who is unlikely to climb Everest (Asch, 2003). It is not necessary to claim that all impairments are negative, or that impairment is only and always negative. But for many, impairment is not neutral, because it involves intrinsic disadvantage. Disabling barriers make impairment more difficult, but even in the absence of barriers, impairment can be problematic.

Limitations of the barrier-free world

In his 1980 monograph developing the social model approach pioneered by UPIAS, Vic Finkelstein wrote: 'Once social barriers to the reintegration of people with physical impairments are removed, the disability itself is eliminated' (Finkelstein, 1980: 33). Finkelstein (1981) created a powerful fable describing a hypothetical village in which all the inhabitants are wheelchair users to illustrate the change of emphasis in the barrier philosophy. Everything is adapted to the villagers' needs, and consequently they are not disadvantaged. They are people with impairments, in other words, but not disabled people. When able-bodied people visit the village, it is they who face problems adapting to the environment. They feel excluded, and they experience physical and psychological difficulties. The fable is a powerful summary of the philosophical change that UPIAS demanded, in the form of what would be later known as the social model of disability.

This focus on barriers was carried through into the Open University reader edited by John Swain and colleagues and entitled *Disabling Barriers, Enabling Environments* (Swain *et al.*, 2004), and into many documents of the disability rights movement. The global goal of disabled people is a barrier-free world in which disabled people are included, not excluded. In practical terms, the barrier-removal mission has radically changed the environment in those countries which have most fully adopted the disability rights critique, for example, the United States of America where barrier removal was mandated by the 1973 Rehabilitation Act, Section 504 and the 1990 Americans with Disabilities Act. At a slower pace, countries such as the United Kingdom have followed suit. The principle of 'reasonable accommodation', enshrined in the Convention on the Rights of Persons with Disabilities, is now a global target that should enable many more individuals to enter the workplace.

The barrier removal philosophy underpins the notion of Universal Design, defined by Ron Mace and others as 'The design of products and environments to be usable by all people, to the greatest extent possible, without the need for adaptation or specialized design' (Centre for Universal Design, 1997). The principles of Universal Design were developed by architects, designers and engineers. For example, users should not be stigmatised or segregated: the same means of use should be provided for all users; information should be in multiple formats and accessible to all; design should be usable with low physical effort; size and space should be appropriate for users with different body sizes, seated or standing. Rob Imrie (2004) has welcomed the development of Universal Design, while expressing caution about its limitations. For example, social and economic relations play a major role in disabling people, and it is not enough to address buildings and products without addressing money and power.

Despite Finkelstein's fable and the development of Universal Design, Design for All and other related concepts, limited conceptual work has been done on the concept of the barrier-free world and the complex interaction of participation and environmental factors (Noreau and Boschen, 2010). There are so many obvious barriers yet to be removed, that perhaps it has not seemed necessary to think too hard about what the inclusive environment might look like, when the utopia is finally achieved. But thinking about a barrier-free utopia is vital for those seeking to conceptualise disability, because the social model is predicated on the assumption that it is possible to remove the barriers that disable people with impairment (although of course the philosophy of barrier removal is not limited to social model perspectives, being present in most social–contextual accounts of disability).

Ironically, the very success of many developed nations in developing inclusive public spaces may provide new evidence that the barriers model is not a sufficient explanation of disability. First, as the obvious and unnecessary barriers are removed, the more stubborn and complex exclusions are left in greater relief, and the deeper moral and political questions about priorities and cost-effectiveness become starker. Second, if disabled people remain poor and disadvantaged, despite social and environmental change, then it suggests that a civil rights or social model philosophy may not be the full solution to the problem of disability. For example, while the United States of America has strong civil rights legislation, which has mandated the most accessible environment in the world, disabled Americans remain disproportionately poor, are more likely to be unemployed, and many are forced to live in segregated nursing homes (Russell, 2002).

Perhaps it is unfair to judge the social model approach on the validity of the concept of the barrier-free world. After all, the social model is about more than physical environments. The BCODP (n.d.) states:

> The barriers disabled people encounter include inaccessible education systems, working environments, inadequate disability benefits, discriminatory health and social support systems, inaccessible transport, houses and public buildings and amenities, and the devaluing of disabled people through negative images in the media.

Architectural and communications barrier removal is often easier than the removal of social and economic barriers. Progress on many of these latter issues has been much slower to achieve, which may explain the persisting poverty of disabled people. After all, minority ethnic groups and women have faced few if any architectural barriers, yet still remain disadvantaged and excluded due to institutional discrimination, the glass ceiling and other insidious social and economic disadvantages. Seeking to reclaim a relational interpretation, Carol Thomas highlights the ways in which the early social model literature stresses oppression as the defining feature of disability. For example, following UPIAS' definition of disability as restriction, quoted earlier, comes the phrase: 'disabled people are therefore an oppressed group in society'. Thomas (2004a) claims that rather than focusing on barriers, social model perspectives should focus on relations of oppression.

Conceding that physical obstacles are only a part of the oppression which disabled people face, a focus on environmental barriers is justified for two reasons. First, creating an accessible environment would reduce social exclusion. Second, the physical obstacles approach to understanding how people are disabled has a powerful symbolic role. The conventional view of disabled people focuses on what people with impairments cannot do, physically, for example, not being able to walk or see or hear. The social model has stressed that this deficit approach is wrong, because using a wheelchair or Braille or sign language is not inferior to the majority approaches to mobility or communication, just different. Using a wheelchair only becomes a problem because the world has been badly designed or unfairly built. In other words, ideas about performance, deficit and access are key to the popular understandings of disability that the social model seeks to challenge. Problems with the notion of barrier removal therefore provide objections to the social model concept itself.

Problems with the barrier-free utopia

Nature

The claim that people are disabled by society, not by their bodies, has been effective in highlighting the human–created obstacles to participation in society. Yet outside the city, the social model seems harder to implement. Wheelchair users are disabled by sandy beaches and rocky mountains. People with visual impairments may be unable to see a sunset, and people with hearing impairments will miss out on the sounds of birds, wind and waves. It is hard to blame the natural environment on social arrangements.

Of course, benign social arrangements can mitigate some of these exclusions (Tregaskis, 2004b). A paved path or wooden walkway can enable people with mobility restrictions to access nature reserves, sites of natural beauty and historic monuments. A special beach wheelchair is sometimes made available at beach resorts. The use of video cameras and audio description will go some way to opening up inaccessible nature. Yet inevitably people with impairments will always be disadvantaged by their bodies: they will not be able to climb every mountain or visit every beach. Even if it were practically possible, it would defeat the very idea of wilderness to create roads and other access facilities to unspoilt and inaccessible landscapes.

In urban areas, it is possible to make both private homes and public buildings accessible. Yet if a wheelchair user lives on top of a hill, then they will face major barriers to getting around their local environment, as I have found to my dismay since I became paralysed. Some cities, for example, San Francisco and Bristol, are innately less accessible than others, for example, Berlin or Cambridge. Equally, wheelchair users in the Nordic countries are regularly disabled by snowfall, whereas their counterparts in southerly latitudes can negotiate the streets throughout the winter months.

Incompatibility

Implicit in the notion of a barrier-free world is the idea that Universal Design can liberate all. Yet, while in each case a solution to an access barrier can often be found, taken as a totality, it may be impossible to create one environment that is accessible to all potential users. The Principles of Universal Design are unarguable taken separately, but may create conflict when aggregated.

For example, wheelchair users demand level access. Yet people with mobility issues who do not use wheelchairs may find that steps are safer and easier for them than ramps. Blind people may find that kerb cuts that liberate wheelchair users make it difficult for them to differentiate pavement from road, and leave them vulnerable to walking into the path of a vehicle. Wheelchair users may have problems with tactile paving that gives locational cues to visually impaired people (Grey-Thompson, 2005). Partially sighted people may request large text on white background: people with dyslexia may prefer black print on yellow paper. Some people will prefer rooms to be dim, others will prefer them to be brightly lit.

Moreover, different people with the same impairment may require different accommodation, both because everyone experiences their own impairment differently, and because each impairment comes in different forms, and because different people have different preferences for solving impairment problems. Surveying 1000 Americans' views on domestic adaptation, Stark found:

> The solution to environmental problems is highly individual for each person and will result from a plan that includes multiple strategies (including architectural modification, assistive technology, programmatic support, and personal support), and considers the perspective of the individual.
>
> *(2001: 47)*

An Australian study in Queensland found that purpose-built residential accommodation for young disabled adults still offered varying challenges, depending on impairment and personal ways of doing things. Big rooms that were good for wheelchair mobility were also hard to heat (Muenchberger *et al.*, 2012).

Some people with visual impairment prefer to access information in large print, others use Braille, and others prefer to access information on audio tape or as a digital file. In other words, fully accessible information would come in a range of different formats, suitable for different users (French, 1993; Imrie, 2004: 282). Full accessibility might mean making every library book available in every format. When consideration is given to expense, person time and storage space, this solution seems inefficient and impractical. In practice, an easier solution would be to use computer technology: new books could be provided to the library as computer files, and a machine could output the information via a voice synthesiser, or a broiler, or a computer screen, depending on the individual preference of the visually impaired or indeed dyslexic user. Such an approach would make some of the information contained in the library accessible on demand, and possibly give the disabled user equal access to the non-disabled user. Disabled users would achieve the same ends as non-disabled users, but via separate and specific and possibly segregated means. This may contain the spirit of a barrier-free environment, but perhaps not the universal utopia that some rhetoric imagines. Measures of this kind begin to sound like a response to special needs, not an inclusive and non-discriminatory universal provision.

Practicality

The library example begins to highlight problems of practicality that may mean that it is impossible to remove every obstacle. For example, it may be considered a poor use of resources to provide books in multiple formats, if this reduces the budget for buying new books. It may be more practical to undertake to make any book available if specifically requested within a reasonable time frame. This again moves closer to special and separate provision than the concept of a barrier-free world, but may seem to many authorities to be a reasonable and practical compromise.

Principles may be less useful than pragmatism when solutions are sought to buildings and facilities that were constructed in an era when the participation of disabled people was never considered. For example, the New York subway and the London Underground are largely inaccessible to wheelchair users, unlike the more modern transit systems in Washington, DC, and Newcastle, UK, each of which was built with elevators and ramps to accommodate the full range of users. Clearly, principles of Universal Design demand that new buildings are barrier-free. But are authorities obliged to make existing facilities accessible, where retro-fitting would impose huge costs and simpler measures to facilitate the independent transport of disabled people could be found? For example, Transport for London runs almost 100 per cent accessible buses (although I and others are sadly aware that the electronic ramps do not always work). Consequently, disabled people can use public transport, but usually cannot make a choice between Underground and bus transport. They can achieve the same ends as non-disabled people but do not have the same freedom of means. The transport system is not fully accessible, but arguably it is accessible enough to ensure dignified, non-segregated transit.

Fully accessible and barrier-free facilities are an important goal, but there are huge difficulties in achieving them. For example, finding accessible facilities for the annual UK disability studies conferences has proved extremely difficult. Financial constraints mean that a university campus is the only realistic possibility. It is far from straightforward to find a campus that can accommodate up to 200 disabled people. In practice, access is often a compromise, and depends on good will and flexibility. For example, proposals for making social events more accessible for workers who are blind or have low vision seem to contradict what happens in leisure situations – people not showing round their holiday photographs, not changing out of their work clothes into party outfits (Naraine and Lindsay, 2011).

Barrier removal means rebuilding society

The implications of creating a fully accessible society are very far-reaching. For example, it might mean not just accessible transport, information and public buildings, but also accessible private homes. At the moment, it is a struggle for many disabled people to find accessible accommodation. This is a major civil rights issue, and a indictment of the failure of many societies to remove barriers or to build effective provision. Land is scarce, and hence at a premium, in the United Kingdom. Single-storey dwellings are rare, and disproportionately expensive. Many bungalows are designed with older people in mind, and as a consequence do not have the number of bedrooms or size of rooms to suit either a young family, or someone manoeuvring a wheelchair. Even those with access to finance find it difficult to locate a suitable property for purchase. It is not far-fetched to think that something could be done about this. Developers could be encouraged to build a higher number of single-storey or accessible homes within new build developments. It could be made a condition of receiving planning permission, or subsidies could be made available to reduce the cost of such dwellings. Housing associations are another way of making low-cost accessible houses available. In this way, it could be made much easier for disabled people to find appropriate accommodation (Madigan and Milner, 1999).

But in an ideal barrier-free world, a disabled person would not just be able to rely on her own home being fully accessible, but would also be able to visit her friends (Emens, 2009). The minimum requirement would be able to enter the ground floor and have access to a toilet, in order to have a drink or a meal together. Brief consideration of the UK shows how difficult it would be to achieve this. Most of the housing stock in the UK is not new-build, and the vast majority presents barriers to people who use wheelchairs. A major transformation seems unlikely, but with political will, new-build homes could be forced to conform to Lifetime Housing standards. However, for the foreseeable future, a wheelchair user will find that most of her friends and relatives live in homes which she is unable to access.

Thinking about other disabled people, there are similar problems. Some people experience impairments that cause pain and fatigue, such as CFS/ME. Barrier-free environments and mobility aids may make it easier for them to negotiate the world. But they may still be immensely limited, and perhaps unable to participate directly in social or economic activities. Even in a barrier-free world, they may remain confined largely to their own homes, or unable to work for more than a few hours a day and hence excluded from the world of work, even if they have the intellectual abilities to contribute.

Imagining how a barrier-free world might be achieved for people with learning difficulties is difficult. Short of a global catastrophe that returned Western society to medieval levels of economic and social organisation, it would be impossible, and indeed undesirable, to recreate a world in which literacy and numeracy were not important attributes for economic independence and advancement. Clearly, many people with learning difficulties have basic literacy and numeracy skills, and there are good examples of people living independently and engaging in paid work. Creating better sheltered and supported employment possibilities to enable people with learning difficulties to benefit from the income, self-esteem and social integration which jobs provide should be a priority for any disability policy (Gosling and Cotterill, 2000). Yet a significant proportion of people with learning difficulties have little prospect of performing even basic work tasks (Vehmas, 2010).

Thinking more specifically still, Judy Singer (1999) asks what barrier removal might mean for people with social impairments such as autism. If someone's impairment makes interaction with others difficult, it is difficult to see how the mainstream world could be adapted to accommodate him alongside other people. People could be educated to become more accepting and supportive of people with autism. This would remove one source of distress and cruelty. But someone with autism may find even the most well-meaning and respectful crowd of people still a disturbing and confusing invasion. With imagination, perhaps facilities could have special sessions reserved for people with social impairments, where people could shop or swim or learn without feeling crowded or disturbed by the presence of others. Efforts can be made to reduce the sensory features that make workplaces inaccessible to people with autism (Young, 2012) or to ensure that everyone said what they meant (Wheeler, 2011). But again, this begins to sound less like barrier-free provision, and more like the specialised and perhaps even segregated provision of solutions for special needs. Conversely, while society undoubtedly creates difficulties for people on the autistic spectrum, not all these difficulties should be conceptualised as oppression or discrimination.

Advocating enabling spatial organisation, Peter Freund (2001) asks how much difference can be accommodated. While limitations of the body will always remain restricting, he argues that there are many unexplored avenues for accommodating different 'mind-bodies'. This reconstruction of space would benefit many bodies, not just those with impairments. I find Freund's analysis helpful, and it is not my intention to oppose barrier removal in practice. But on a theoretical level, the barrier-removal solution to disability does not fully succeed, and this failure undermines the tenets of the social model. Neil Levy (2002: 139) argues that for a social causation model of disability to work, two conditions must apply: first, it must be possible to alter social arrangements so as to remove disadvantage and, second, there must be no compelling reason why social arrangements could not be altered. Resource constraints are sometimes a compelling reason preventing the removal of barriers. The specifics of impairment also create disadvantage that no inclusive social arrangements can mitigate. In these situations provision of alternative ways of accessing facilities or services can often be both appropriate and acceptable.

The disability rights movement has always worked for inclusive provision and a barrier-free world. But barrier removal is not an end in itself. It is a means to an end. The aim of barrier removal is to facilitate the participation and improve the quality of life of people with impairment. In many cases, barrier removal and inclusive provision are the most appropriate and cost-effective way of achieving that end, with the added advantage of minimising segregation of disabled from non-disabled people. But sometimes, separate or alternative provision for disabled people may be a more appropriate way of enabling them to achieve their ends and goals. For example, for people with autism, that might be about providing spaces and opportunities for them to work, shop, learn or socialise where there are fewer people, fewer disturbing sounds or images, less disruption and more routine. For people with learning difficulties, that might be about supported living or working situations, or learning opportunities, or alternatives to employment which give a sense of value, purpose and fulfilment to their lives.

Conclusion

The materialist account of disability makes a distinction between impairment and disability; claims that disability can be removed by social change; and downplays the role of impairment in the lives of disabled people. In this chapter, I have argued against each of these points. My claim is that, even in the most accessible world practical, there will always be residual disadvantage attached to many impairments. If people suffer from fatigue, there is a limited amount that can be done to help: motorised scooters and other aids may help increase the range and scope of activities, but ultimately the individual will be disadvantaged, when compared to others. Sally French, in her discussion of visual impairment, argues that providing adapted equipment and information to people with visual impairment does not remove disabling barriers, and may even make them worse by removing human contact (French, 1993: 19).

The concepts of a barrier-free world and of Universal Design are immensely valuable in highlighting the many ways in which unnecessary barriers and thoughtless planning disadvantage many people with impairment, or people who have dependants, or who are old or injured. Most would accept that there is a moral and political imperative to do much more to promote inclusion, although the legal scholar Adam Samaha has argued that the social creation of disability, on its own, does not have policy implications (Samaha, 2007): the social model shows causes of disadvantage but a wider normative framework is required to generate responses. But even granted this philosophical point, there are major practical and intrinsic obstacles to solving the problem of disability solely or perhaps even chiefly through barrier removal. As Michael Bury has argued: 'The reduction of barriers to participation does not amount to abolishing disability as a whole' (1997: 137).

Underlying the idea of a barrier-free world is an attempt to show that impairments can be irrelevant, and to make equal disabled and non-disabled people. Those who adopt the social creationist approach are relativist, in that they claim that having an impairment is a different but equal form of embodiment to not having an impairment. From a social model perspective, it is not the form of embodiment which is the problem, but the failure of the social world to accommodate to that form of embodiment by removing barriers. Various examples or folktales are deployed to illustrate this insight. For example, Michael Oliver has claimed: 'An aeroplane is a mobility aid for non-flyers in exactly the same way as a wheelchair is a mobility aid for non-walkers' (1996: 108). This sort of statement is amusing, provocative, and forces people to attend to the ways in which we take certain things for granted. But it cannot be taken seriously. Not being able to fly is not the equivalent of not being able to walk. While both aeroplanes and wheelchairs enable individuals to overcome the natural restrictions of their bodies, walking is part of normal species functioning for human beings (Boorse, 1977), whereas flying is not. There is no symmetry or equality between the situation of the non-flyer and the non-walker. A wheelchair is not just one travel option for a paralysed person: it is an essential facilitator.

A second example is the frequent reference to Nora Groce's historical study of Martha's Vineyard (Groce, 1985). In this isolated community in America, hearing loss was comparatively common (1 in 155 as compared to 1 in 5728 in the wider world), deaf people were not a separate community and 'everyone spoke sign language'. The common interpretation of this study is that because Deaf people could communicate with all their neighbours, they did not experience disabling barriers, and hearing impairment was not a problem. Like Oliver's flyers and wheelers, this is a suggestive and valuable lesson for those who refuse to accept that disability can be normalised. But it is not evidence that a barrier-free environment eliminates disability and equalises non-disabled and disabled people. Deaf Vineyarders may have flourished in their isolated community, but unless all their hearing companions were to forgo speech, they would still miss out on some social interaction. Hearing people would have had the advantage of two forms of communication, speech and sign language, whereas Deaf people would have been limited to one form of communication, however effective. They would not have had the same choices as their hearing companions to leave the community and trade or travel off-island. They would have been disadvantaged in experiencing and negotiating the natural world because of the lack of one of their major senses.

Finkelstein's utopian village provides a third example, and is similarly an illusory solution to the disability problem. Moreover, by equating able-bodied with disabled people, it glosses a real disadvantage. No village for wheelchair users would be inaccessible to non-disabled people, for the simple reason that non-disabled people always have the choice to use wheelchairs, just as hearing people have the choice to learn sign language. Again, there is no symmetry. These examples imply something important about the difference between disabled people and non-disabled people. Disabled people have less flexibility and fewer choices than non-disabled people. As Janet Radcliffe Richards (2002) has put it, an ability cannot be turned into a disability, just as no change of values turns a disability into an ability. An accessible environment minimises the inconvenience of impairment, but does not equalise disabled people with non-disabled people.

Those who defend the strong social model, and see no reason for it to be revised or replaced, will remain un-persuaded. In particular, they will claim that my analysis creates a 'straw person': I have misinterpreted the social model, and given an inaccurate picture of how people in the British disability movement really think and operate. Nobody seeks to deny the body or impairment, they say, except for a few over-zealous disability equality trainers. Nobody is opposed to medical intervention (Oliver, 2004; Oliver and Barnes, 2012). The impairment/disability distinction is only 'a simplified representation of a complex social reality' (Oliver and Barnes, 2012: 23). There are no crude dichotomies.

There are three responses to this defence. First, I have cited examples above – and there are many more – where the public position and campaigns of the disability movement have promoted exactly the sorts of positions and distinctions which I criticise. Academic defenders of the social model are trying to have it both ways. They protest that they are not promoting crude dichotomies, in one breath, whereas, in the other, they do exactly what they are disavowing. There is a lack of consistency in thinking (Grönvik, 2007). While some of the leading exponents of the social model now claim to operate a less rigid approach, they still simultaneously reinforce the 'strong' social model.

Second, it may be true that in private, activists do not consistently think or talk in terms of the social model. For example, many disability rights campaigners concede that behind closed doors they talk about aches and pains and urinary tract infections, even while they deny any relevance of the body while they are out campaigning. Yet this inconsistency is surely wrong: if the public rhetoric says one thing, while everyone behaves privately in a more complex way, then perhaps it is time to re-examine the rhetoric and speak more accurately. For example, Kirsten Stalker et al. (1999) found that many voluntary organisations that claimed to support the social model, in practice used concepts that were incompatible with it. Rather than condemning these inconsistencies, I would applaud the pragmatism of people working in the field: the problem is the limitations of a model that is hard to operationalise. Similarly, many researchers espouse the social model in the introduction to their paper, and then continue with a much more nuanced and multi-factorial approach when they come to presenting and analysing their evidence (Grönvik, 2007; Söder, 2009).

Alternatively, defenders of the social model orthodoxy argue that it is unfair to criticise the inadequacies of the social model, because it is not a fully-fledged social theory. For example, Vic Finkelstein said:

> In my view juvenile criticisms of the social model of disability arise because it is frequently used as if it explains our situation rather than as a tool for gaining insight into the way that society disables us ... The social model does not explain what disability is. For an explanation we would need a social theory of disability.
>
> *(2001: 10)*

Similarly, Michael Oliver has argued that 'the social model of disability is a practical tool, not a theory, an idea or a concept' (2004: 30) and that 'models are ways of translating ideas into practice' (ibid.: 19). Oliver also suggests that 'it seems superfluous to criticise the social model for not being something that it has never claimed to be' (ibid.: 24). Most recently, Oliver and Barnes state: 'Almost to the point of boredom, we have constantly stated that the social model is a tool to be used to produce changes in society and is not and was never intended to be a social theory' (2012: 7). It is hard to know how to respond to these defences of the social model. Perhaps, by referring to it as a tool, these materialist disability theorists mean that we should merely 'take the hint' and focus on the environmental and social factors that disable people, and ignore the rest of the lives of people with impairments. But then, on reading their work, it is clear that something more grandiose is being attempted, for example, a strong argument about the role of capitalism in disabling people (Finkelstein, 1980; Oliver and Barnes, 2012: 100); an account of disability identity (Oliver and Barnes, 2012: 112); an explanation for the origins of mental illness (ibid.: 113). For a simple tool, the social model is being used to explain a considerable number of things. At a conference once, Mike Oliver quoted the old American labour movement song, 'If I had a hammer', to advocate for the benefits of the social model; in response, I cited the even older proverb: 'Give a man a hammer, and all he sees is nails.'

The social model certainly provides a definition of disability. According to the *Concise Oxford Dictionary*, 'definition' means 'stating precise form of thing or meaning of word' while the most relevant definition of 'model' is as 'simplified description of system'. The distinctions between the social model as definition, as explanation, as a tool for insight, as a tool for practice, or as a social theory do not seem significant to me. Llewellyn and Hogan (2000) argue that a model is usually a small-scale theory to promote understanding and generate new research hypotheses. But they suggest that the social model of disability seeks to have a larger application, and it is misleading to see it as a model: instead, it should be seen as a theoretical system:

> A system is a general theory in the grand sense, it seeks to describe what the subject of study is about, as well as commenting on the methods that should be employed to research into it. A system, then, needs to be inclusive in that it seeks to account for a wide range of phenomena, organises the available data and offers an account of this.
>
> *(ibid.: 164)*

This seems exactly to describe the strong social model project.

Social model advocates freely criticise accounts of disability that are not based on the social model. Yet they resist criticism on the basis that the social model is not a social theory or an explanation or an idea. Again, advocates of the social creationist approach are trying to have it both ways. After at least thirty years of writing about the social model and applying the social model, it is hard to deny that the social model provides a theoretical system or paradigm, however much this label is abjured. Above all, it hardly matters whether the British social model is a system, model, paradigm, idea, definition or even tool. What matters is that the strong social model overstates the social creation of disability, and fails to give an adequate account of the complexities of disabled people's lives.

3

CULTURAL DISABILITY STUDIES

When a second edition of this book was proposed, reviewers suggested that I engage with 'Critical Disability Studies', not just the British social model perspective. The former approach seems closely related to the dominant North American approach to researching and theorising disability, which has often adopted the label 'Cultural Disability Studies'. Initially, I thought to aggregate this diverse group of theorists within an overall category of 'social constructionist' approaches to disability, given that they share a scepticism towards the nature of reality. However, while this post-structuralist and postmodernist informed approach does operate a form of social constructionism, it is different from the classic social constructionism of Peter Berger and Thomas Luckmann (1966). I do not think the term 'Critical Disability Studies' sufficiently distinguishes these theorists from either the materialist or the Critical Realist approaches, each of which also has a critical attitude to the status quo and wants to question assumptions (Shildrick, 2012). Hence the title of 'Cultural Disability Studies' for this chapter, in which I will explore whether this tradition offers hope for a better understanding of disability and, more importantly, for improving the lives of people with disabilities.

Cultural Disability Studies is part of what I have previously called 'the family of social approaches': they adopt a version of the social model, but usually differentiate themselves from the British materialist approach. They tend to be more interested in cultural representations than in economic questions. They are strongly influenced by post-structuralist and postmodernist authors such as Michel Foucault, Judith Butler, Gilles Deleuze and Félix Guattari. Among prominent contributors, I am thinking of academics such as Rosemarie Garland Thomson, Sharon

Snyder and David Mitchell, Shelley Tremain, Dan Goodley, Fiona Kumari Campbell, and most recently Rob McRuer. Lennard Davis sometimes appears to be in the constructionist camp, but more recently has followed his own path (Davis, 2002), rejecting the social constructionist approach as dated, and scorning the work of Michel Foucault. Helen Meekosha has rallied behind the 'Critical Disability Studies' banner and shares many of the commitments of these other cultural theorists.

I have considerable sympathies with the Cultural Disability Studies approach, because I once lamented the lack of theorisation within disability studies of the British materialist kind. Specifically, I was dismayed by the modernist reliance on crude dichotomies (social model versus medical model, impairment versus disability, disability studies versus medical sociology), and the neglect of culture and identity as issues for enquiry. I also found myself researching alongside the late Mairian Corker (Mairian Scott-Hill). She contributed an admirably clear and well-argued chapter on Derrida and other post-structuralist thinkers to the Disability Reader which I edited (Corker, 1998), and we went on to edit a collection on *Disability/Postmodernity* (Shakespeare and Corker, 2002). In my own doctoral thesis, I explored Foucauldian and feminist thought.

Thus, when Helen Meekosha and Russell Shuttleworth describe how Critical Disability Studies moves away from simplistic binaries, and how the struggle for social justice 'is not simply social, economic and political, but also psychological, cultural, discursive and carnal' (Meekosha and Shuttleworth, 2009: 50), this seems, on the face of it, very promising. Margrit Shildrick (2012: 32) specifies the following features, none of which I would wish to contest: emphasis on embodiment; awareness of the cultural imaginary; deconstruction of binary thought in favour of fluidity of all categories; and recognition of the importance of emotion and affect.

Another valuable aspect of the Cultural Disability Studies approach compared to Materialist Disability Studies is the greater openness to making parallels with other oppressed groups, with the concept 'disablism' paralleling hetero/sexism and racism (Goodley, 2011: 9). If not taken too far, these connections between experiences of oppression and marginalisation can be very intellectual rich and fruitful. It also enables disability studies writers to deploy a whole arsenal of conceptual big hitters. Thus just about everyone uses feminist theory, Fiona Kumari Campbell uses critical race theory (2009: 37), Rob McRuer uses queer theory. Dan Goodley tells us that: 'Queer contests the able individual, disputes the psychological, geographical and cultural normative centre and breaks fixed binaries of "straight/gay", "dis/abled". Disabled, female and dark bodies are no longer seen as incomplete, vulnerable or incompetent bodies' (2011: 41).

Queer theory challenges the division into straight and gay, hetero- and homo-sexual, and highlights how gender and sexuality can be more fluid. Queer is a contested concept within lesbian and gay activism, and for those to whom it is acceptable, it is predominantly a term of identity and cultural politics. Conversely, disability categories emerge from the need to diagnose and treat disease, and to allocate welfare services and benefits. While activists can self-identify in whatever way they choose, it is hard to see how a Queer theory perspective will illuminate medicine or social policy.

This hints at the dangers of a too-easy elision. It's not enough simply to substitute the term 'disability' for the term 'gender/race/sexuality': hence, compulsory able-bodiedness instead of compulsory heterosexuality, crip for queer, and so on. Rather than just playing with words, theorists have to make a case, with evidence, for the similarities between race, gender, sexuality and disability. These are sometimes analogous, but not always. Pushed too far, all of these parallels collapse because of the underlying false analogy that I highlighted in Chapter 2. Gender, race and sexuality have minimal biological underpinning. However, disability always has a biological dimension that usually entails limitation or incapacity, and sometimes frailty and pain. These aspects of disability can be modified or mitigated by environmental change or social intervention, but often cannot be entirely removed. They are not just a matter of culture or language.

Analysis of cultural representations and language

Cultural Disability Studies is a prime example of what has been called the 'cultural turn'. This refers to how academics in the social and cultural sciences turned to language in the 1970s and to discourse in the 1980s. The great benefit of the Cultural Disability Studies approaches is that they explore not just material social relations, but also cultural imagery. As Sharon Snyder and David Mitchell point out, 'Rather than lacking a term exclusively referring to "social disadvantage", the cultural model has an understanding that impairment is both human variation encountering environmental obstacles and socially mediated difference that lends group identity and phenomenological perspective' (2006: 10).

Although some British social model writers (e.g. Barnes, 1992; Darke, 1998) have discussed cultural representations, in general, the social creationist approach to disability studies has not developed extensive or sophisticated accounts of cultural imagery and language. Indeed, often the reliance on materialist understandings of the world means that culture has to be analysed through economic categories: the theory that ideas about disability reflect underlying material social relations (Oliver and Barnes, 2012: 99). In the first decades of British disability studies, some authors developed promising analyses drawing on psychoanalytical and other social theories (Hevey, 1992; Shakespeare, 1994; Corker and French, 1999), but at first these approaches did not become mainstream in the disability studies field.

Within Cultural Disability Studies, by contrast, there is a considerable interest in the role disability plays in cinema or in the classic novels of the Western canon (Davis, 1995; Thomson, 1996; Snyder and Mitchell, 2006), and many humanities scholars, particularly in North America, have written about cultural phenomena such as the freak show (Thomson, 1996), etc. More recently, British scholars have been inspired by North American work to produce their own accounts (Bolt, 2012), and the launch of the *Journal of Literary and Cultural Disability* is an example of that welcome development.

The impact of this work is to show how disability is not simply about having a medical condition, but is about how medical conditions come freighted with meaning and symbolism and connotation. Thus, Lennard Davis brings the focus on texts and discourses back to the definition of disability itself: 'Disability is not so much the lack of a sense or the presence of a physical or mental impairment as it is the reception and construction of that difference' (2002: 50).

An exploration of how disability is regarded differently across cultures and times helps establish that disability is locally variable, at the least, and entirely relative and contingent, at most (Bickenbach, 2009).

One of the benefits of the approach is in displacing disability from the impaired body: disability becomes about discourse, not about abnormality (Goodley, 2011: 109). Or as Sharon Snyder and David Mitchell state, a cultural model is 'a politicized self-naming strategy that distances people with disabilities from dominant definitions of incapacity and dysfunction' (Snyder and Mitchell, 2006: 9). Indeed, the corollary of the focus on negative cultural representations and cultural variability is that disabled people and their allies can also create alternative ways of thinking about and depicting disability, which are challenging to traditional stereotypical ideas, and potentially affirming and liberatory, or at least destabilising. Rosemary Garland Thomson considers culture to have impacts on the material world: 'I suggest that representation informs the identity – and often the fate – of real people with extraordinary bodies' (Thomson, 1996: 15). While this must be true to some extent, the full impact of cultural representations – especially those emanating from high culture, let alone obscure culture products – remains to be proven. There is an extensive debate over the effects of culture on society. Nobody would invest in advertising if it did not influence consumer behaviour, but at the same time, viewers and readers are not simply dupes of the messages that they see in fictional and non-fictional media and culture. So representations usually have a somewhat indirect effect on the fates of disabled people.

Another valuable dimension of the cultural analysis is exploring the attitudes of non-disabled people and the notion of able-bodiedness. As Margrit Shildrick (2012) suggests, this is about exploring why the exclusion of disabled people happens, as opposed to simply the how. At the beginning of my own academic career, I suggested that one explanation for negative cultural representations of disability was that disabled people became dustbins of disavowal for the aspects of embodiment which nondisabled people found troubling (Shakespeare, 1994). More recently, Dan Goodley has provided a psychoanalytical gloss on that idea: 'Disabled people become projection objects in the psychoanalytical splitting of good/bad, able/unable, whole/fragmented selves' (Goodley, 2011: 97). This process perhaps helps explain the ubiquity of images of disability in art and media: 'The disabled body provides a metaphorical "crutch" for the sustenance of "abled" culture: it becomes a body that sparks cultural fascination but also rejection' (ibid.: 59). This connects to Rob McRuer's new theoretical coinage 'compulsory able-bodiedness': 'A system of compulsory able-bodiedness repeatedly demands that people with disabilities embody for others an affirmative answer to the unspoken question, "Yes, but in the end, wouldn't you rather be more like me?"' (McRuer, 2006: 9). Picking up on this, Dan Goodley claims: 'The disabled individual queers and crips the normative pitch of the autonomous citizen' (Goodley, 2011: 79).

Conversely, Fiona Kumari Campbell promises to explore the contours of what she calls Ableism, defined as: 'a network of beliefs, processes and practices that produces a particular kind of self and body (the corporeal standard) that is projected as the perfect, species-typical and therefore essential and fully human' (Campbell, 2009: 5). Indeed, she calls for a shift from 'disability studies' to 'studies in ableism', which refers to 'the production of the abled-body as part of a tussle over ordering, a desire to create order from an assumed disorder; a flimsy but often convincing attempt to shore up the so-called optimal ontologies' (ibid.: 197).

Propping up a notion of able-bodiedness is difficult, given that ordinary human bodies are forever letting one down, becoming ill, tired or dysfunctional, especially with ageing. Lennard Davis builds on the idea, expressed by Irving Zola originally, that everyone is impaired. Davis suggests that impairment is the rule, not the exception: 'the only universal is the experience of the limitation of the body' (Davis, 2002: 32) and he sees this concept as a way of going beyond postmodernity:

> The dismodern era ushers in the concept that difference is what all of us have in common. That identity is not fixed but malleable. That technology is not separate but part of the body. That dependence, not individual independence, is the rule.
>
> *(ibid.: 26)*

These are all exciting ways of thinking about disability and culture, and to some extent they coincide with ideas from the feminist ethic of care that I will discuss later. However, while welcoming research and debate on cultural representations of disability, there is a balance to be struck. In my view, disability studies should make space for cultural and historical investigations, but alongside empirical social research on the lives of disabled people and the disabling barriers that they experience.

When Dan Goodley writes, 'Poststructuralism replaces truth with discourse and scrutinizes the latter' (2011: 104), he highlights the unfortunate fact that Cultural Disability Studies writers generally seem much more interested in texts and discourses than in the ordinary lives of disabled people. For example, disability studies in North America is dominated by the humanities, and seems to have little space for sociological work. Almost all the leading authors – Davis, Thomson, McRuer, Mitchell, Snyder – are working in the humanities. This means they are more likely to write about representations than they are about material conditions such as poverty or unemployment. To take an example, a recent collection on sex and disability was dominated by chapters that analysed texts or discourses: only about a quarter of the book contained any sort of empirical social research (McRuer and Mollow, 2012). But the problem for disabled people is not just negative images of sex and disability, it is the limited opportunities to form relationships, the lack of access to sex education, the failures of reproductive healthcare, the likelihood of children being removed from parents with intellectual disabilities, as I will outline later in this book. Similarly, Rob McRuer spends 10 pages of the introduction to his (2006) book, *Crip Theory*, analysing one minor Hollywood film, *As Good As It Gets*, which seems an inadequate response to the considerable social and economic challenges facing the world's billion disabled people.

While accepting that Rosemarie Garland Thomson, quoted above, is not wrong in stating that cultural representations inform real lives – at least to some extent – I would hypothesise that even the best book or film review is unlikely to be as powerful as hearing the voices of disabled people themselves, or reading empirical evidence about disadvantage. For example, her book, *Staring* (Thomson, 2009), is a sophisticated cultural analysis of the role of the gaze in culture, and contains an analysis of various literary and artistic treatments of staring, as well as of the work of disabled performers who have made art out of their unusual physiques or physiognomies. But in everyday life, as my team discovered when we interviewed people with restricted growth (Shakespeare *et al.*, 2009), staring at people who have visible differences or impairments is part of disabling social relations. To try and escape the impact of staring and name-calling, people may stop leaving their houses or may avoid certain places – the vicinity of schools, areas with lots of drunken people (Gravell, 2012). This lived experience of staring as a negative and cruel interaction is largely absent from this eloquent book on staring and disability in culture.

In thinking about the role of cultural analysis and cultural challenge, it may be relevant to turn to Nancy Fraser (2000), who distinguishes between the strategies of recognition and redistribution (see, for example, Fraser and Honneth, 2003), as part of a challenge to postmodern approaches. Cultural Disability Studies helps greatly to expand and explore our understandings of recognition, but has almost nothing to say about the pressing problems of redistribution. Contrast this with the recent analysis of newspaper reporting about disability conducted by the Strathclyde Centre for Disability Research and the Glasgow Media Group (Briant *et al.*, 2012). Researchers compared representations in 2010–11 to 2004–5, and ran focus groups with the general public. They concluded that there was a new and politicised reporting of disability that is much less sympathetic than the past, and with an increased focus on disability benefit and fraud and the representation of disabled people as an economic burden. Focus group members believed that fraud rates were much higher than they actually are, thinking that up to 70 per cent of disabled claimants were fraudulent, and citing newspaper articles in evidence. Here, the issues of representation and redistribution – cultural and economic dimensions of disability – are shown to connect and reinforce each other.

The absence of empirical research is partly to be explained by the fact that leading Cultural Disability Studies authors are scholars in the humanities, not the social sciences, for which they cannot, in fairness, be blamed. However, it should be noted that the lack of empirical evidence usually does not stop these authors making sweeping claims and generalisations. For example, Fiona Kumari Campbell talks extensively about law. But she does not offer close readings of legal texts – laws or judgments or cases – to substantiate her claims. Rob McRuer does offer interesting readings of films and other cultural phenomena. But these texts and the occasional first-person testimony seem insufficient evidence to substantiate far-reaching claims, for example, about compulsory able-bodiedness.

Another clue as to the source of the problem lies in the claim by Helen Meekosha and Russell Shuttleworth, drawing on Horkheimer, that critical social theory is irreducible to facts: 'While critical social theory is not averse to strategically employing quantitative approaches, it views the workings of society and culture as much more dynamic than what can be captured quantitatively' (Meekosha and Shuttleworth, 2009: 52). It is hard to know how to answer this. It is true that quantitative data has to be supplemented by qualitative data, and by interpretation. However, all these forms of knowledge aspire to truth about society. Assertions are being made about the workings of society by Cultural Disability Studies authors, and yet they are unable to test their theories empirically. Particularly when those assertions are rather sweeping, most readers could easily instance examples from his or her experience where the assertion is false. Either way, there is no means of testing the truth of the comment.

A specific dimension of this is that empirical research often enquires about the life experiences of disabled people in general, or of a particular group of people with disabilities – people with intellectual disabilities, for example, or people with restricted growth. But if a theorist is wedded to a radical deconstruction of categories, as I discuss below, then it might make no sense to ask about 'disability' or 'intellectual disabilities' – all such entities are arbitrary. If you are demolishing the distinction between disabled people and non-disabled people, it is hard then to operationalise those categories in quantitative research (Söder, 2009: 73). Of course, for many post-structuralist and postmodernist thinkers, there is a scepticism towards the possibility of knowing anything definitive about the world – indeed, there is no world, outside of language. But I would say that some form of realism is indispensable in critical social science:

> For our knowledge to be fallible, it must be capable of being mistaken, and for it to be mistaken there must be something independent of any particular claim, such that there is something it can be mistaken about.
>
> *(Sayer, 2011: 47)*

Without evidence, there is no reason to accept the truth of what anyone says. If we agree with an author's assumptions and implicit values, we might read her with approval. If we are unsure or sceptical, there is nothing to persuade us of the value of her arguments.

The problems that arise from Cultural Disability Studies' reliance on social constructionism are also found in other areas of the social sciences, let alone the humanities. The UK sociologist Ian Craib once described social constructionism as a form of social psychosis (Craib, 1997). Rather than engage with the world as it is, too many academics would rather deconstruct the terminology people use. He called this a manic defence. For example, rather than research poverty, research ways of talking about poverty. Rather than research the lives of disabled people, research how 'disability' has been constructed at different times and in different places. None of these forms of intellectual work are wrong, *per se* – indeed, they are often extremely interesting. But the priorities of academics may sometimes be questionable. Andrew Sayer highlights the risk of critical social science becoming too reflexive (Sayer, 2011: 241). He discusses how in his academic work, Michel Foucault refuses to evaluate or tell others what to do, but perpetually questions, while in his own life he did take positions and was an activist, for example, in the field of mental health.

From this perspective, the considerable attention to terminology and language is interesting, but perhaps a case of putting the cart before the horse. Words certainly connote the shifting social construction of different groups – thus, the shift from idiot to mental retardation to mental deficiency to intellectual disability, to learning difficulty, or from mongol to Down syndrome. Or alternatively, one could explore how different Chinese ideograms describe disability (Stone, 1997). These different terms do signify different eras, different frames of reference. Words or ideograms do reinforce negative ways of thinking – for example, 'retarded' or 'broken' will make it more likely that those referred to are negatively valued. But the uncomfortable truth is that using the term 'learning difficulty' as opposed to 'mental handicap' does not necessarily mean an enlightened way of thinking. As Hans Reinders writes:

> Negative connotations do not reside in words but in the mind. Negative connotations are attached to words because of how people think about disability; thus, without changing their habits of thinking, people will use new words just as they used the old ones.
>
> *(2008: 46)*

For Andrew Sayer, respect and inclusion are not about words or thoughts but about social justice:

> While we can signal respect through how we talk to others, what we say about them, words are rarely sufficient ... Expressions of equality of recognition which are not backed up by equality of treatment and distribution of resources and opportunities are likely to appear hypocritical.
>
> *(2011: 210)*

It is unlikely that any Cultural Disability Studies author would disagree with this. Indeed, this is why Helen Meekosha, Russell Shuttleworth, Margrit Shildrick and others position themselves as 'Critical Disability Studies'. Shildrick (2012: 35) argues that the equality model and the social model do not go far enough, and that the ethical task is to 'mobilize both discursive analysis and substantive intervention'. Yet exactly how much political impact has postmodern discursive analysis ever had on the thought processes of ordinary people? The trouble is, to steal from Barry Barnes, that in practice these perspectives sometimes come across as 'very slightly critical disability studies'.

Deconstruction of the disability category

A particularly helpful dimension of the Cultural Disability Studies approach is the attention to the disability category itself. Lennard Davis (2002) describes postmodernism as the solvent that dissolves all categories. Following post-structuralists and postmodernists who deconstructed the notion of homosexuality or asked what a woman was, it is an obvious move to explore the historical emergence of the notion of disability (Davis, 1995), and to investigate contemporary processes of defining and diagnosing impairment (Areheart, 2011). This begins from the very sensible recognition that disability is extremely diverse (Shildrick, 2012). But soon, not only does the rigid dualism between disabled and non-disabled break down, but post-structuralist and postmodernist approaches are also seen to problematise essentialist notions of disability identity (Corker, 1998) and even the minority group approach to disability politics (Liggett, 1988).

Is impairment natural?

The comparison with feminism is instructive. The early 1970s distinction between sex and gender has been widely criticised by feminist theorists, for creating a dangerous dualism of social gender and biological sex. Scholars such as Judith Butler (1990) who have abandoned the sex/gender distinction do not do so in order to return to the traditional idea that woman's being is biological. Instead, it is observed that sex itself is already social. This opens up the possibilities of seeing how sexual difference has been conceptualised in different eras. John Hood-Williams concludes his discussion of the problems of dualism by saying:

> The sex/gender distinction dramatically advanced understanding in an under-theorised area and, for over twenty years, it has provided

a problematic which enabled a rich stream of studies to be undertaken, but it is now time to think beyond its confines.

(1996: 14)

Because of my own scepticism about the impairment/disability distinction in the social creationist approach, I initially welcomed the potential theoretical enrichment of disability thinking. In the field of social con-structionist disability studies, a landmark intervention came when Shelley Tremain (2002, 2005), working in the Foucauldian tradition, echoed the Judith Butler move. For Tremain, the famous UPIAS distinction between impairment and disability endangers critical work in disability studies. She objects, probably rightly, that the early disability activists conceded too much in seeing disability as a social creation, but leaving impairment as a biological or medical concept. For her, the category of impairment itself is discursively constructed – not just individual impairments. Butler argues that what we think of as sex is always seen through a gendered lens: 'Perhaps this construct called "sex" is as culturally constructed as gender ... with the consequence that the distinction between sex and gender turns out to be no distinction at all' (Butler, 1990: 7). Tremain wants to perform a similar magical reveal on the impairment/disability binary: 'Impairment has been disability all along. Disciplinary practices in which the subject is inducted and divided from others produce the illusion of impairment as their pre-discursive antecedent in order to multiply, divide and expand their regulatory effects' (Tremain, 2002: 42). 'Power' has duped us into taking impairment for granted.

Cultural Disability Studies thinkers do valuable work in showing the historical emergence of particular disability categories. Thinkers such as Lennard Davis (1995, 2002) trace the emergence of normality in the early nineteenth century, and with it, the idea of abnormality, of which disability is a prime example. Disability is about corporeal deviance, the failure to conform to 'corporeal rules' (Thomson, 1997: 6). This process goes beyond language or professional power to structure everyday life:

How societies divide 'normal' and 'abnormal' bodies is central to the production and sustenance of what it means to be human in society. It defines access to nations and communities. It determines choice and participation in civic life. It determines what constitutes 'rational' men and women and who should have the right to be part of society and who should not.

(Meekosha and Shuttleworth, 2009: 65)

Scholars pay attention to how particular ideas about disease emerge at different times. In other words, how does a category become legitimate? In particular, medical conditions, such as anorexia, CFS/ME, hyperactivity, autism, are the classic contested categories which social constructionists tend to focus on. It is not hard to imagine that impairment categories are not real, but are invented. You have only to think of notions such as 'Special Educational Needs', 'Emotional Behavioural Difficulties', 'Autistic spectrum disorder' or, most notoriously, 'Attention Deficit Hyperactivity Disorder'. The frequent implication here is that diagnostic labels cannot be trusted, because they are changeable: different professionals do not agree about a particular individual's diagnosis, and diagnoses change with fashions. Conditions such as 'hysteria' and 'ADHD' are what Ian Hacking (1999) calls 'transitional diagnoses', fashionable in a particular place and time. Moreover, there is undoubtedly a tendency for 'identity spread' or 'diagnostic overshadowing', whereby the diagnosis becomes the most important thing, and the individuality of the child or adult is ignored or lost. All of this is true, and it is necessary to expose and criticise failures of diagnosis and of professional response to diagnosis.

But the dangerous error is to confuse diagnosis with impairment. For example, Areheart's paper developing a Judith Butler-style approach to the impairment/disability divide is typical. He states:

> Diagnosis is a core element for structuring and understanding disability. Indeed, without diagnoses, many disabilities would not be under-stood as such by either the person diagnosed or by others ... In short, impairments understood as the physical traits associated with disabilities, seem little more than diagnoses.
>
> *(Areheart, 2011: 362)*

Having reduced impairment to diagnosis, it is not hard for him to show that diagnosis is a culturally and socially contingent process, using similar criticisms to those just outlined. So, he is able to conclude: 'Yet, in a very real sense, an impairment does not exist until we agree that it does – until it is created' (ibid.: 364). He gives the example of anorexia, which he takes to be a transient mental illness associated with norms of feminine beauty (ibid.: 368). This may or may not be true, but there are strong reasons for thinking that Saint Catherine of Siena and Mary Queen of Scots both had the disease, and they lived many centuries before the heyday of anorexia. Diagnosis is not the same as disease.

Yes, sometimes a cluster of symptoms is redefined as an impairment, as happened with the discovery of osteoporosis as a preventable disease. The cluster of symptoms associated with phenomena like schizophrenia or autism are heterogenous, poorly understood, and may actually be multiple conditions (Happé, 1994). Sometimes too, as with visual impairment, there is a continuum ranging from average visual acuity through to what is legally classified as blindness and beyond. But none of this uncertainty, heterogeneity and gradation implies that there is no underlying biological impairment causing a decrement in species-typical functioning. When Areheart seeks to trace the social origins of a diagnosis of depression, he confuses the cultural process of consultation and diagnosis with the lived experience of the underlying biological disorder:

> The very formation of depression as an impairment thus depends upon patients' internalisation of their distress and later articulation to a medical professional. In this sense, the diagnosis of depression involves an aggregation of social norms, a person's view of her own symptoms, and a narrative dispensed to the medical professional. Any effort to isolate the part of depression that is biological impairment (as opposed to social disablement) would seem artificial at best.
>
> *(Areheart, 2011: 371)*

It is true that when an impairment or disease category comes into being, and when it is applied to an individual, this may have implications for how people with that condition are understood, and how particular individuals are perceived and reacted to. Both the process of categorisation and ascription, and the reaction of the person to being so described, have consequences. In his classic article, 'Making up people', Ian Hacking (1986) shows how such categorisations and diagnoses alter the possibilities for identity and personhood. But again, this does not mean that the underlying condition does not have a reality.

To take another example, Dan Goodley shows how Down syndrome has had different names and implications at different times, concluding that Down syndrome is 'a phenomenon created through signification' (2011: 117). He is absolutely right to point to the different cultural and political meanings and social consequences of what we now know as Down syndrome, all of which affect the lived experience of Down syndrome person (Wright, 2011). But this does not mean that Down syndrome, as an organic impairment, is different now from what it was when it was first identified in 1866, or indeed, what it was when Goya painted people with Down syndrome in Madrid in the early nineteenth century: it is an intellectual impairment caused by having three copies of chromosome 21, and always was. The error that Goodley and other social constructionist disability studies scholars make is to confuse objects, and ideas about objects. The idea of Down syndrome is a social construct, but Down syndrome is not a social construct (Hacking, 1999: 14).

In drawing attention to the historical process whereby categories emerge and become official (for example, through the famous *Diagnostic and Statistical Manual of the American Psychological Association*), Cultural Disability Studies scholars sometimes seem to slip into a version of functionalism. By this, I mean, that categories of disease are claimed to exist because they serve certain functions – for particular groups, or for corporate interests. Sometimes, this slips into what feels like conspiracy theory. Thus Fiona Kumari Campbell states: 'Inscribing certain bodies in terms of deficiency and essential inadequacy privileges a particular understanding of normalcy that is commensurate with the interests of dominant groups (and the assumed interests of subordinated groups)' (2009: 11).

Dan Goodley claims that medicalisation of distress is linked to pharmaceutical industries and implies that their funding influences government health policies (2011: 115). I assume that conditions such as Attention Deficit Hyperactivity Disorder are the obvious focus here, with the concomitant rise in the prescription of Ritalin, although the critique also has relevance to mental illnesses such as anxiety disorders, depression, or schizophrenia, where one of the predominant clinical responses is the prescription of life-long medication. However, to say that certain corporate interests benefit from a particular scientific claim is not to say that the underlying category of illness or impairment does not exist, unless one is totally committed to a conspiracy theory. It does suggest a suspicion is merited, towards the existence of the category, and towards its application to particular individuals, and the treatments which it legitimates.

Cultural Disability Studies theorists seem to have particular difficulty with the idea that anything could be partly biological, genetic or otherwise innate. They often seem wedded to a blank slate notion of human embodiment. Alternatively, there is a relativist approach that prefers to see deficits as differences: Fiona Kumari Campbell tells us we should not evaluatively rank ontological differences (2009: 14). This often necessitates relocating the problem from the body to the external world, which is the conventional social model move. Thus, while Fiona Kumari Campbell accepts that impairments can cause tiredness and pain, 'the primary source of harm is external to the person, situated in the realm of belief' (ibid.: 16), while a critical account of the diagnosis of Asperger's syndrome claims that: 'The distress of the individual is real enough, it's just that the causes are likely to be found as much if not more outside the labeled person as within their supposedly internal psychobiological world' (Moloney, 2010: 139).

In Chapter 2, I challenged this externalisation of impairment effects. There is ample historical evidence that conditions such as hyperactivity and anorexia, let alone schizophrenia and depression, are not modern inventions but have been found across cultures and historical times. Obviously, the experience and the responses are different, because these phenomena are understood in different ways across time and place. But the underlying biomedical or cognitive phenomenon has a remarkable continuity. Similarly Julian Leff (2001) shows how the prevalance of schizophrenia is consistent in different countries. Genetic and cognitive psychological research shows that many of these conditions are strongly heritable, pointing to an underlying biological factor (Cross Disorder Group of the Psychiatric Genomics Consortium, 2013). This is not to say that external social and environmental factors are not relevant. But they often interact with intrinsic biological differences in the individual.

The argument about the contingency of categories is strongest when it relates to conditions that are on a spectrum, where the process of marking a cut-off can be shown to be contingent. For example, visual acuity is on a scale – 20/20 is the normal vision, whereas 20/200 is the legal definition of blindness. A person with 20/200 vision will still be able to see something – they are not totally blind in the sense of completely lacking that faculty. Again, 20/190 vision is only a little better sight, but is not socially legitimated as blindness.

Where the blindness example demonstrates the philosophical problem – how to mark a dividing line when there is no obvious point where things change – at least people accept the existence of blindness. In the case of intellectual disability, the very concept itself is contested (Goodley, 2011: 29) and, indeed, the example of 'mild intellectual disability' is where the social constructionist critique feels strongest. Mild intellectual disability comprises up to three-quarters of all intellectual disability, and is defined as two standard deviations below average intelligence (as measured by an IQ test where the average is 100) (Kittay and Carlson, 2010). Note that what is being described here is not Down syndrome or Fragile X or any of the other known causes of profound to moderate intellectual disability, but a mild deficiency in cognition. Note that the people so labelled are broadly competent and can live independently, or with minimal support. Prior to the arrival of intelligence testing, the social constructionists argue they would probably not have been identified as a problematic category of person: 'Underpining these cultural formations is a testing culture based around a spurious (at worst), culturally relative (at best), concept of (low) intelligence' (Goodley, 2011: 58). Perhaps someone with mild intellectual disability might have been regarded as a bit simple, at worst as 'village idiot', or they may not have been disadvantaged at all, at a time or in a culture where literacy and intellectual knowledge in general were not prioritised. In an agrarian context, not being able to read or follow complicated instructions is not such a problem. Today, in a knowledge economy where most people live independently, these folks are scrutinised, problematised, overprotected and devalued, as the work of scholars such as Dan Goodley, Cathy Boxall, Andrea Hollomotz, Griet Roets and others highlight. The competence they do have is ignored or denied, and they are seen as vulnerable and in need of surveillance (Hollomotz, 2011). It is these processes that lead Dan Goodley and others to argue that intellectual disabilities are created by cultural and political forces, an ideological construction which emerges from 'mass education, differentiation, testing and auditing' (Goodley, 2011: 59; see also Roets, 2009).

While I have sympathy for this approach, I do not subscribe to the idea that there is a plot to exclude people with learning difficulties or that disciplinary power has created the problem. Prior to the development of intelligence testing, people with below average intelligence were considered to be different (Wright and Digby, 1996). It seems to me plausible that there was always an underlying difference. Some people are at the low end of the intelligence continuum, however you choose to measure it. In earlier centuries, this was not such a social problem, because people could flourish in the mainstream, supported by their family. In a modern society, these folk cannot pass exams or learn to work in a knowledge economy. Nor do they always manage to live successfully on their own. Therefore, a process is needed to identify people who are now in danger of exclusion, and support them to maximise their abilities, and then help them make a productive contribution within their capacities, and to live a full and valued existence. Most high-income countries have undoubtedly failed to achieve these progressive intentions. Worse, labelling has been associated with devaluing and with a failure to see the strengths of people with learning difficulties, and to respect and include them But the answer, in my view, is not to claim that there is no problem, and that if it was not for the social interventions, folks with mild intellectual disabilities would be fine. They would not. They would almost certainly be in many more difficulties and dangers than they are now.

We have to concede that the biomedical sciences are historically and culturally located. Ways of thinking about illness and impairment change and develop over time. But this is a different claim to suggesting that there is no underlying reality that these sciences are trying, however crudely to capture. Moreover, disability status is inherently uncertain, polymorphous and contested: many people with impairments neither of think of themselves as disabled, nor are thought of that way by others. Impairments, as I will argue, vary greatly in the nature and extent of their impact on a person. Consequently, the disability experience is very varied and disability as an aggregate of different health conditions or impairments is yet more contingent as a category. The binary divide that Cultural Disability Studies theorists (Campbell, 2009: 5; Meekosha and Shuttleworth, 2009: 65) want to demolish for us may not be very binary in the first place.

Diagnosis as biopower

A particular theme in the deconstruction of the disability category, as in the work of Areheart (2011), is an attention to diagnosis as the pre-eminent moment where an individual becomes inscribed with a particular impairment:

> Diagnosis is a core element for structuring and understanding disability. Indeed, without diagnoses, many disabilities would not be understood as such by either the person diagnosed or by others. [...] in short, impairments understood as the traits associated with disabilities seem little more than diagnoses.
>
> *(Areheart, 2011: 362)*

In a related claim, it has been suggested that diagnosis becomes a form of oppression (Snyder and Mitchell, 2006: 193). This could be linked to the process of assessment within a welfare system, which also often depends on medical legitimation. Fiona Kumari Campbell cites examples of claiming welfare benefits or legal redress under anti-discrimination legislation, where the disabled individual has to take up a victim position which undermines their sense of self (Campbell, 2009: 40, see also Goodley, 2011: 723). A similar argument is made by Margrit Shildrick (1997) when she discusses the process of claiming Disability Living Allowance, where the claimant has to maximise their own incompetence and present themselves as incapable, in order to get the benefits to which they should be entitled.

Nick Watson and Simo Vehmas (forthcoming) point out that categories of impairment and illness play a positive role in allocating services, including welfare benefits, psychological and social support. It is unfeasible that someone could be entitled to public services simply because they decide they want them. A process is needed to legitimate and allocate support in a welfare state. Medical diagnosis and welfare assessment are the prime means by which an individual gets a disabled parking badge, a welfare benefit to cover the extra costs of a condition, or access to a disability pension if they are unable to work. In school, a diagnosis is the necessary confirmation that there is a real difference, and that the individual is not lazy or naughty but has a specific medical condition that influences their behaviour or performance. As a result, they may be entitled to remedial help, classroom assistance, extra time in an exam, or special information and communication technology. Far from being a sinister apparatus of power/knowledge, as the Foucauldians point out, this can be a liberating and empowering process which facilitates functioning and inclusion. When teachers fail to accept medicalisation, then the child gets blamed for her behaviour (Farrugia, 2009).

There are good reasons for scepticism about the process of diagnosis and assessment in practice, as recent debates about British welfare reform and the role of ATOS indicate. Within medicine and psychology, actually existing diagnosis may sometimes be mistaken and even oppressive. The treatments – electroshock therapy, hypnosis, Ritalin – may be crude, may be over-prescribed, and may have damaging side effects. But the undoubted problems of diagnosis suggest to me that we need to strive for better understandings of impairment and illness, and to be more careful both about how we diagnose, and how we respond to people who are diagnosed. It does not suggest to me that diagnosis is inevitably oppressive, or that we should simply ignore impairment. We should not throw the baby out with the bathwater.

Underlying these arguments about the role of categories and of diagnosis seems to be a common assumption that interventions designed to alleviate the difficulties of disability are malign, not helpful. For example, Shelley Tremain draws on Foucault's concept of power/knowledge to show how ideas about disability are produced in particular constellations of governmentality:

> For during the last two centuries, in particular, a vast apparatus, erected to secure the well-being of the general population, has caused the contemporary disabled subject to emerge into discourse and social existence … These (and a host of other) practices, procedures and policies have created, classified, codified, managed, and controlled social anomalies through which some people have been divided from others and objectivised as (for instance) physically impaired, insane, handicapped, mentally ill, retarded, and deaf.
>
> *(Tremain, 2005: 5)*

Here she refers to Foucault's conception of the productive nature of disciplinary power, as opposed to the prohibitive sovereign power that is wielded by nation-states. Helen Meekosha and Russell Shuttleworth explain the benefits of this new genealogical approach to the history of disability: 'What makes Foucault's ideas so useful to CDS is that they perform a radical de-familiarisation of modern institutions and practices as caring and benevolent and reveal technologies and procedures that classify, normalize, manage and control anomalous body-subjects' (Meekosha and Shuttleworth, 2009: 57).

In researching how professional knowledge and practice have been experienced as disempowering and alienating, these theoretical approaches are extremely useful. Revealing the shadow side of care (Shakespeare, 2000), or how 'helping hinders', is another classic Foucauldian radical challenge.

In particular, as Dan Goodley (2011: 29) goes on to say, institutions such as schools play a key role in defining children as impaired through labelling. Thus, Goodley draws on Foucault's idea of biopower to suggests that diagnoses are constructing, not simply describing, the objects of their investigations (ibid.: 114). In other words, there is only discursive power/knowledge being operated by professional experts imposing their standards of normality and deviance, there is no ontological or material reality to these impairments. Not just schools, but any setting can be a place where disability is concocted – schools, long-stay hospitals, clinics, workplaces, universities, community groups, rehabilitation centres and families: 'Institutions engender disability discourse that can, quite literally, be a matter of life and death' (ibid.: 162).

The implication is almost that if it were not for clinics, hospitals, schools, day centres and other settings, intellectual disability would not exist – or at least, would not be a problem. Again, it seems to me that the critique is overstated. Intellectual disability is ontologically real (Vehmas and Mäkelä, 2008). For mild intellectual disability, it may be that the main problem is social treatment. For moderate and profound intellectual disability, it is harder to maintain that the intrinsic deficit is not the main source of difficulty (Vehmas, 2010). Recent empirical evidence in the case of autism disproves the claim that diagnosis is a social determinant of health outcomes: there appear to have been neither beneficial nor negative effects for children who received a diagnosis (Russell et al., 2012).

In the Foucauldian approach, almost any intervention can be questioned. So Margrit Shildrick maintains that: 'We can identify a thoroughgoing governmentality at the heart of policy initiatives – as with rehabilitation programmes or the use of prosthetics – that indicate they are never as positively progressive as they claim or may seem' (2012: 38). Presumably, the problem with helping people to walk or talk is that this reinforces the normative assumption that walking is better than wheeling, or that communication is preferable to silence. While it is always healthy to be sceptical and sometimes very necessary to criticise institutions and professionals in health, welfare and educational services, the suspicion seems overstated (cf. Shakespeare, 2010). Power may be inescapable, but sometimes it is deployed with positive effects. The 85 per cent of disabled people in the world who do not get the wheelchairs or prosthetics or orthotics that they require would probably willingly accept a bit of governmentality (WHO, 2011). Closer to home, the Department of Health's *Valuing People* document (Department of Health, 2001) marked a sea-change in the learning disability field – although, no doubt, it could also be deconstructed, using the concept of biopower as a theoretical scalpel. Post-structuralists and postmodernists seem almost like American Tea Party activists in rejecting government/ality. Sayer points out that the problem with a Foucauldian approach is that it does not distinguish between negative and positive uses of power, adopting instead a 'vaguely dystopian view of the world' (2011: 242). Many workers and services are doing extremely progressive, productive and positive work, which enhances the lives of children and adults with disabilities and promotes their flourishing. And whatever they do, intellectual disability and other forms of disability remain a predicament for individuals, families and society, which cannot be wished away with some fancy postmodern footwork.

Undermining disability identity

In Chapter 5, I will return to the issue of categories and identities in more detail. However, it should be noted here that while Cultural Disability Studies writers may be keen to destabilise categories and dissolve away the material effects of illness and impairment, disabled people may have a different viewpoint. Thus, Susan Wendell (1996) criticises the relativism of postmodern feminists, saying that her impaired body experience cannot be changed by seeing it as a creative expression of her subjectivity, because the impairment limits her freedom. Similarly, when Dan Goodley states confidently that: '"Unliveable pain" for one person might be an "ordinary bodily experience" for another' (2011: 119), he may be referring to different pain thresholds or cultural forms of expressing pain, or he may simply have never experienced what many people with impairments experience. In this context, I confess to a certain discomfort when it comes to non-disabled researchers like Lennard Davis, Dan Goodley or Rob McRuer telling me, who has two rather painful and disabling impairments, that impairment does not exist or is only the product of discourse. Diagnosis is not my problem, and nor is the label which you give to my skeletal dysplasia/restricted growth/ dwarfism/achondroplasia, let alone my spinal cord injury and consequent neuropathic pain. My problem is my physical embodiment and my experience of negative symptoms arising from impairment.

Faced with the question of whether non-disabled people have the right to theorise about disability, it is all too easy for academics to respond by challenging the ontological basis of the category. Rob McRuer, who writes about wearing an 'HIV Positive' tee shirt when he is not HIV+, is as paradoxical as ever: 'I find it more important to raise issues about what it means, for the purposes of solidarity, to come out as something you are – at least in some ways – not' (McRuer, 2006: 57). As I wrote in the previous edition of this book, I have no objection to non-disabled people researching or theorising disability, and it is also the case that disabled scholars are themselves challenging the ontology of disability. But Dan Goodley quotes Simi Linton (1998: 357), with whom I am in agreement on this point: 'It is incumbent on non-disabled scholars to pay particular attention to issues of their own identity, their own privilege as non-disabled people, and the relationship of these factors to their scholarship.' Academics who want to make comments about the impact of impairment, might do well to base their analysis on empirical evidence about how disabled people feel about their embodiment.

Cultural Disability Studies scholars tend to be more comfortable discussing the personal experience of disability than impairment, to use the social creationist dichotomy. For example, when it comes to everyday interactions with nondisabled people, Dan Goodley helpfully cites Arlie Hochschild's (1983) concept of emotional labour to explore how disabled people face the strain of being conciliatory in the face of ignorance and prejudice:

> Disabled people learn to respond to the expectations of non-disabled culture – the demanding public – in ways that range from acting as the passive disabled bystander, the grateful recipient of others' support, the non-problematic receiver of others' disabling attitudes. Maintaining this emotional labour can be psychologically testing.
>
> *(Goodley, 2011: 92)*

Fiona Kumari Campbell highlights the importance of being disabled, but again more in terms of social response to what she calls the 'spectre of ableism' (Campbell, 2009: 122) than living with impairment. As with Snyder and Mitchell (2006: 8), she is alive to the possibility of 'internalised ableism', which used to be known as 'internalised oppression' or even false consciousness.

Ordinary disabled people do not generally see their lives in terms of the high theory that these academics espouse (Priestley *et al.*, 2010). Nor do they feel happy to elide the matter of impairment and its physical and mental impacts, which is a daily reality for many disabled people. Rather than wanting to dissolve identities and undermine the subject, as Butler or Foucault would have it, the disability category, and the identity that goes with it, as I shall discuss in a later chapter, are a potential source of resistance. The 'temporary and partial affinities' that Shildrick (2012: 33), following Donna Haraway (1988), wishes disabled people to celebrate do not offer the robust sense of identity and collectivity to which many people aspire. As Wendell (1996) suggests, disabled people themselves may be keen to hold onto their identities. Thus, Simi Linton has written: 'I'm not willing or interested in erasing the line between disabled and nondisabled people, as long as disabled people are devalued and discriminated against, and as long as naming the category serves to draw attention to that treatment' (1998: 13). The replacement of essentialism by constructionism risks leaving the activist with scant identity to rely on (Davis, 2002: 13).

Cultural Disability Studies is rather vague about political action and resistance. Fiona Kumari Campbell is critical of the legal project of disability rights (Campbell, 2009:12), and shares with Margrit Shildrick (2012: 35) a scepticism of the equality model, but neither offers much alternative. Rob McRuer lauds the disability activists at the World Social Forum in Mumbai, but says little else about how discourses can be challenged. Helen Meekosha and Russell Shuttleworth (2009) reiterate that the goal is autonomy and social participation, and mention the need for praxis and emancipation from hegemonic and hierarchical ideologies, but offer no practical detail of how their theoretical stance contributes to this. Dan Goodley (2011) puts his faith in radical humanism, but is not clear about how to make this stance compatible with the ways in which Foucault and others demolish the idea of the autonomous and self-possessed subject. The reduction of everything to discourse can mean that the truth of life as a disabled person is denied, and the possibilities of resistance are eroded. Norman Geras (1995: 110) warns:

> [I]f truth is wholly relativized or internalized to particular discourses or language games or social practices, there is no injustice. The victims and protestors of any *putative* injustice are deprived of their last and often best weapon, that of telling what really happened.

Deconstructing social constructionism

It is my firm belief that nobody should be allowed to write from a social constructionist perspective if they have not first read the philosopher Ian

Hacking's excellent clarification – and demolition – *The Social Construction of What?* (1999). In this regard, I note that while Snyder and Mitchell (2006) and Davis (2002) do cite Hacking, recent texts by Goodley (2011), Meekosha and Shuttleworth (2009), Campbell (2009) and McRuer (2006) do not.

Hacking points out how social constructionism has often – but by no means always – been liberating, because it suggests that phenomena like disability are not fixed and natural, but historically and cultural contingent and can thus potentially be changed. Social constructionism is radical and sets itself against the status quo (see also Shakespeare, 1998b; Shakespeare and Erickson, 2000).

But Hacking feels that 'social construction' language is both over-used and wrongly used. He cautions us to be much more disciplined about both the 'social' and the 'constructed' in the phrase 'socially constructed'. The term 'social' is usually redundant, because phenomena such as 'special education' and 'welfare' and 'divorce' are always social, they do not occur in nature. The term 'construction' literally suggests a process of making over time, or a product, and should perhaps be reserved for such instances. Specifically referring to ideas about disability, Hacking cautions us against using the word 'construction' when we might mean 'construal', as in a way of understanding something (Hacking, 1999: 39).

Hacking distinguishes between interactive kinds – where institutions and practices develop to respond to new categories such as hyperactive children – and indifferent kinds, where human action makes no difference to the phenomenon – like quarks (ibid.: 103ff).

> People, including children, are agents, they act, as the philosophers say, under descriptions. The courses of action they choose, and indeed their ways of being, are by no means independent of the available descriptions under which they may act. Likewise. We experience ourselves in the world as being persons of various kinds.
>
> *(ibid.: 103)*

Note that he is not saying, as a consequence, that hyperactivity or ADHD are not real phenomena. In general, classifications in the natural sciences are indifferent kinds, while classifications in social sciences are interactive kinds (ibid.: 108). There is a parallel here to John Searle's distinction between brute facts and institutional facts (discussed in Vehmas, 2012). Some medical conditions, such as multiple sclerosis or spinal cord injury, are natural kinds, which are indifferent to human classification. Hacking suggests that other conditions – such as 'mental retardation' or schizophrenia or autism – are both interactive kinds and indifferent kinds (he also points out that each of these categories subsumes multiple types of condition). He explains this by using the linguistic theories of Hilary Putnam, suggesting that the different meanings for, in his example, autism, constitute a vector – the class of things falling under the term.

Put more simply, the label of Trisomy 21 or Down syndrome or idiocy changes, but the underlying genotype to which the terms attach does not. Diagnosis should not be confused with impairment. Down syndrome is an interactive kind because as our reactions to and social and medical responses to a disease entity change over time, this will change the experience of the disease – enable us to live with it, or to participate in society with it – which means that it is then a different thing to be a person with Down syndrome. There may even be bio-looping, for example, if it is discovered that a different diet changes the symptoms of Down syndrome, then the condition itself changes. Down syndrome, however, remains an indifferent kind, because the disease itself remains the same. One might equally say it is both socially constructed and also real, although I would prefer to say that a natural kind is being socially mediated.

It should be noted that whether something is an interactive or indifferent kind does not have immediate implications for treatment: a pharmaceutical approach or psychodynamic approach or social approach may each be appropriate to different conditions. Moreover, one person may have an organic impairment and receive a diagnosis (say, ADHD). Another person may have an organic impairment and never be diagnosed. A third person may be diagnosed, but may not have the organic impairment (Shakespeare and Erickson, 2000). This is relevant to the upsurge in diagnoses and consequent pharmaceutical treatments of ADHD: not all the children so diagnosed have the condition. So, it is valid and indeed very important to be sceptical about labelling and sceptical about categories. But it is very dangerous indeed to consider that this means impairments do not exist or do not matter.

> The human world is an interpreted, construed world. Yet it would be intellectually and politically disastrous to conclude that impairments are not primarily or even secondarily physical facts and that nothing exists until it is spoken or written about.
>
> *(Vehmas, 2012: 299)*

Conclusion

All too often, in my view, Cultural Disability Studies seems more concerned with speaking to academic audiences than in advancing the liberation of disabled people. The reliance on theory reflects the predominant emphasis on carving out a new pedagogical domain, a discipline or sub-discipline, alongside gender studies, post-colonial studies, queer studies and other highly theorised zones of the academy. These texts are often opaque. The language seems redolent of the heyday of French post-structuralist and postmodernist theory, and thus not just inaccessible but also rather dated. The reader is liable to get conceptual indigestion from what Goodley, praising Campbell, calls 'a wonderful Smörgåsbord of theories' (Campbell, 2009: xi). Meekosha and Shuttleworth, who have a gift for writing clearly themselves, state, wisely, that: 'the task is always to balance the activist's cry for accessible conceptualisation with the scholar's understanding of the complex, interwoven but continually changing fabric of human societies' (2009: 64).

But the problem is that some Cultural Disability Studies theorists do not achieve the right balance, and leave their readers mystified and probably alienated. The liberatory promise of disability studies risks being ossified into a fascination with theory for its own sake, which is very much the same trajectory that feminism travelled in the 1980s, and Marxism did in mid-century.

Cultural Disability Studies is an exciting, if sometimes esoteric, body of theory. It does valuable work in opening up cultural representations and discourses to critical examination. However, it is oriented more towards the academy than towards activism. It is hard to see practically how it could be operationalised. The concept of governmentality, taken too far, engenders a suspicion towards almost all interventions. Moreover, the project of destabilising impairment is ultimately counter-productive. It does not help individuals make sense of their real physical or mental predicaments. Challenging processes of diagnosis and definition is welcome, but a realist approach to the world, grounded in empirical research, appears to me more helpful, both politically and at an individual level.

4

CRITICAL REALIST APPROACHES TO DISABILITY

From the preceding two chapters, my position has become evident. Rather than setting medical model versus social model, I think it is more fruitful to distinguish reductionist accounts and multi-factorial accounts, and I favour the latter. Existing perspectives have benefits and weaknesses. Chronic illness perspectives in medical sociology offer helpful empirical evidence exploring how the impact of illness or impairment affects a person's sense of self and their relations with others but fail to situate disability in wider economic and political structures (Thomas, 2007). Materialist disability studies highlight how social barriers disable people with impairments but fail to account for impairment, either as personal experience or as causal explanation for disadvantage. This, together with its crude dichotomies, makes it hard to operationalise 'strong' social model approaches in social research. Cultural disability studies tell us that dichotomies are unhelpful, and draw attention to how cultural and historical variations differ in ways of classifying and describing impairment, and explore psychological explanations for why impairment is threatening to non-disabled people (Shildrick, 2012). However, they lack a strong political commitment, and this approach too is hard to operationalise in social research. In this chapter, I want to sketch how an alternative social approach to disability might reconcile different factors, avoid the perils of either biological or social or cultural determinism, and serve as the basis for a progressive politics.

I am unashamedly eclectic and pragmatic in my theoretical allegiances, finding a plurality of approaches beneficial in the analysis of disability. For example, feminism offers the concept of the personal being political and exciting work on the feminist ethic of care. The work of Nancy Fraser (1995, 2000) and Axel Honneth (1995) has proved powerful in analysing the demands of radical social movements, and exploring the inter-personal dimensions of oppression. Most recently, Andrew Sayer's book *Why Things Matter to People* (Sayer, 2011) does an excellent job of articulating why social science cannot be divorced from normative ethics. Like Sayer, I find the Aristotelian virtue ethics approach to be particularly fruitful, together with the work of Amartya Sen (1992) and Martha Nussbaum (2006) on the capabilities approach.

I find the critical realist perspective to be the most helpful and straightforward way of understanding the social world, because it allows for complexity. Critical realism means acceptance of an external reality: rather than resorting to relativism or extreme constructionism, critical realism attends to the independent existence of bodies which sometimes hurt, regardless of what we may think or say about those bodies. Roy Bhaskar, in his seminal work outlining the realist theory of science, asserts: 'Things exist and act independently of our descriptions, but we can only know them under particular descriptions' (Bhaskar, 1975: 250). In other words, critical realists distinguish between ontology (what exists) and epistemology (our ideas about what exists). They believe that there are objects independent of knowledge: labels describe, rather than constitute, disease. In other words, while different cultures have different views or beliefs or attitudes to disability, impairment has always existed and has its own experiential reality. Cultural sensitivity is required, but relativism is corrosive (Bickenbach, 2009).

In disability research, strong statements from the critical realist perspective have been made by Simon Williams (1999) and Berthe Danermark (Danermark and Gellerstedt, 2004), and more recently by Nick Watson (2012). Each seeks to avoid arguments over medical model versus social model perspectives by demanding an analysis that gives weight to different causal levels in the complex disability experience. For example, Williams concludes: 'Disability ... is an emergent property, located, temporally speaking, in terms of the interplay between the biological reality of physiological impairment, structural conditioning (i.e. enablements/constraints) and socio-cultural interaction/elaboration' (1999: 810).

Whereas Danermark and Gellerstedt suggest:

> This implies that injustices to disabled people can be understood neither as generated by solely cultural mechanisms (cultural reductionism) nor by socio-economic mechanisms (economic reductionism) nor by biological mechanisms (biological reductionism). In sum, only by taking different levels, mechanisms and contexts into account, can disability as a phenomenon be analytically approached.
>
> *(2004: 350)*

Nick Watson (2012: 101) quotes Collier (1998) in calling it a stratified or laminated system and cites Bhaskar and Danermark (2006) who distinguish between the following:

- physical
- biological
- psychological
- psychosocial and emotional
- socio–economic
- cultural
- normative.

The mechanisms working at different levels cannot be reduced to each other, which means that critical realism offers a non–reductionist perspective, in which neither culture, nor economics nor biology dominates: 'In sum, only by taking different levels, mechanisms and contexts into account, can disability as a phenomenon be analytically approached' (Danermark and Gellerstedt, 2010: 350). The critical realist perspective appears to offer a good basis on which to elaborate a workable understanding of disability, which combines the best aspects of traditional approaches, strong social model approaches, and social constructionist approaches.

Disability as an interaction

According to those who follow the social model (Oliver, 1990; Barnes, 1998b), traditional accounts of disability have been individual and medical in their focus. The alternative social model of disability is a structural and social approach, emphasising barriers and oppression. While the UK disability movement has endorsed the social model perspective, academic dissenting voices have been raised both within (Morris, 1991; French, 1993; Crow, 1996) and outside (Williams, 1999) the disability studies community. These criticisms have centred on the failure of the social model to recognise the role of impairment, as well as the ability of the social model to encompass the range of different impairment/disability experiences.

The approach to disability that I propose to adopt suggests that disability is always an interaction between individual and structural factors. Rather than getting fixated on defining disability as a deficit or a structural disadvantage or alternatively a product of cultural discourse, a holistic understanding is required. Put simply, the experience of a disabled person results from the relationship between factors intrinsic to the individual, and extrinsic factors arising from the wider context in which she finds herself. Among the intrinsic factors are issues such as: the nature and severity of her impairment, her own attitudes to it, her personal qualities and abilities, and her personality. I accept that contextual factors will influence these intrinsic factors: impairment may be caused by poverty or war; personality may be influenced by upbringing and culture, etc. Among the contextual factors are: the attitudes and reactions of others, the extent to which the environment is enabling or disabling, and wider cultural, social and economic issues relevant to disability in that society. Understanding and measuring the impact of environmental factors on participation turn out to be harder in practice than it is in theory (Noreau and Boschen, 2010).

The difference between my interactional approach and the social model is that while I acknowledge the importance of environments and contexts, including discrimination and prejudice, I do not simply define disability *as* the external disabling barriers or oppression. I thus avoid what Mårten Söder calls 'contextual essentialism'. The problems associated with disability cannot be entirely eliminated by any imaginable form of social arrangements, as I showed earlier. The priority for a progressive disability politics is to engage with impairment, not to ignore it.

The difference between my approach and what social creationists would describe as the medical model is that I do not explain disability *as* impairment, and I do not see impairment as determining. My approach is non-reductionist, because I accept that limitations are always experienced as an inter-play of impairment with particular contexts and environments. Impairment is a necessary but not sufficient factor in the complex interplay of issues that results in disability. Social modellists would claim that so-called 'medical modellists' assume that 'people are disabled by their bodies', whereas they say instead that 'people are disabled by society, not by their bodies'. I would argue that 'people are disabled by society *and* by their bodies'.

There are similarities between my interactional approach and the relational model adopted by Carol Thomas (1999, 2007). She developed her amended version of the social model as a result of the qualitative research she carried out with disabled women. This led her to add the concept of 'impairment effects' to the dualistic conception of impairment and disability that Oliver had outlined. This concept allows Thomas to account for individual limitations that arise from impairment, rather than from social oppression. Thomas has also made two other innovations. First, she argued that disability (by which she means social oppression) has psycho-emotional effects. This I agree with, although I would add that impairment itself also has psycho-emotional effects.

Second, she argued that the original UPIAS approach should be understood relationally, and that disability should be defined in terms of oppression rather than barriers. She distinguishes (Thomas, 2004a, 2004b) between what she sees as the original UPIAS social relational understanding and the subsequent social model of disability. Thomas equates the social model with a stress on barriers to activity and believes that it is this that has caused the confusion over impairment.

In my opinion, Thomas has falsely made a distinction between a social oppression and a social barriers version of the social model. Both aspects co-exist in both the UPIAS formulation and the subsequent development of the social model. Thomas appears to be trying to refine, develop and tweak the social model to deal with the absences, limitations and confusions to which it leads. While she now suggests that the social model should be set to one side (Thomas, 2004b: 33), she does not want to abandon it. Although for her, it is not a 'credible social interpretation of disability', she believes it is of symbolic importance both because it differentiates disability studies from medical sociology, and orients disability studies to the disability movement.

Thomas and I both agree that a relational approach to understanding disability is needed. By relational, I mean that the disability is a relationship between intrinsic factors (impairment, personality, motivation, etc.) and extrinsic factors (environments, support systems, oppression, etc.). However, Thomas uses the term 'social relational' to refer to the relationship of 'those socially constructed as problematically different because of a significant bodily and/or cognitive variation from the norm and those who meet the cultural criteria of embodied normality' (ibid.: 28). While recognition of the role of power is important for any theory of disability, in my view, Thomas' approach is fatally flawed because it defines disability (and hence disabled people) in terms of oppression: 'Disability is a form of social oppression involving the social imposition of restrictions of activity on people with impairments and the socially engendered undermining of their psycho–emotional wellbeing' (Thomas, 1999: 60).

There are a number of problems with this claim:

1 Thomas reproduces the circularity within the traditional social model. If disability is defined in terms of oppression, then this puts social researchers in a difficult position. When researching disability, they are committed to finding that disabled people are oppressed, by definition. The only question is the extent to which disabled people are oppressed. Anders Gustavsson (2004: 67) quotes Mårten Söder, arguing that this circular reasoning is a particular danger of either clinical or contextual essentialism.

2 It seems that Thomas is further committed to separating two categories: the set of people with impairment (who may experience impairment effects) and, within that group, the subset of disabled people (meaning people with impairment who experience oppressive social reactions in addition to their impairment effects). For example, I may not consider myself to be oppressed much of the time: I certainly have impairments, and sometimes environments, policies or social reactions are oppressive and damaging to my psycho-emotional well-being. Often, however, they are not. In other words, in some situations, I am a person with impairment, and in other situations, I am a disabled person, according to Thomas' definitions. This seems impractical and confusing.

3 Many disabled people, much of the time, actually experience positive responses from non-disabled people. For example, they may receive support from non-disabled relatives, friends, or strangers who assist them in daily activities. Or they may experience positive benefit from statutory or voluntary services. To define disability entirely in terms of oppression risks obscuring the positive dimension of social relations which enable people with impairment.

Note the difference between the impairment/disability distinction, and the sex/gender distinction with which it is often compared. Feminists (e.g. Oakley, 1972) distinguished between biological sex (male/female) and socio-cultural gender (masculine/feminine). They argued that to be a man or woman in a particular historical and cultural context was a social, not biological experience. Yet they did not claim that gender equalled oppression, even though they provided evidence that women had historically been oppressed in different ways. Gender was socio-cultural, and often associated with oppression. Compare Thomas' view of disability: impairment is defined, in the social model, as an individual biological attribute (corresponding to sex for the feminists). But the social model does not define disability as the socio-cultural experience of impairment. Instead, disability is defined *as* oppression – or in Thomas' phrase 'forms of oppressive social reaction visited upon people with impairments' (2004a: 579).

Thomas argues (ibid.) that I am committed to a commonplace meaning of disability as 'not being able to do things' and as 'restricted activity'. I deny her interpretation of the position outlined in Shakespeare and Watson (2001a). Then, as now, I define disability as the outcome of the interaction between individual and contextual factors, which includes impairment, personality, individual attitudes, environment, policy, and culture. Rather than reserving the word 'disability' for 'impairment effects' or oppression or barriers, I would rather use the term broadly to describe the whole interplay of different factors that make up the experience of people with impairments (much as 'disability' is used in the WHO *International Classification of Functioning, Disability and Health* [WHO, 2001]). Impairment is a necessary but not sufficient element in the disability relationship. Disability is always the combination of a certain set of physical or mental attributes, in a particular physical environment, within a specified social relationship, played out within a broader cultural and political context, which combines to create the experience of disability for any individual or group of individuals (Sim *et al.*, 1998).

I would not claim to have a wholly new and original understanding of disability. The obviousness of my conception is one of its merits, and others have argued very similar things (Williams, 1999; Danermark and Gellerstedt, 2004; Gabel and Peters, 2004; Woolf, 2010). For example, the Nordic relational approach corresponds closely to my understanding of disability: Anders Gustavsson talks about the relative interactionist perspective as an alternative to essentialism: 'a theoretical perspective that rejects assumptions about any primordial analytical level and rather takes a programmatic position in favor of studying disability on several different analytical levels' (2004: 62).

A Dutch research team (van den Ven *et al.*, 2005) came to a similar conclusion based on qualitative research. They concluded:

> An individual with a disability should be willing to function in society and adopt an attitude towards others in society in such a way that they can join in with activities and people in society. On the other hand society should take actions to make functioning in society possible for people with disabilities. In other words, society should be inclusive with respect to people with disabilities by passing laws on anti-discrimination, ensuring accessibility of buildings and arranging appropriate care facilities for people with disabilities.
>
> *(ibid.: 324)*

These authors, like myself, balance medical and social aspects. They refer to three issues which influence integration: (1) individual factors, which include personality and skills as well as impairment; (2) societal factors, referring to accessibility, attitudes, etc.; and (3) factors within the system of support, by which they mean social support, professional care and assistive devices. The inter-relation of these three sets of factors determine or produce disability. This research team adopt a conception of integration adopted by this research team that I also find helpful. They highlight five elements:

1   Functioning in an ordinary way without getting special attention or being singled out as a result of disability.
2   Mixing with others and not being ignored in friendship and networks.
3   Taking part in and contributing to society whether through paid work or volunteering.
4   Trying to realise one's potential, which may need help from others.
5   Being director of one's life.

This approach seems adequate to the complexity and diversity of disabled people and their aspirations, and a helpful basis for future research.

Thomas (2004a) is right to suggest that there are continuities between my own understanding and that of Williams or Bury, or indeed of the WHO's *International Classification of Functioning, Disability and Health* (ICF). The medico–psycho–social model that lies at the heart of the ICF helps us understand the complexity of disability. Some disability rights commentators have rejected the new WHO framework as being no more than a rebadging of the discredited *International Classification of Impairments, Disabilities and Handicaps* (Pfeiffer, 1998, 2000; Hurst, 2000). This seems wrong: the new approach does recognise the role of the environment in causing restriction (Imrie, 2004). It does not use the term 'disability' to refer to impairment, functional limitation, or indeed environmental barriers, but uses it to describe the entire process:

> The locus of the problem and the focus of intervention are situated not solely within the individuals, but also within their physical, social and attitudinal environments. The label of disability becomes a description of the outcome of the interaction of the individual and the environnment and not merely a label applied to a person.
>
> *(Bornman, 2004: 186)*

Following Zola (1989), the ICF framers take a universal approach, recognising (with Cultural Disability Studies) that the entire population is at risk of impairment and its consequences (Bickenbach *et al.*, 1999; Bickenbach, 2012).

However, Rob Imrie (2004) is correct to note that the ICF is theoretically underdeveloped. Unlike critical realism, the ICF takes the reality of health conditions for granted. Mårten Söder (2009) argues that the ICF sees biology as determining, whereas critical realism sees causal mechanisms for observable phenomena in the complex interplay of factors at different levels. Furthermore, because the developers of the classification could never reach agreement, the final version of the ICF fudges the difference between 'activity limitations' and 'participation restrictions', which makes it harder to understand and operationalise than the straightforward ICIDH approach (Bickenbach, 2012; Davis *et al.*, 2012). 'Impairment' and 'activity limitations' are also not always clearly distinguished, and arguably the concept of impairment should have been excluded from this classification and left to the International Classification of Disease (ICD). Perhaps for these reasons, in practice, some users of the ICF slip back into the ICIDH distinctions between impairment, disability and handicap.

An interactional model is able to account for the range and diversity of disability experiences. For example, there can be variation depending on the nature and extent of the impairment. Simo Vehmas (2010) has written about Steve, a man with profound intellectual impairments. Steve cannot communicate or live independently, let alone work. However, he can respond to certain stimuli and can express pleasure and pain. Vehmas argues that Steve will not be helped by initiatives such as independent living, civil rights or barrier removal: they will not make a significant difference to his life, because his impairment is very limiting. Eva Feder Kittay (1999) has made the same point about her daughter Sesha (see also MacIntyre, 1999). Any social theory of disability has to avoid the error of conflating and simplifying the variety of disabled people's different experiences, or of trivialising life with severe impairment (e.g. McRuer, 2006: 31). Impairment is scalar and multi-dimensional, and differences in impairment contribute to the level of social disadvantage that individuals face (Davis *et al.*, 2012).

Failure to appreciate the impairment continuum contributes to some of the sterile arguments about the nature of disability. It appears to me that some of those who see disability as a tragedy that should be prevented at all costs are seeing only the most severe end of the continuum. And some of those who deny that impairment can be problematic and see disability as just another difference are seeing only the milder end of the continuum. In other words, the two camps are talking at cross-purposes: because they imagine different cases when they discuss disability, they are unable to come to agreement about how disability should be understood or defined. Any adequate theory of disability has to be able to account for minor differences such as Deafness or cleft lip and palate, and very severe differences such as Epidermolysis Bullosa or profound intellectual impairment.

A related phenomenon is the distinction that disability studies theorists have attempted to draw between chronic illness and impairment. This appears to be an attempt to reject the critique of medical sociologists such as Michael Bury, Gareth Williams and Michael Kelly (Barnes and Mercer, 1996; Thomas, 2007). It also shores up the social model by emphasising disabled people who have static conditions that do not degenerate or need medical care. But in practice, it is hard to say that people with multiple sclerosis, HIV/AIDS, or cystic fibrosis are not disabled people, and it has been important to include such conditions in disability discrimination legislation (see also Hughes, 2009). Any adequate account of disability has to include people who have degenerative chronic illnesses such as diabetes or arthritis, as well as people with 'classic' impairments. For some individuals, impairment is a major limiting factor, which renders any social manipulation or barrier removal almost irrelevant. For others, impairment itself causes little restriction: it is the reaction of others that causes problems of exclusion and disadvantage. The interactional model can allow for this variation.

One of the reasons why disability rights activists and disability studies have been unwilling to look too closely at the issue of impairment differences is perhaps the fear of reinforcing a hierarchy of disability. There is a reluctance to imply that some disabled people are better or more worthy than others. Yet it seems to me inescapable that some forms of impairments are more limiting than others. Some disabled people are very restricted by their impairments, and others are not. A precise ranking of impairment is of course impossible, because it depends on subjective or cultural judgements as to how different factors are weighted: presence of pain, reduced life expectancy, visibility, mobility, and other aspects would presumably be viewed differently by different people. It seems likely that, in general, disabled people come to terms with their own personal circumstances, while often thinking of other impairments as harder to deal with: the human capacity for accommodation and adaptation to adverse circumstances is extraordinary (Albrecht and Devlieger, 1999; Shakespeare, 2013). Despite the reluctance to admit it, there are many instances of disabled people themselves adopting a hierarchy of impairment (Deal, 2003). Needless to say, differences in the significance of impairment are not of moral or political relevance. All disabled people are of equal worth and are entitled to the same human rights, and the same human flourishing.

None of these claims contradict two important points which disability studies has asserted strongly. First, non-disabled people generally perceive impairment to be far more negative and limiting than those who experience it directly (Young, 1997; Mackenzie and Scully, 2008). Second, social barriers and social oppression are major factors in the lives of people with impairment, and for many disabled people cause more problems than their impairment. A key dimension of disability is the extent to which a society removes barriers and enables people to participate, regardless of their individual differences. The value of the social model tradition is in highlighting oppression and exclusion, issues that have been neglected in all previous research on disability. Yet impairment almost always plays some role in the lives of disabled people, even if social arrangements or cultural context minimise the exclusion or disadvantage.

As the Dutch research highlights, the interactional approach also makes space for an often-neglected aspect of disablement: personal attitudes and motivation. It is not just the extent or nature of impairment, or the extent of the barriers and oppression, that dictates the extent of disadvantage. For example, people with very similar impairments in the same society have different experiences, depending on their attitudes and reactions to their situation, as we discovered in our research with people with restricted growth (Shakespeare *et al.*, 2009). Enabling disabled people to take a more positive approach and enhancing their self-esteem and self-confidence may sometimes transform their lives as much as providing better facilities or access to medical treatments. Joining a self-advocacy or disability rights group can change an individual's attitudes to themselves and their situation, enabling them to take control of their lives and become more effective.

The interactional approach also highlights the different ways in which the situation of disabled people can be improved. Traditional approaches to disability stress medical cure and rehabilitation. Social model approaches stress barrier removal and anti-discrimination legislation. For example, Michael Oliver has suggested that:

> The social model is not an attempt to deal with the personal restrictions of impairment but the social barriers of disability ... [It is a] pragmatic attempt to identify and address issues that can be changed through collective action rather than medical or professional treatment.
>
> *(1996: 38)*

And more recently: 'While medical and rehabilitative interventions may be appropriate to treat disease and illness, it is increasingly apparent that they are of little use for the treatment of disability' (Oliver and Barnes, 2012: 19). However, the reality is that disabled people are affected by physical and psychological problems as well as by external barriers. I am sure that Oliver and Barnes would identify exclusion from employment as a form of disabling barrier. This can be addressed at the structural level by putting in place anti-discrimination legislation and enabling welfare support such as Access to Work; at the individual level, providing medical and vocational rehabilitation to the individual will increase their likelihood of finding a job. A theory that addresses only external barriers is an incomplete response to the challenge of disability, just as substituting personal solutions for the required social change and barrier removal is also unacceptable. Multiple approaches are needed.

If the importance of intervening at multiple levels is accepted, this not only allows for the recuperation of psychological support, to deal with both impairment-related and social exclusion-related complexities, but it also reminds us of the importance of health. The health needs of disabled people are rarely taken into account in disability studies. Yet evidence shows that disabled people have higher unmet needs than non-disabled people – three times higher, according to a Canadian survey, for adults (McColl *et al.*, 2010). Analysis of the WHO World Health Survey reveals that disabled people were twice as likely to find healthcare provider skills or equipment inadequate, three times more likely to be denied care, and four times as likely to be treated badly (WHO, 2011). People with learning difficulties are particularly at risk of poor healthcare (Redley *et al.*, 2012). Failure to meet general or impairment-related health needs is itself a disabling barrier, which implicitly challenges Bill Hughes' comment:

> The central point that arises from the social model critique of medicine is that medicine is impotent when it comes to the amelioration of disability. It may have some efficacy when in relation to impairment. It cannot, however, be regarded as an ally when it comes to the abrogation of disabling barriers and the discrimination, exclusion and oppression that come from them.
>
> *(2009: 678)*

Ensuring better access to healthcare will enable individuals with impairments to be less excluded and have a better quality of life.

An interactional approach allows for the different levels of experience, ranging from the medical, through the psychological, to the environmental, economic, and political. Rather than dismissing individual interventions as reactionary and structural change as progressive, this approach allows each option to be discussed on its merits. An interactional approach would suggest there are many different factors which could be addressed to improve quality of life: coaching or therapy to improve self-esteem; medical intervention to restore functioning or reduce pain; aids and adaptations; barrier removal; anti-discrimination and attitudinal change; better benefits and services. Given the multiple and non-contradictory options for intervention, a debate is needed as to which approach is the most appropriate or cost-effective for different impairments or specific individuals. There can be no prior assumption that one approach is automatically preferable in all cases. The notion of *appropriate interventions* suggests that judgements about how to improve individual situations are complex, and should be based on evidence, nor ideology. I agree with Jonathan Woolf when he argues: 'Where medical intervention is cheap, quick, safe, and effective, it seems the obvious way to address disability' (2010: 151). But cases such as limb-lengthening, cochlear implants and cosmetic surgery for children with Down's syndrome, let alone the Ashley case, illustrate the contested nature of these decisions. Evaluations of particular new technologies are also relevant, for example, the Ibot wheelchairs that can negotiate steps and raise individuals to reach high and make eye contact. Such assistive technology overcomes architectural barriers: but is investment in very expensive individual solutions a distraction from campaigning for universal design?

Ubiquity of impairment

The interactional approach to understanding disability as a complex and multi-factorial phenomenon necessitates coming to terms with impairment. Critiquing the social model, I argued that impairment was both personally significant and causally relevant and so had to be adequately theorised in any social theory of disability. In response to social constructionist approaches, I suggest that impairment is both real and more problematic than average embodiment. Whereas Margrit Shildrick hopes:

> Perhaps if there were more recognition that there is no single acceptable mode of embodiment, and that all bodies are unstable and vulnerable, then rather than being labeled as deficient, the bodies that are further from normative standards would be revalued as simply different.
>
> *(2012: 40)*

I want to say that impairment and illness is often experienced not just as difference, but as difficulty and limitation and pain and suffering. Disability entails a decrement in health (WHO, 2001). Having an impairment is not like being gay or from a different culture: the solution is not just revaluing diversity.

Until now, only two alternatives for conceptualising impairment have been available: (1) the traditional approach, what Michael Oliver calls the 'medical tragedy theory'; and (2) the denial or neglect of impairment within materialist and constructionist approaches. I would argue that impairment and illness should not be regarded as the end of the world, tragic and pathological. But neither are these bodily experiences irrelevant, or just another difference. Many disabled people are unable to view impairment as neutral, as Michael Oliver and Bob Sapey concede in the second edition of *Social Work with Disabled People*:

> Some disabled people do experience the onset of impairments as a personal tragedy which, while not invalidating the argument that they are being excluded from a range of activities by a disabling environment, does mean it would be inappropriate to deny that impairment can be experienced in this way.
>
> *(Oliver and Sapey, 1999: 26)*

Instead of the polarised and one-dimensional accounts in both traditional research and disability studies, a nuanced attitude is needed, rooted in empirical evidence from disabled people, and involving a fundamental ambivalence. Disability studies needs to capture the fact that impairment may not be neutral, but neither is it always all-defining and terrible (Shakespeare, 2013).

One way of capturing the complexity of impairment is to view it as a *predicament*. The *Concise Oxford Dictionary* defines predicament as 'an unpleasant, trying or dangerous situation'. Although still negative, this does not have the inescapable emphasis of 'tragedy'. The notion of 'trying' perhaps captures the difficulties which many impairments present. They make life harder, although they can be overcome. The added burdens of social oppression and social exclusion, which turn impairment into disadvantage, need to be removed: this seems to me very much the spirit of the original UPIAS approach to disability. Everything possible needs to be provided to make coping with impairment easier. But even with the removal of barriers and the provision of support, impairment will remain problematic for many disabled people.

For example, I have restricted growth. This is a very visible impairment, but is comparatively minor. Before the first edition of this book in 2006, the main effect in daily life was that many people stared at me. This is because the vast majority of people do not have restricted growth and are unfamiliar with people with restricted growth. For them, and particularly for children, dwarfs are fascinating (Shakespeare *et al.*, 2009). Education may reduce but is unlikely ever to eliminate this basic curiosity. Therefore, I will always be stared at. This is not pleasant, even if people are not actually hostile. I cannot escape the awareness of my abnormal embodiment, however much I am happy and successful as an individual. But I do not think these reactions can easily be explained away as oppression. They are a fact of life, like the vulnerability to back problems that is another dimension of the impairment. Since 2008,

I have had a spinal cord injury, which makes me reliant on a wheelchair, which makes my life much harder, even in a totally accessible environment. I also have constant neuropathic pain from the spinal lesion. No amount of civil rights or social inclusion will entirely remove these dimensions of my predicament as a dwarf: they are a predicament, even though my life remains happy and fulfilled.

Similarly, many of the persistent environmental barriers discussed previously might better be theorised as predicaments. The predicament of impairment – the intrinsic difficulties of engaging with the world, the pains and sufferings and limitations of the body – means that impairment is not neutral. It may bring insights and experiences that are positive, and for some these may even outweigh the disadvantages. But that does not mean that we should not try and minimise the number of people who are impaired, or the extent to which they are impaired: I would very much like to turn back the clock to before the onset of my paraplegia.

It is not only impairment that is a predicament. For example, Zygmunt Bauman argues that: 'The postmodern mind is reconciled to the idea that the messiness of the human predicament is here to stay, This is, in the broadest of outlines, what can be called postmodern wisdom' (Bauman, 1993: 245). Other aspects of embodiment – for example, the pains of menstruation or childbirth for women – could also be understood through the predicament concept, as could the inevitability and tragedy of death. To call something a predicament is to understand it as a difficulty, and as a challenge, and as something that we might want to minimise but which we cannot ultimately avoid. As Sebastiano Timpanaro suggests: 'Physical ill ... cannot be ascribed solely to bad social arrangements: it has its zone of autonomous and invincible reality' (Timpanaro, 1975: 20). But this is not to fall into the trap of regarding impairment as a tragedy or an identity-defining flaw.

Some people will object to what appears to be a negative approach to impairment, and to my implicit support for a Boorse-derived concept of species-typical functioning (Boorse, 1977). They should note that I am not denigrating disabled people, nor claiming that impairment makes disabled people second-class citizens or less worthy of support and respect. Disability is a decrement in health, but not in moral value. Disabled people are often inferior to non-disabled people in terms of health, function or ability, but they are not less in terms of moral worth, political equality or human rights, as I stated earlier. The suffering and happiness of disabled people matter just as much as that of non-disabled people.

If impairment truly was neutral – or beneficial – then we could have no objection to someone who deliberately impaired a child. If impairment was just another difference, then, as John Harris (1993, 2001) points out, there would be nothing wrong with painlessly altering a baby so they could no longer see, or could no longer hear, or had to use a wheelchair. Even if no suffering or pain were caused in the process, we would surely consider such actions irresponsible and immoral. Something would have been lost (see Asch and Wasserman, 2010, for an eloquent presentation of a different view, from within disability studies). The implication of this must be that impairment prevention should have an important role in social responses to disability (Shakespeare, 2013). This does not undermine the worth or citizenship of existing disabled people. It suggests that because impairment causes predicaments and is limiting in various ways, we should take steps to prevent or mitigate it, where possible, as I will discuss in Part II of this book.

Furthermore, the connection to other embodiment predicaments underlines a commonplace observation which was central to the work of Irving Zola (1989), and which has great significance for a post-social model approach to disability (see also Bickenbach *et al.*, 1999). Impairment is a universal phenomenon, in the sense that every human being has limitations and vulnerabilities (Sutherland, 1981), and ultimately is mortal. Across their life course, almost everyone experiences impairment and limitation. Impairment is more likely to be acquired than be congenital: ageing is particularly associated with increased levels of impairment. The ubiquity of impairment is underscored by the Human Genome Project that has shown that everyone has approximately hundreds of mutations in their genome, many of which may predispose the individual to illness or impairment (Scully, 2008). In this sense, genetic diagnosis is toxic knowledge, which has the power to turn healthy people into pre-impaired people.

To claim that 'everyone is impaired' should not lead to any trivialising of impairment or the experience of disabled people. As I have argued above, impairments differ in their impact. It is important to appreciate and respect those real differences – particularly in the extent to which people are affected by suffering and restriction (Vehmas, 2010). At the extreme, as Alasdair MacIntyre argues, are very severely impaired people: 'such that they can never be more than passive members of the community, not recognizing, not speaking or not speaking intelligibly, suffering, but not acting' (1999: 127). It would be wrong to neglect the particular needs that arise from these different differences.

Not everyone is impaired all the time. Taking a life course view of impairment highlights the ways that impairment is manifested over time: disabled children grow up to be non-disabled adults, non-disabled people become impaired through accident or in old age. Impairments can be variable and episodic: sometimes people recover, and sometimes impairments worsen. The nature and meaning of impairment are not given in any one moment. Not all people with impairment have the same needs, or are disadvantaged to the same extent. Different environments mitigate or accentuate disability and disadvantage. Moreover, different people experience different levels of social disadvantage or social exclusion, because society is geared to accommodate people with certain impairments, but not others. Everyone may be impaired, but not everyone is oppressed: the argument about the ubiquity of impairment does not in any way obscure oppressive practices and social relations, contra Helen Meekosha and Russell Shuttleworth's claim (2009).

The benefits of regarding every human being as living with the predicament of impairment are that it forces us to pay attention to what we have in common; it counsels us to accept the inextricable limitation of life, rather than to deny or fight against it; it suggests the need to re-evaluate disabled people; it focuses attention on the social aspects of disability. For example, if everyone is impaired, why are certain impairments remedied or accepted, and others not? How can we minimise the impact of impairment on functioning? Why does impairment result in exclusion in some cases and not others? These processes and choices are largely social and structural and can be changed. In policy terms, a universal approach would use the range of human variation as the basis for universal design, and aim for justice in the distribution of resources and opportunities. Particularly in the context of an ageing population, a universal approach becomes a policy imperative. Disabled people should not be expected to identify themselves as members of a particular group, or as incompetent in stigmatised ways, in order to qualify for provision, but needs should be seen as distributed among the whole population, albeit unequally.

Conclusion

The complex reality of impairment suggests that equalising the situation for disabled people will necessarily be more complex and difficult than equalising the situation for women and other minorities. In the previous chapters, I argued that there were differences between disability, on the one hand, and race, gender and sexuality on the other, because disability was connected to intrinsic disadvantage. As Jerome Bickenbach et al. (1999) have argued, disabled people experience both restrictions of negative freedom – in the form of discrimination which prevents them achieving their potential – but also restrictions of positive freedom because they cannot participate freely in society:

The denial of opportunities and resources is an issue, not of discrimination, but of distributive injustice – an unfair distribution of social resources and opportunities that results in limitations of participation in all areas of social life.

(ibid.: 110)

Ending disablism – unfair discrimination against disabled people – will not solve all the problems of disabled people. Even if environments and transports were accessible and there was no unfair discrimination on the basis of disability, many disabled people would still be disadvantaged. For example, it is well known that some impairments generate extra costs – heating, equipment, diet (Smith *et al.*, 2005). Many disabled people require personal assistance or care. And while many disabled people could work just as productively as non-disabled people once discrimination was fully removed, this does not apply to all disabled people. Some disabled people are unable to work a seven-hour day or a five-day week, due to fatigue. Some disabled people are unable to work at the intensity or productivity of non-disabled workers. Some disabled people are very limited in the types of tasks they are able to perform. And of course, some disabled people are entirely unable to work.

This problem has been noted by several commentators. For example, Henley (2001) discusses the ways in which the emphasis on normalisation in policy towards people describes how efforts to promote employment of people with learning difficulties in the 1980s led to the closing of day centres and other projects. In 1984, the King's Fund published *An Ordinary Working Life*, which stated that paid employment for all people with learning difficulties was an achievable aim (ibid.: 940). While many more people with learning difficulties undoubtedly can work than were working at the time, it is unrealistic to suggest that this is an option for all:

The lesson to be learnt from the past is that the policy of pursuing total inclusion for all people with learning disabilities and encouraging the decimation of all forms of specialist service support in the process has, in practice, proved to be fundamentally flawed.

(ibid.: 946)

This is a point that was also recognised, from a materialist perspective, by Paul Abberley (2001: 131). At the start of the disability movement, Paul Hunt (1966) challenged the social policy focus on work, arguing that disabled people outside the labour market contributed to society in different ways, not least by challenging utilitarian values.

Analysing the first version of the British Disability Discrimination Act, Gooding argues that more is required than treating everyone the same (2000: 536). Society's failure to meet the needs of disabled people cannot be accounted for simply by the concept of disablism. The strategy of promoting employment, while very desirable, will also leave a residuum of unemployed and unemployable disabled people. Disability includes intrinsic limitation and disadvantage. Societies will need to address this, by making additional investment to equalise the situation between disabled and non-disabled people – not just equal opportunities, but redistribution.

While disability studies and disability rights movements have criticised individual and medical approaches to disability, the focus on civil rights still implies a liberal solution to the disability problem (Russell, 2002). Anti-discrimination law and independent living solutions seem to suggest that the market will provide, if only disabled people are enabled to exercise choices free of unfair discrimination. But market approaches often restrict, rather than increasing choice to disabled people (Williams, 1983; Wilson *et al.*, 2000). An individual, market-based solution, by failing to acknowledge persistent inequalities in physical and mental capacities, cannot liberate all disabled people.

Human beings are not all the same, and do not all have the same capabilities and limitations. Need is variable, and disabled people are among those who need more from others and from their society. Alasdair MacIntyre begins to explore the political implications of this reality:

> a form of political society in which it is taken for granted that disability and dependence on others are something that all of us experience at certain times in our lives and this to unpredictable degrees, and that consequently our interest in how the needs of the disabled are adequately voiced and met is not a special interest, the interest of one particular group rather than of others, but rather the interest of the whole political society, an interest that is integral to their conception of their common good.
>
> *(1999: 130)*

This approach, which is also found in the feminist ethic of care thinkers (Tronto, 1993) and can be related to the capabilities approach (Sen, 1992; Nussbaum, 2006), seems as radical, and more adequate, than the 'strong' social model denial of the persistence of impairment as a factor in creating disadvantage. The capabilities approach is based on corporeal need, not the idea of autonomous rationality that is central to the Kantian and contractarian conception of liberal rights (Vehmas, 2012). Impairment is not usually a matter of individual responsibility: it arises from the random effect of genes or disease, or the socially created costs of work, warfare, poverty, or from the nature effects of the ageing process. If disabled people have equal moral worth to non-disabled people – and are viewed politically as equal citizens – then justice demands social arrangements that compensate for both the natural lottery and socially caused injury. Creating a level playing field is not enough: redistribution is required to promote true social inclusion.

5

THE POLITICS OF DISABILITY IDENTITY

Introduction

There is a strong consensus in the disability studies literature that the disability movement has been a very positive force, both in the collective ability to lever political change, and in the benefits to individual participants (Driedger, 1989; Gilson *et al.*, 1997; Charlton 1998; Branfield, 1999; Peters *et al.*, 2009): 'A confident, positive disability identity within a broad, inclusive disability community has emerged. The benefit to disabled people to determine and relate their own stories is increasingly evident' (Gilson *et al.*, 1997: 16). Many disability studies researchers – including myself – have been active in, or have emerged out of, the disability rights struggle. The principle of emancipatory research (Mercer, 2002) suggests that disability studies should be accountable to the priorities and organisations of disabled people. Perhaps this very closeness leads to an unquestioning acceptance of the benefits of political affiliation and an affirmatory reading of disability identity politics. For example, Jane Campbell and Michael Oliver's social history of the disability movement gives a largely positive account of the political developments of the 1970s and 1980s. The growth of political consciousness and collective organisation was welcomed by many contributors to their book, particularly because it built the self-esteem of individual participants. The social model came as an immense liberation (Hasler, 1993; Campbell and Oliver, 1996: 117). Conscientisisation (Freire, 1972) through disability rights analysis changes a person's self-conception. As James Charlton suggests:

> The critical consciousness that emerges from this position may lead some people to adopt the disability activist subject position which can involve street level political action or challenging and

transforming the organisations for the disabled to become organisations of disabled people and so on. In this sense, to name disability as
social oppression is not the defeated wailings of victims, but the
clarion call of social change agents.

(1998: 192)

One example of this mobilisation is provided by the Deaf community.
During the 1970s, Deaf people began organising as a social movement,
challenging the idea that they were impaired, and defining themselves
increasingly as a linguistic minority, using the model of ethnicity. In this
period, slogans such as Deaf Pride and Deaf Power became popular.
One of the culminations of this new Deaf identity and political consciousness came with the successful 1988 Deaf President Now protest at
Gallaudet University. After the appointment of a hearing President at
this university for the Deaf, students exploded into political action,
closing down the college in order to demand that the Board of Trustees
appoint the first deaf president in the school's history. As two analysts
commented:

> The transformation involved deaf persons: (a) identifying them-
> selves as members of a community sharing common values and
> traits (e.g. sign language) and (b) evaluating the group and its values
> and traits in a positive light. Ironically, as a group's members come
> to value themselves after a long period of self deprecation, the
> consciousness-raising can lead to anger, resentment, and political
> action over the perceived injustices.
>
> *(Rose and Kiger, 1995: 522)*

The same anger can be seen in the direct action of disabled people in
many countries of the world (which is well documented in Charlton, 1998).
  Campbell and Oliver's contributors also stress the role of direct action
and other collective forms of political process, which give disabled people
the feelings of power and validation, and provide a symbolic challenge to
an oppressive and exclusionary society. The implication of these studies
is to suggest that the growth of disability politics has created new social
forms, and new possibilities for individual affiliation and identity. Bill
Hughes *et al.*, reviewing the issues for young disabled people in contemporary culture, claim that: 'The growth of disability pride suggests
that disabled people do not want to be other than they are. They are
not rejecting disability as an identity or trying to escape the biological
realities of impairment' (2005b: 7). My worry with this suggestion is that
it implies that disability identity is a given, and that impairment will

automatically define personal identity. Instead, I would claim that disability politics offers new options for individuals to think about both their impairment, and their position in society. Following Ian Hacking (1986), I suggest that the rise of disability politics has created a new category, a new way of affiliating and identifying, which did not exist before.

Some scholars and activists have actively tried to develop the notion of a disability identity, suggesting that it is appropriate to talk in terms of disability culture, and affirming an ethnic conception of disability identity. Susan Peters (2000) argues that there is a disability culture just as there is a deaf culture. She points to a common language, a shared historical lineage, cohesive social community, and political solidarity. For her, the Independent Living community in Berkeley was the equivalent of Martha's Vineyard for Deaf people. Peters quotes Carol Gill: 'I believe very firmly in disabled culture – and if we don't have one, we should. We need it to survive as an oppressed minority, both physically and emotionally' (Peters, 2000: 584). In the same vein, Fran Branfield has called for a separatist approach to disability research (Branfield, 1998, 1999).

In passing, I note that an interesting feature of the work on disability as a political identity is that it shows that the social barriers approach that is the defining characteristic of the UK social model actually overlaps with, or subsumes, a minority group conception (Shakespeare, 1999b). A social barriers approach does not define a particular group who are to benefit from barrier removal; it implicitly refuses to identify people with impairments as a distinct group. But in the practices of the disability movement, clearly a group emerges of people with impairment who are campaigning both for the removal of barriers, and for better provision for their minority. In other words, rather than seeing a major distinction between US and UK strategies, there is overlap between minority group and barriers theory. US approaches are framed in terms of the minority group approach, but contain an emphasis on social barriers; UK approaches are framed in terms of the barriers approach, but contain a strong element of minority group conception. For example, Michael Oliver's discussion of disability identity suggests that it comprises three elements: (1) having an impairment; (2) experiencing externally imposed restrictions; and (3) self-identification as a disabled person (Oliver, 1996: 5).

In this chapter, I will challenge some of the taken-for-granted assumptions about the benefits of disability identity. First, I will explore the tension between labels and badges. Then I will critically evaluate the extent to which disabled people do identify politically, and the representativeness of the disability movement. Next, I will explore some of the problems with identity politics, particularly in the case of disability, before concluding with an alternative account of emancipatory politics, drawn from the work of Nancy Fraser.

Labels and badges

It is paradoxical that the identification of people with impairment as members of a disabled collective is generally viewed positively, whereas the ascription of group membership – in the form of labelling – is generally viewed negatively in the disability community. Deconstruction of these processes – the difference between a badge and a label – is important in understanding the complexity of identification.

In previous chapters, I showed how scepticism with medical categories is often signalled with scare quotes. Within the field of learning difficulties, the influence of normalisation has led to an opposition to any form of medical or psychological diagnosis or labelling (Gilman *et al.*, 2000; Chappell *et al.*, 2001). Opposition to labelling arises from an awareness of the stigma that can be a consequence of particular labels or diagnoses. When someone is given a label – for example, of learning disability or mental illness – this may trigger other negative associations. The phenomenon of 'identity spread' means that the person's individuality – both their personality, but also other aspects of their identity such as gender, sexuality and ethnicity – can be ignored, as the impairment label becomes the most prominent and relevant feature of their lives, dominating interactions.

There are several reasons to qualify the opposition to labelling. Barbara Riddick (2000) points out that stigma can happen even without labelling. In theory, at least, labelling can happen without stigma. Moreover, for some groups, diagnosis is a very important and valuable process. My colleague Steve Macdonald (2009) researches the experiences of people diagnosed as dyslexic. He argues strongly that diagnosis is valued by his respondents, because it enables them to see themselves not as intellectually limited, but as having a particular brain difference. Moreover, a diagnosis enables people with dyslexia to obtain the computer technology and educational support they need to survive in school and university (ibid.). Similarly, Fox and Kim (2004) argue that people with what they call 'emerging disabilities' – which are often invisible – are struggling to achieve medical acceptance. Such individuals positively welcome a label:

> While many interest groups of persons with disabilities are highly vocal in their desire to disconnect their disability from medical diag-nosis and treatment, groups of persons with disabilities perceived as

emerging stage their early battles for this very turf, hoping that medical acceptance will lead to greater social acceptance.

(ibid.: 334)

Diagnosis for people with hidden impairments gives credibility to their difference, may lead to effective medical or educational support, and also gives protection under anti-discrimination legislation such as the Americans with Disabilities Act. Bill Hughes has discussed how, as well as disability identity, there are also new groups of 'biological citizens', patient activists who campaign for better biomedical provision (Hughes, 2009).

Understanding that an impairment is real, and may have a biological basis, has been liberating for families affected by autism (Farrugia, 2009): in previous generations, parents were blamed for having emotionally deprived their children. But Hodge (2005) reflects on ambivalence about the process of diagnosis in the case of autistic spectrum disorders (see also Wheeler, 2011). Diagnosis can lead to better understanding of the problem and to access to appropriate support mechanisms: resource allocation is label-led. But a diagnosis can also be disempowering for parents, causing them to fear for the future. There is also a danger of seeing the label, not the individual child:

> After his diagnosis the author noticed a big difference in the way he was treated in school and by society in general. He was tolerated, his behaviours were attributed to his AS and attempts were made to support him. As he grew older, however, it soon became apparent that people were not tolerating him, but rather were tolerating the disorder. Every behaviour he exhibited was attributed to his condition and he was defined not as a person, not as an individual, but as a label.
>
> *(ibid.: 848)*

Equally, minimising the extent to which autism is an impairment – seeing it simply as 'an alternative way of being' – could be a denial of the pervasive and sometimes devastating impact of autism on both the child and the family.

Labelling is a complex and paradoxical process (Brown, 1995; Shakespeare and Erickson, 2000). For example, Clarke *et al.* (2005) and other authors have pointed out the contradiction between defining an individual with impairment as normal within family and community, when at the same time that same individual needs to identify as abnormal to get services and benefits (Shildrick, 1997). A similar paradox surrounds political identification as disabled, as I will discuss below: people who would oppose labelling and reject medical diagnoses are, nevertheless, willing to identify politically as disabled and accept a badge or banner. Yet, as I show, many people with impairments do not want to identify either as impaired (with a label) or disabled (with a badge): they want to be seen as ordinary members of society, free of limitation or classification.

Identification as disabled

Notwithstanding the positive disability studies assessment of the disability movement, there are important questions about the extent to which people with impairment identify with the disability movement, or indeed as people with impairment. Despite the visibility of disability rights protest, it has always been a minority activity for disabled people (Campbell and Oliver, 1996). Of course, lack of activism does not necessarily imply lack of affiliation to the values or demands of the disability rights movement. Other liberation movements – such as the women's movement and the lesbian and gay movement – have never mobilised a significant proportion of their communities. Moreover, due to transport barriers and mobility and income restrictions, it is harder for disabled people to mobilise. Therefore it is important to look to other research to understand the extent to which disabled people view themselves as part of a larger minority group. *Disabled for Life?*, a research project undertaken by the Department of Work and Pensions in 2003, found that 52 per cent of DDA-defined disabled people did not define themselves as disabled people: young people were particularly likely to reject this identification. However, this might indicate a reluctance to identify with a stigmatised social label, and an ignorance of the social model redefinition of disability. A 2002 survey of 200 disabled people conducted by the British Council of Disabled People found that only 3 per cent of them had heard of the social model (Rickell, 2006).

Bob Sapey, John Stuart and Glenis Donaldson (Sapey *et al.*, 2005) conducted research in North-west England to explore reasons for the increase in use of wheelchairs, and to investigate perceptions of disability: over 1000 people responded to their survey. Nearly 80 per cent of the respondents agreed that wheelchairs can be liberating for disabled people; 48 per cent of people agreed that the environment around made it hard for them to do many things they wanted in their wheelchair, but 80 per cent of people also agreed that their illness or condition stopped them doing many things they wanted to do, which is far from a social model position. The authors of the study claim that the findings are consistent with the social model of disability, and show that social model analysis is relevant to lived experience. This appears to me to be a rather selective reading of the data, which suggests that both impairment and environment are implicated in the experience of disability, supporting the interactional conception of disability that was proposed in Chapter 4.

Turning to qualitative research, several studies challenge a simplistic social model identification. For example, in Kelly's research with young people with autism, respondents' experiences and affiliations could not straightforwardly be subsumed under the social model and different respondents emphasised different aspects of their experience – not being able to walk, or exclusion from social opportunities, for example (Kelly, 2005: 271). Jane Andrews's research with disabled volunteers found that neither a medical model nor a social model approach satisfactorily explained her data:

> In particular, the volunteers interviewed during the pre-field and pilot stages of the study continually expressed frustration with the medically derived limitations placed upon them as individuals living with various illnesses and impairments. Such limitations appeared to them to be more restrictive than any socially constructed barriers encountered during the normal day-to-day routines of volunteering.
>
> *(Andrews, 2005: 203)*

Nick Watson conducted an in-depth qualitative study with 28 disabled people in Scotland. Despite daily experiences of oppressive practices, only three of the participants incorporated disability within their identity. Instead, they normalised their experience of physical limitation. They were all able to describe experiences of discrimination. But they rejected a political identity as disabled people:

> Being disabled, for many of these informants, is not about celebrating difference or diversity, pride in their identity is not formed through the individuals labelling themselves as different, as disabled, but it is about defining disability in their own terms, under their own terms of reference.
>
> *(Watson, 2002: 521)*

Their wish was to assimilate with the mainstream and negate a demeaning difference. We found a similar response when we did research with young disabled people in the late 1990s: while they could identify exclusionary processes and lack of access as problems, their goal was to be part of the mainstream youth culture, not to identify as disabled (Priestley *et al.*, 1999). Similarly, the people with restricted growth whom my team interviewed did not start to identify as disabled until their health symptoms caused them pain or restricted participation (Thompson *et al.*, 2010).

The implication of early disability activism that people with impairments were oppressed and that salvation lay in collective identification and mobilisation has proved over-optimistic: only a tiny proportion of people with impairments have ever signed up to the radical campaign, and many have actively disowned it. Many people do not want to see themselves as disabled, either in terms of the medical model or the social model, such as the respondents to our restricted growth research (ibid.). They certainly downplay the significance of their impairments. But they also resist seeing themselves as part of the disability movement or identifying with a political conception of disability (see also the research reported in Scully, 2008). Probably the majority of people with impairments or chronic illnesses regard themselves as 'really normal', refusing to allow their health condition, or responses to it, to dominate their lives. Recognising this, the former UK Disability Rights Commission shifted away from using the term disabled people, referring instead to 'people who have rights under the Disability Discrimination Act' (Fletcher, 2006). The refusal to define oneself by impairment or disability has sometimes been seen as 'internalised oppression' or 'false consciousness' by radicals in the disability movement. Yet this attitude can be patronising and oppressive. After all, the denial of disability is implicitly based on the rejection of the idea of an exclusive 'normality', and a refusal to be categorised. This approach may be rather individualist, and may overlook the problems of discrimination and prejudice, but surely it is a legitimate alternative to a minority group approach.

Is the disability movement representative?

Above, I argued that the majority of disabled people do not identify with the social model or in terms of a disability identity. A related issue is the extent to which the disability rights movement is representative of the disabled population as a whole. The disability movement in many countries is dominated by a somewhat restricted section of the impaired population. For example, in Western countries, approximately half of all people with impairments are over the age of 50. Yet most activists enter the movement at a much younger age, and older people who have impairments neither make up a significant proportion of the movement, nor are likely to identify with a civil rights perspective.

Again, there have been persistent questions about the role and involvement of particular impairment groups. For example, people with learning difficulties may have been excluded because their particular access and language issues have not been properly understood, or because they have not been welcomed, or because social model theory has not effectively incorporated intellectual impairments (Chappell, 1998; Chappell *et al.*, 2001; Stalker, 2012). Some disabled people have sought to bolster their own status as people with physical impairments, at the expense of those with intellectual impairments. People with mental health conditions often resist affiliation, not wishing to add another stigmatised identity – disabled – to their existing stigma of mental illness (Beresford, 2012). Another example is the Deaf community, who have resisted identification with the mainstream disability movement. Often this is because Deaf people see themselves as a linguistic minority, not as people defined by a medical condition. Of course, some radical disabled people themselves have rejected a medical identity, so perhaps the problem is less one of definition, and more about separate cultures (Corker, 1999). More of a problem is that dominant disability rights demands – such as inclusive education for all disabled children – are rejected by Deaf communities who want their children separately educated via the medium of Sign Language. Deaf politics found it easier to adopt a straightforward identity politics model, as the movements for Deaf Pride and Deaf Power demonstrate. Rose and Kiger (1995) use the work of the social psychologist Henri Tajfel (1978) to explore the process of a hitherto excluded community acquiring a 'voice' through social action to enhance the interests of a minority group, which comes to see itself as oppressed minority. To bolster their self-image, a group exaggerates and values its members' distinctiveness. A sense of injustice and resistance leads to increased identification with the group, which also promotes the self-esteem of its members. Yet more recently, Deaf politics has become more complex, not least through cochlear implantation. Jackie Leach Scully (2012) demonstrates how even this paradigmatic case of cultural identity has become questionable, with the growing diversity of experiences of deafness.

Aside from differences of impairment and age, other social cleavages are also evident in disability politics, which has failed to account for the diversity of identity (Vernon, 1996, 1999). Feminists have often criticised the disability movement for sexism and the exclusion of women's issues. Minority ethnic communities have sometimes felt ignored by disability groups that are dominated by the majority population. Lesbian and gay disabled people have experienced homophobia, or have felt unwelcome in disability organisations that have taken on radical disabled perspectives, but may be very conventional in terms of sexual politics. Finally, access to economic and social power is a strong determinant of the life-experience of disabled people in general (Shakespeare, 2010), and also influences involvement in disability politics: many leaders of the movement have come from privileged socio-economic contexts. Nor, as Gary Albrecht suggests, have civil rights approaches benefited poorer disabled people, who are less savvy about lobbying (Albrecht, 1992: 300).

If the disability movement (and disability studies) have not been fully representative of the variety of disabled people's experiences, then perhaps this suggests another reason for the inadequacies of the social model approach. The activists of UPIAS were predominantly people with physical impairments, mainly wheelchair users. Their conceptualisation of disability may have reflected the specificity of their own experience. For example, people with spinal cord injury, once stabilised, do not suffer degenerating chronic illness. There may be neuropathic pain, and vulnerability to pressure sores or urinary infections, but these may seem like management and hygiene issues. To a wheelchair user, their health may not be the problem, whereas the lack of physical access and the prejudices of employers and professionals might well be. In other words, the social model possibly works from the perspective of someone with a stable physical impairment. But had the original UPIAS ideological discussions included people with mental health issues, people with learning difficulties, or even people whose physical impairments involved more intrinsic suffering, then perhaps a richer and more complex understanding of the nature of disability might have resulted.

Challenges to disability identity

Disability identity politics has been very powerful, but also contradictory and incoherent. This may derive from the heterogeneity of disabled people's experience. As Jerome Bickenbach et al. (1999) note, the analogy between racial minorities and disabled people breaks down at many important points, because of the diversity of the disability experience: 'There is no unifying culture, language or set of experiences; people with disabilities are not homogenous, nor is there much prospect for transdisability solidarity' (ibid.: 1181). A pure barriers approach does not specify a group of subjects who could adopt a political identity as disabled. But, equally, the basis of disabled identity could not be located in impairment. The social model was based on the irrelevance of impairment to the definition of disability. Moreover, impairment is negatively valued socially. Slogans such as 'glad to be gay', 'black is beautiful' do not have an equivalent in the disability movement. Therefore, the basis of identity had to be found in shared resistance to oppression, similar to the feminist slogan 'sisterhood is powerful'. Without a basis in impairment, disability identity becomes voluntaristic and difficult to define or police. Disabled people become classed as the category of people who identify as having experienced disability oppression. For example, Simi Linton suggests: 'The question of who "qualifies" as disabled is as answerable or as confounding as questions about any identity status. One simple response might be that you are disabled if you say you are' (1998: 12). Self-identifying as disabled has been taken as key by British scholars and activists also (Campbell and Oliver, 1996).

However, this approach would include some people who happen to like the idea of being members of a disabled minority group, but in objective terms are not oppressed in any way. It would also exclude some people who may objectively experience oppression, but subjectively refuse to identify as such. It may also include people who may experience forms of social exclusion based on physical difference, but would not traditionally be seen as disabled. For example, one writer asks whether a fat woman can call herself disabled:

> Many fat people suffer poor self-esteem, we grow up fearing our own bodies in shame, public ridicule and social ostracism, and the cultural fear and hatred of us can ruin our lives. I believe that self-defining as 'disabled' enables us to take ourselves seriously and demand that others do also.
>
> *(Cooper, 1997: 33)*

In developing a social model approach to fatness, Cooper shows how defining disability in terms of social barriers or social oppression, rather than a biological impairment, opens up the category to a range of other social excluded or devalued groups: what about anorexic women (Tierney, 2001)? If 'disabled people' emerge as a result of individual political action or group affiliation, it becomes an artificial, contingent and ultimately unsatisfactory grouping.

A deeper set of challenges question the form that disability identity takes, particularly the ethnic or cultural conception of disability. For example, Humphrey (1999, 2000) has challenged the separatism of identity-based approaches. Researching disability identity in the context of a trades union disability network, she argues that self-definition is problematic, because self-defined people may be suspected of not really being disabled. Failure to discuss impairment benefits those with visible impairments, and makes it harder to discuss impairment-related needs:

> [T]he social model as operationalised within the UNISON group has both reified the disability identity and reduced it to particular

kinds of impairments – physical, immutable, tangible and 'severe' ones – in a way which can deter many people from adopting a disabled identity and participating in a disability community.

(Humphrey, 2000: 69)

Humphrey also criticises the opposition of disabled to non-disabled people that results from an exclusive version of disability identity, which cannot account for those who inhabit both disabled and non-disabled worlds, and which can result in separatism (ibid.: 81).

The notion of disability identity raises particular problems. But any resort to identity politics is problematic (Scully, 2008). The logic of identity politics can prove counter-productive. At one level, this arises from the inexhaustible number of possible identities. Lennard Davis argues that identity politics is self-defeating, because ultimately everyone has an identity: 'The list of identities will only grow larger, tied to an ever expanding idea of inclusiveness. After all, when all identities are finally included, there will be no identity' (Davis, 2002: 88). As Phil Lee argues, socially constructed identities are 'contestable and subject to change; sub- and splinter groups emerge, as different aspects of the identity are prioritized' (2002: 151).

But the more significant problem with a minority group approach to disability was first identified by Helen Liggett (1988) and draws on Foucauldian ideas, discussed in an earlier chapter. Disability politics, by its very nature, often rests on a fairly unreflexive acceptance of the disabled/non-disabled distinction. Disabled people are seen as those who identify as such. Disabled leadership is seen as vital. But Liggett argues:

> From an interpretative point of view the minority group approach is double edged because it means enlarging the discursive practices which participate in the constitution of disability ... [I]n order to participate in their own management, disabled people have had to participate as disabled. Even among the politically active, the price of being heard is understanding that it is the disabled who are speaking.
>
> *(ibid.: 271ff)*

This relates to what Denise Riley has called 'the dangerous intimacy between subjectification and subjection' (1988: 17). A minority group approach demands a dichotomy between disabled and non-disabled people, reinforcing differentness, rather than promoting assimilation. As Galvin argues:

> By claiming an identity which has been created through the pro-
> cesses of hierarchical differentiation and exclusion, subjugated peoples
> reinforce their own oppression and restrict their hopes to the belief
> that they can demonstrate how positive it is to be identified as such.
>
> *(2003: 682)*

To be an activist – whether as a gay person, or a woman, or a disabled
person – is to make the label into a badge, to make the ghetto into an
oppositional culture. Yet what about those, like the disabled people
cited earlier, who wish to be ordinary, not different? Post-structuralists
such as Diane Fuss (1989) argue that an essentialist theory of identity,
however attractive, is ultimately not a secure foundation for politics.

However, there is potentially a higher price to adopting the disability
label than just to highlight separateness and difference. A more serious
problem, within the disability context, is that building an identity around
oppression leads the minority group into taking up a victim position
(Takala, 2009). In this sense, a social model of disability can be as
negative as a medical model of disability. Whereas the latter sees disabled
people as victims of their flawed bodies or brains, the former sees disabled people as prisoners of an oppressive and excluding society. In both
versions, the agency of disabled people is denied and the scope for
positive engagement with either impairment or society is diminished.

Building identity on victimhood leads to the recital of a litany of
oppression and woe. For example, the editors of the revised edition
of the seminal *Disabling Barriers, Enabling Environments* claim that in the
ten years since the first edition, nothing has changed: 'Despite major
changes in legislation, for instance, the dominant picture remains one of
discrimination, prejudice, injustice and poverty, often rationalised on the
grounds of supposed progress for disabled people' (Swain *et al.*, 2004: 1).

Mike Oliver and Colin Barnes sound a similar lament in the second
edition of *The New Politics of Disablement*: '[T]he individual and tragic
view of disability continues to hold sway in almost all policy and social
interactions' (Oliver and Barnes, 2012: 14).

I think that some of the considerable attention given to hate crime is
part of this generalised tendency to stress the victimhood of disabled
people (Quarmby, 2011; Roulstone and Mason-Bish, 2013). This way
of thinking serves to obscure the progress that has been made in recent
decades, often due to the political mobilisation of disabled people
themselves. It is true that disabled people continue to do less well than
the majority of society, and there is much to be done to ensure equality
and inclusion. At the time of writing, a savage attack on the living
standards of disabled people is underway (www.wearespartacus.org.uk),

in the form of tightened eligibility criteria for Personal Independence Payment (formerly Disability Living Allowance) and Employment Support Allowance (formerly Inacapacity Benefit), together with a cultural backlash that associates disabled benefit claimants with scroungers (Strathclyde Centre for Disability Research, 2012). But notwithstanding these very serious problems with welfare reform, conditions for disabled people have improved in other ways over the last twenty years, thanks to the Disability Discrimination Acts and Equality Act and other initiatives.

Office of Disability Issues statistics (2013) state that between 2002–12, the employment gap between disabled and non-disabled people reduced by 10 percentage points. Between 2005/6 and 2010/11, the numbers attaining five or more GCSE A–C pass rates have increased from approximately 20 per cent to approximately 60 per cent for special educational needs students without a statement of special educational needs, and from approximately 9 per cent to approximately 25 per cent for students who do have a statement of special educational need. Between 2004/5 and 2011/12, the number of accessible buses increased from 52 per cent to 88 per cent of buses. For people with learning difficulties, the government's *Valuing People* White Paper (Department of Health, 2001), drafted with the participation of people with learning difficulties themselves, has put the principles of rights, independence, choice and inclusion at the centre of policy. Although many other statistics and policies are still woeful, there are some signs of progress.

Denying progress is as misguided as overlooking the continuing problems. The consequence of taking up a victim position and of exaggerating the differences and the polarity between the minority group and the mainstream is that politics can become more extreme, separatist, vanguardist and aggressive. The politics of coalition (Lee, 2002: 158) becomes less likely.

The victim position can be reassuring for individuals. It explains that any problems they might encounter, or failure they experience, has resulted from oppression, not from any fault of their own. It gives an excuse for not trying, because all efforts are doomed, and all change is illusory. The victim position also makes the success of other people who seemingly share your status become very threatening. If some disabled people have achieved their goals, or have managed to be successful in a disabling society, then this undermines the victimhood analysis. For this reason, it becomes important to disown or condemn the 'tall poppies' who have succeeded.

Underlying identity politics, the social model can play an important psychological role for disabled people. It is a powerful way of denying both the relevance and the negativity of impairment. Activists can maintain that their problems are not their deficits of body or mind, but are due to the society in which they live. By combining with others who share this belief, their own self-image is reinforced, and they can achieve solidarity and self-respect. The social model became ideologically dominant precisely because it moved away from the individual and the personal and the psychological. This may explain how difficult it has been for social model perspectives to engage with the question of impairment: how could an identity-sustaining theory include what had been disavowed?

At the heart of the social model approach to disability is a kind of denial. Social model theory enables disabled people to deny the relevance of their impaired bodies or brains, and seek equality with non-disabled people on the basis of similarity. What divides disabled from non-disabled people, in this formulation, is the imposition of social oppression and social exclusion. Moreover, the identity politics that is fuelled by this ideology paradoxically depends on strengthening the coherence and separateness of the disability group. Disabled people are contrasted with non-disabled people. Non-disabled people and the non-disabled world are increasingly seen as oppressive and hostile. Those who claim to help disabled people – professionals, charities, governments – are rejected. A strong political identity, which should be a means to an end, has become an end in itself. Rather than looking outward, the disability movement has often turned inwards. Rather than building bridges with other groups or seeking the integration of its members within society, the vanguard of the disability movement has often been separatist, promoting a notion of 'us', the disabled people, against 'them', the non-disabled oppressors (Holdsworth, 1993; Branfield, 1998, 1999). For disability activists, this has been powerful and motivating, but as the basis for disability politics, it has been counter-productive.

Affirmation approaches

Radical social model perspectives stress oppression as the basis for identity. Arguably, this still leaves disabled people in a pathologised situation. While the causation has shifted from the impaired body to the exclusionary society, disabled people are still rendered as victims, rather than agents. The bulk of disability studies literature casts disabled people in a negative light, and discusses the woes of bodies that don't work, in a society that does not care. This is not only depressing for disabled readers, but it also does not accurately capture the lives of disabled people and their families, which are almost always more positive than these accounts suggest. Government statements on disability focus not on positive flourishing, but on shifting disabled people from a negative state to a neutral state: the full range of human emotions and aspirations, including the positive, are not reflected in discourse (Sunderland *et al.*, 2009).

John Swain and Sally French (2000) have suggested a new conception of disability, which they term an affirmation model. This combines a focus on the political benefits of identifying with a collectivity, but also a redefinition of the nature of impairment. For example, impairment is seen to bring benefits such as being able to escape role restrictions and social expectations, the possibility of empathy with others and better relationships:

> In affirming a positive identity of being impaired, disabled people are actively repudiating the dominant value of normality. The changes for individuals are not just a transforming of consciousness as to the meaning of 'disability', but an assertion of the value and validity of life as a person with an impairment.
>
> *(ibid.: 578)*

For Swain and French, the role of disability culture – for example, disability arts cabarets – is central to this process. An affirmation approach to disability highlights the possibilities of political and cultural resistance, solidarity and meaning making. It rejects the discourses of either tragedy or oppression, and celebrates ordinary everyday life.

For people on the autistic spectrum who identify as neuro-diverse, an affirmation model is about celebrating the difference that their condition offers them, not as deficit, but as a different way of being and relating to the world (Chamak, 2008; Wheeler, 2011), which has its own strengths. This means that an affirmation approach is very relevant and useful. Psychologist Brian Watermeyer suggests that what is needed is: 'a vehement recognition of disabled subjectivity not as an incomplete analogue of non-disabled life, but as novel, complete, unitary and of clear human relevance' (2009: 100).

Affirmation also seems relevant to people with learning difficulties other than autism. The self-advocacy movement offers people a place where they can meet friends, feel affirmed, and celebrate their lives. Opposition to labelling is very strong among self-advocates, who wish to be treated as individuals, not to be defined in terms of what is wrong with them:

> The value of the self-advocacy movement lies in how it enables people with 'learning difficulties' to critically challenge the power of the dominant master narrative about them. With support from each other and their advisors, self-advocates resist stereotypes and

challenge pervasive power takeovers on all their selves as 'unable', 'deviant' and 'impaired' beings in particular ways.

(Roets, 2009: 697)

While respecting and welcoming the positive work of the self-advocacy community, it is also the case that people with learning difficulties generally reject a sense of themselves as being different or vulnerable (e.g. Hollomotz, 2011: 117). Robert Edgerton (1984) famously called this 'the cloak of competence', the rejection of stigmatisation. I think an attitude of respectful ambivalence towards the identity claims of self-advocates is necessary: the fact that they do not interpret their lives using the language of intellectual impairment does not mean that they are correct.

The idea of affirmation is also relevant to non-disabled people with a disabled family member. Bryony Beresford (1994) stresses that parents of disabled children should not be seen as only or predominantly suffering from grief and stress and burden. As with Rannveig Traustadottir's research, she talks about how parents gain a sense of satisfaction and purpose, have a better sense of proportion, learn skills, have pride in their achievements and love for their child. Another study explored the positive aspects of having a disabled sibling, rather than the tradition of seeing this as a source of strain and stigma. The respondents highlighted the close and unique bond, the strong sense of family unity, the positive reaction from friends (Guse and Harvey, 2010).

It seems to me that balance is required in any account of disability, and these affirmation accounts re-balance away from the emphasis on victimhood or incapacity. As will be evident from the previous chapter, I would not agree when Swain and French (2000) seek to challenge the idea of impairment as a problem: for most disabled people, impairment is often a difficulty. I would question the extent to which impairment has value for many disabled people. It does not seem to me that affirmation approaches constitute a new model. However, these ideas do counsel scholars and activists alike to ensure balance in representations of the lives of disabled people and their families. A model has to be complex enough to encompass the positive aspects of life with a health condition, and allow for the possibilities of adaptation and flourishing (Amundson, 2010).

Post-identity politics

Nancy Fraser (1995) has argued that radical social movements often combine a challenge to socio-economic injustice with a challenge to cultural injustice. She distinguishes between the politics of redistribution and the politics of recognition. What she calls 'bivalent collectivities' 'suffer both socioeconomic maldistribution and cultural misrecognition in forms where neither of these injustices is an indirect effect of the other, but where both are primary and co-original': in these cases, remedies for the two injustices may pull in different directions. She calls for transformational remedies – which deconstruct groupings and promote solidarity – rather than affirmative remedies, which leave deep structures intact and may even stigmatise the disadvantaged class. She also recognises that the politics of recognition can have negative effects, forcing individuals to conform to group culture and discouraging debate: 'The overall effect is to impose a single, drastically simplified group identity which denies the complexity of people's lives, the multiplicity of their identifications and the cross pulls of their various affiliations' (ibid.: 112).

For her, this version of identity politics can become repressive, intolerant and conformist, all adjectives which might be applied to the radical disability rights movement, which has exactly encouraged the separatism and group enclaves which Fraser fears.

The alternative which Fraser proposes is to seek recognition, not as a member of a disadvantaged group, but in terms of individual status: 'To view recognition as a matter of status means examining institutionalised patterns of cultural value for their effects on the relative standing of social actors' (ibid.: 113). Rather than valorising group specificity and promoting essentialism, her social status approach to recognition may lead to a 'non-identitarian politics': 'Redressing misrecognition now means changing social institutions – or, more specifically, changing the interaction-regulating values that impede parity of recognition at all relevant institutional sites' (ibid.: 115).

While supportive of Fraser's approach, Berthe Danermark and L.C. Gellerstedt (2004) criticise Fraser for her lack of focus on face-to-face encounters. Like several other recent disability theorists, they look to the work of Axel Honneth (1995) to combine the different levels of misrecognition and injustice. Drawing on Mead and Hegel, Honneth looks at individual, social and cultural dimensions:

> This implies that injustices to disabled people can be understood neither as generated by solely cultural mechanisms (cultural reductionism) nor by socio-economic mechanisms (economic reductionism) nor by biological mechanisms (biological reductionism). In sum, only by taking different levels, mechanisms and contexts into account, can disability as a phenomenon be analytically approached.
>
> *(Danermark and Gellerstedt, 2004: 350)*

These different approaches may offer elements in a post–identity, post–social model disability politics. Such a re-conception is necessary to offer an alternative to the prison of identity politics, which leads to the politics of victimhood, and the celebration of failure. Many disabled people will prefer to seek what they have in common with non-disabled people, promoting inclusion and equal status, not separatism. The goal of disability politics should be to make impairment and disability irrelevant wherever possible, not to seek out and celebrate a separatist notion of disability pride based on an ethnic conception of disability identity.

PART II
APPLICATIONS

6

QUESTIONING PRENATAL DIAGNOSIS

We have become the kinds of people who think of our present and our future in terms of the quality of our individual biological lives ... we have entered the age of vital politics, or biological ethics and genetic responsibility.

(Rose, 2001: 21–22)

This chapter explores disability rights arguments about prenatal diagnosis (PND), challenging the basis on which objections have been expressed by activists and academics. However, I should state at the outset that my reluctance to accept certain arguments from disability rights critics of prenatal diagnosis does not entail support for prenatal diagnosis as it is currently practised. Nor do my arguments in this chapter imply acceptance of the positions of bioethicists, such as John Harris (1985, 1992) or Peter Singer (1993). These utilitarian philosophers have argued strongly for screening, and even challenged opposition to infanticide in certain situations (Kuhse and Singer, 1985; Singer, 1993). Elsewhere, my colleague Simo Vehmas (2003a, 2003b, 2004) has developed a strong and well-argued philosophical critique of the assumptions and arguments about disability in this mainstream bioethical literature. While I have always tried to criticise both genetic practices and discourses about genetics and disability (Shakespeare, 1995a, 1998a, 1999a, 2005a), in this chapter I continue the revisionist work established earlier in this volume by critically analysing the basis of the disability rights critique.

Within the disability rights movement, there has been considerable concern about the scientific and societal enthusiasm for genetic research in contemporary Western societies (Shakespeare, 1995a; Rock, 1996; Saxton, 2000; Asch, 2001, 2003; Goggin and Newell, 2005). Disabled activists and authors have always been prominent among those opposing developments in human genetics and reproductive medicine. But these critical and cautionary voices of disabled people and their families have not always sufficiently figured within the policy and media debate about the impact of antenatal diagnosis on society. Looking at disability rights objections to antenatal diagnosis and selective termination, there are two linked themes: (1) a powerful narrative about eugenics, common in activist responses; and (2) a more subtle claim about discrimination, coming through disability bioethics. In this and the succeeding section I will discuss these themes, and show why I believe that they cannot entirely be sustained.

Is prenatal diagnosis eugenic?

The eugenic narrative suggests that new genetic technologies combine twenty-first-century science with early twentieth-century-eugenic ideology. Particularly in activist literature, genetics sometimes becomes rendered as a coherent and consistent plot to eliminate disabled people. For example, a bioethics supplement of the international disability rights newsletter *Disability Awareness in Action* talked about disabled people as: 'the target group for a "search and destroy" mission, both before and after birth, incorporating highly effective technologies' (DAA, 1997: 1). The Nazi or fascist comparison is a frequent feature of critiques of this kind:

> Disabled people know only too well they are not welcomed in society, but the active promotion of abortion on the grounds of disability and determining that euthanasia is a viable proposition for the disabled foetus/child – is fascism.
>
> *(Rock, 1996: 124)*

In the publicity for her recent film and installation 'Resistance', the disabled artist Liz Crow again made the comparison between the historical experience of Nazi euthanasia and the modern context of prenatal diagnosis and selective termination: 'We move to today, where rising hate crime, increased pre-natal screening and abortion and a race to assisted suicide challenge the worth of disabled people's lives and even their right to exist' (www.roaring-girl.com, n.d.).

No discussion of genetics should ignore the historical experience of Nazi euthanasia and eugenics. It is an important starting point for contemporary evaluations. For example, many have raised the spectre of Nazi eugenics as a reminder of what can go wrong with attempts to improve the health of the population (Bailey, 1996: 144). This seems legitimate. It should be remembered that eugenic ideas were both common and widely supported in Europe and North America prior to 1945 (Kerr and Shakespeare, 2002). Sterilisation laws were adopted in parts of Canada, the United States (Kevles, 1985) and all the Nordic countries (Broberg and Roll-Hansen, 1996), as well as in Germany. Under the Nazis, disabled people were persecuted with ruthless efficiency (Gallagher, 1995). Sterilisation was carried out on 5 per cent of the population, and on the outbreak of war a ferocious euthanasia programme led to the death of 200,000–275,000 people, the majority with mental illness or learning difficulties (Burleigh, 1994). Medical professionals were at the forefront of Nazi eugenic and euthanasia programmes (Lifton, 1986).

However, making direct analogies between Nazi programmes and contemporary policy and practice (DAA, 1997: 1) makes for highly effective rhetoric but dubious argument, as historian Michael Burleigh suggests (1998: 145). While there are many problematic aspects to the extension of antenatal screening, it is unhelpful and insulting to see most clinicians as fascists or megalomaniacs. Modern democracies do not have sterilisation laws equivalent to those which all Nordic countries and many US states adopted and implemented between 1911 and 1960 (Kevles, 1985; Broberg and Roll-Hansen, 1996). Ideas about 'racial hygiene' and Social Darwinism are no longer acceptable in the mainstream. Contemporary clinical genetics is aimed at preventing and treating genuine illness, rather than 'purifying the population' or eliminating racial and social minorities. When disability rights critics rhetorically resort to the Nazi analogy, it becomes easier for scientists, ethicists and policy-makers to ignore the valid element of the disability critique, and even to exclude disabled people from debates as 'irrational' and 'emotive'.

Moreover, the plot discourse imparts an intentionality and coherence to contemporary policy on reproduction which it does not necessarily possess (Shakespeare, 1999a). The conspiratorialism feeds the idea of a plan by the state, abetted by science, to eliminate all disabled people. But genetic advances are incremental, haphazard, contested and complex. Despite the hyperbole of some genetic researchers, the science is limited, incomplete and uncertain. Few congenital conditions are detectable through mass antenatal screening, despite evidence that some prospective parents think that all types of anomalies can be detected (Skirton and Barr, 2010). Approximately 2 per cent of all births are affected by congenital abnormality, whereas disabled people comprise up to 20 per cent of the population, suggesting that genetic screening could never seriously reduce the incidence of disability. While there are public health policies that will undoubtedly have the indirect consequence of reducing the numbers of babies born with certain impairments (in particular Down syndrome and neural tube defects), the mechanism is more complicated than a negative eugenic programme. There is no government plan to eliminate disabled people.

In particular, consumer demand plays a significant role in the adoption of testing in pregnancy, and the principle of patient autonomy is central to the modern practice of genetics and obstetrics. Rather than coercive eugenics, individual choice is the mechanism by which antenatal screening is implemented (Hampton, 2005), with professionals such as midwives committed to nondirective counselling (Ahmed *et al.*, 2012). The role of prospective parents has largely been ignored by disability rights critics of genetics. Often it is prospective parents, not clinicians, who are the active agents in choosing to terminate pregnancy. Acceptance of antenatal screening varies, and there is some evidence that it has declined. Recent UK studies have found as few as 28 per cent (Shantha *et al.*, 2009) and on average 60 per cent of pregnant women accepted second trimester screening, with 56.5 per cent (Tringham *et al.*, 2011) and 95 per cent (Tsouroufli, 2011) accepting the new forms of first trimester combined screening. In the latter study, 49 per cent of women had made up their minds what to do before the offer of screening (Williams *et al.*, 2005; Tsouroufli, 2011).

When disabled activists argue that: 'Disabled people are under threat for their existence in our modern technological societies. Medical science feels able to flex its muscles and power to abolish all life where the unborn foetus may be imperfect or impaired' (Rock, 1996: 121) or:

> Disabled people as a distinct group are specifically targeted before they are born. Access to prenatal diagnosis has for many years been driven by the goal of getting rid of certain groups of disabled people, for example those with Down syndrome or spina bifida.
>
> *(DAA, 1997: 1)*

they are producing a narrative which locates control firmly with doctors, not pregnant women, and which suggests that screening is motivated by a eugenic urge to eliminate disabled people. This plot narrative grossly simplifies and misrepresents the complexities of the antenatal encounter and obscures the way in which women, and their partners, take responsibility for difficult decisions about their pregnancies (Statham *et al.*, 2001).

Paul (1992) shows that the debate about the eugenic nature of contemporary genetics is not ultimately resolvable, because the term 'eugenics' has so many meanings. 'Eugenics' literally means 'well born', and could be broadly defined as any attempt to improve the quality of future generations. But at this level of generality, eugenics includes all those areas of welfare policy which are directed towards improving the well-being of children and families. Eugenics could be defined more narrowly as attempts to influence the distribution of particular undesired genes in the population. This is closer to the common understanding of the term. But conceptually and in practice, this also could imply a range of approaches. Historians distinguish between positive eugenics and negative eugenics (Kevles, 1985). The former involves encouraging reproduction of individuals with preferred characteristics. The latter involves discouraging reproduction of individuals with undesirable characteristics. Another key distinction is between a eugenics which relies on voluntary action, influenced by education and advice, and a coercive eugenics, based on legal controls or paternalistic professional practices (Caplan *et al.*, 1999).

Regardless of emphasis and method, each of these approaches implies eugenic intentions: an agent with eugenic goals who acts to further those goals. In contemporary biomedicine, it is rare to find explicitly eugenic values or programmes promoted (although see Rogers, 1999, for an example). However, another approach would define eugenics in terms of outcomes, rather than the presence of a eugenic agent, or an explicitly eugenic agenda. This approach highlights how, as a result of particular social policies and individual choices, eugenic outcomes (a reduction in the births affected by particular conditions) may result. This is what Philip Kitcher (1997) calls '*laissez-faire* eugenics' and what Simon Hampton (2005) describes as 'family eugenics'. Many contemporary bioethicists have argued that this form of eugenics is not objectionable, so long as there is no coercion involved (e.g., Caplan *et al.*, 1999). For some, eugenics of this voluntary, consumer or *laissez-faire* type should be positively endorsed as a moral and social practice (Harris, 1992). However, in my own work, I have tried to highlight the limitations on choice (Shakespeare, 1998a, 2005a), suggesting that, even in the absence of explicitly eugenic intentions, eugenics may be an 'emergent property' arising out of the thousands of interactions, implicit expectations, subtle influences and restricted choices in which prospective parents find themselves (McLaughlin, 2003; Hampton, 2005).

The complexities of these issues undermine the sloganising which equates genetics with eugenics, or doctors with Nazis. Eugenics has become a powerful slur word to denounce contemporary practices, but it carries no commonly agreed meaning apart from the general implication that anything eugenic must be bad, because of the historic abuses carried out in the name of eugenics (Wikler, 1999). Complacency about the context in which reproductive decisions are made is misguided. But polemic and conspiracy theory are also misplaced (King, 1999). It is offensive both to physicians and to those prospective parents who agonise long and hard about testing and termination, to use highly emotive rhetoric to denounce modern antenatal screening, and those who hold different moral positions on abortion or disability.

Is prenatal diagnosis discriminatory?

The second theme of the disability rights critique eschews the rhetoric of eugenics and conspiracy, and focuses on the meanings and implications of individual choices and biomedical practices (Parens and Asch, 2000). For example, it is sometimes claimed that prenatal diagnosis discriminates against foetuses with impairments. A pregnancy that would have continued to term if the foetus had been unaffected is aborted because the foetus has, or is believed to have, a condition which would lead to impairment. Adrienne Asch and David Wasserman have criticised what they call the synecdoche entailed in trait-based selection: 'To reject a parental relationship with a future child on the basis of knowledge of a single characteristic is to allow that characteristic to obscure or eclipse all other features of the future child' (2010: 201).

Or it may be claimed that prenatal diagnosis discriminates against disabled children and adults, because it sends the message that it would have been better if they, too, had not been born. This argument is often called 'the expressivist objection', because it suggests that genetic diagnosis and selective abortion 'express' discriminatory or negative views towards disabled people. Adrienne Asch writes: 'I believe it will be very difficult for most families to consider bringing children with diagnosable disabilities into the world if they know that the society believes their births should have been prevented' (2003: 340). One of the strengths of the expressivist objection is that it forces us to attend to the language of prenatal diagnosis, and the wider messages which it conveys. There are many examples of highly prejudicial language being used about disabled people in the literature on genetics and screening, for example, 'culprit chromosomes' and 'random tragedies' (Shakespeare, 1999a). A second important dimension of the expressivist objection is that it captures the extent to which impairment is part of the identity of many disabled people, particularly those with congenital conditions: whereas non-disabled commentators see impairment as a separate aspect (like having influenza), disabled people argue that it is an important aspect of who they are (Edwards, 2004, 2005).

The expressivist objection also highlights the emotional impact of screening programmes on disabled people, and often on those who love and support them. It can be very difficult to accept that a genetic test or screening technology has been developed which might have prevented one's own birth. A person with a congenital impairment immediately imagines whether their own parents would have taken advantage of the technology. It brings up fears about rejection and not being wanted by one's family or society. It makes one think of a society in which one did not exist. All of these are painful and threatening thoughts, made worse by the very negative language in which these technologies are discussed and promoted: as Steve Edwards suggests, 'the moral wrongness of the practice stems from the harmful effects it has' (2004: 419).

Yet there is a logical contradiction in this emotional response. Any disabled person has already been born. Prior to being born, the disabled person does not exist in any meaningful sense. During the mother's pregnancy, a cluster of developing cells existed, but not a person with identity, experiences and feelings. The response 'I would not have been born' has an emotional resonance, but cannot be understood in strictly rational terms, because before anyone is born, there is no 'I' not to be born. The more logical response is to think 'this technology might prevent future people like myself being born' or 'this may lead to a world in which there are fewer people with conditions like mine'. This may still be experienced as regrettable and distressing, but has less personal resonance than the idea of non-existence.

Moreover, there are many circumstances in which one could imagine a situation in which one would not have been born, as John Harris (1992) and others argue. For example, I would not have been born if my parents had not met; if they had used contraception; if they had made love a month later; indeed, had they made love a millisecond later, I would not have been born. According to Saul Kripke's zygotic principle, each individual is the unique result of one sperm fertilising one egg (unless they are a monozygotic twin), and any other combination or moment of conception would have resulted in a different person – a brother or sister, but not me (Kripke, 1980).

The expressivist objection seems to apply to any technology which limits possible births: contraception or sterilisation expresses negative valuation of large families, or people with single parents. But the expressivists reply, the point about antenatal diagnosis is that it specifies a class of people who are to be avoided. It is the characteristics of the potential child which are diagnosed and which the parents endeavour to avoid. Asch and Wasserman write: 'Any trait-based selection conflicts with the ideals of unqualified welcome and inclusiveness to which prospective parents and society as a whole should aspire' (2010: 201).

It is the message which screening sends about disability that is so problematic. We need then to turn to the question of whether seeking to prevent disability necessarily expresses a negative valuation of existing disabled people.

Is it always wrong to prevent impairment?

Contrary to the expressivist objection, I do not believe that attempts to prevent impairment necessarily send negative messages about disabled people (Shakespeare, 2013). It is not inconsistent to support the rights of existing disabled people, while seeking to prevent more people becoming impaired (Durkin and Gottlieb, 2009). For example, any public health programme attempts to minimise the number of people who are disabled. Inoculation of babies or mine clearance schemes are all intended to stop people becoming impaired, but do not therefore imply that people with polio or missing limbs are second-class citizens. Of course, there are ways of promoting these morally positive endeavours that do rebound negatively on perceptions of disability. For example, in the late 1990s there was a British anti-drink driving campaign which used footage of a severely brain-damaged man. The hard-hitting message of the advertisement was that viewers risked ending up as a pathetic vegetable if they drove a vehicle under the influence of alcohol. An important piece of health information was conveyed in a way which expressed very negative attitudes towards people with brain injury.

But, in general, most people would accept that because impairment is not a neutral state, but a condition that is generally unwelcome and best avoided, attempts to reduce the numbers of disabled children being born are acceptable, if they are promoted in ways that do not threaten existing disabled children and adults. For example, cerebral palsy is associated with premature births and complications during delivery that cause anoxia, and hence brain damage. Obstetric and neonatal specialists attempt to reduce the incidence of cerebral palsy through improving care of mothers and babies. These efforts do not express a negative valuation of people with cerebral palsy, or have implications for their rights or potentiality. Another example is the policy of promoting folic acid as a dietary supplement. Folate is proven to reduce the incidence of spina bifida during early foetal development. If it was added to flour, as happens in USA, the numbers of pregnancies affected by spina bifida and other malformations would reduce dramatically. This would seem to be straightforwardly a good outcome.

It may be that disability activists who experience spina bifida or cerebral palsy object to these policies. Long ago, at a Congress of Rehabilitation

International in Oslo, I met a Ugandan woman who told me that disability activists in her country had criticised polio immunisation programmes, on the grounds that these expressed negative attitudes to disability. Such criticisms seem misguided. Many people with polio, cerebral palsy and spina bifida are indeed happy, well adjusted and successful. All people with these conditions are deserving of rights and respect. But this does not have implications for measures to prevent future people experiencing conditions that can be associated with discomfort and restriction. Impairment is bad, although life with impairment can be good (Shakespeare, 2013). Impairment prevention does not imply negative valuation of people who already have an impairment, and the two policies – impairment prevention and disability rights – are not incompatible.

However, there is an important distinction that needs to be made. In philosophical terms, these examples are 'same number cases' (Parfit, 1984). Often bioethicists talk in hypothetical terms about a situation in which someone could take a pill, which would prevent or cause impairment in their future child, or perhaps avoid impairment by waiting a month to conceive. In these cases, it is commonly argued that the prospective parent has a moral duty to take the course of action that would result in the healthy, unaffected child. Interventions such as folate supplementation, or obstetric and neonatatal care do not prevent the birth of a particular foetus, but instead prevent that foetus being born with impairment. As with inoculation, these practices are about preventing impairment in future people, not preventing potential people who are impaired. As Ruth Bailey observes, to think of prenatal diagnosis in exactly the same terms as these other forms of impairment prevention is wrong:

> This obscures the fundamental difference between prenatal testing and any other way of preventing illness, namely that the 'treatment' which follows prenatal testing – abortion – 'cures' the condition by eliminating the foetus rather than by stopping the condition occurring in the first place.
>
> *(1996: 149)*

In other words, the force of the expressivist objection does not seem directed against the reduction of impairment *per se*, but against reduction of impairment using abortion as the method. It is this that might send the message that 'it is better to be dead than disabled' and thus expresses a negative valuation of, or misrecognition or disrespect towards, the lives of disabled people. Therefore, we need to examine arguments about the acceptability of termination of pregnancy.

Is it wrong to terminate pregnancy when the foetus is impaired?

The morality of abortion is complex and contested, and full discussion is beyond the scope of this chapter (see Warren, 1993, for fuller discussion of different positions on abortion). However, I want briefly to explain why I cannot accept the two most extreme responses to the problem, namely the position which argues life starts at conception – and so all abortion is wrong – and the position which says abortion is permissible until birth (on the grounds of a woman's autonomy, or that a baby is not a person).

Some people, including some motivated by disability rights arguments, are opposed to abortion in all circumstances. They do not distinguish between cases where the foetus is disabled, and cases where the foetus is unaffected. They believe that abortion is wrong in all circumstances, because the foetus is a living human being, which is entitled to the rights and respect due to other human beings. Just as it is wrong to kill a baby, child or adult human being, so it is wrong to kill an embryo or foetus as it develops in the womb. Abortion, or embryo research, from this perspective, is murder.

The polar opposite view to the anti-abortionist position is held by those feminists and others who stress a woman's right to choose what happens to her body (Sharp and Earle, 2002). The foetus is part of the woman, and therefore the woman is the only person who has the right to decide what happens to the pregnancy. Either the foetus has no rights, because it is not a person, or the rights of the foetus are trumped by the rights of the woman in whose womb the foetus is developing. The maximalist feminist position suggests that a woman has the right to abortion on demand at any stage up until birth, for any reason.

However, many disability rights commentators take a third position, because while they support the feminist principle of reproductive autonomy, they are anxious about selective termination of impaired foetuses (Asch, 2000; Saxton, 2000). They argue that abortion is allowable if a woman does not want to be pregnant. However, it is not allowable if a woman does not want to be pregnant with this particular foetus. In other words, abortion rights should extend to the choice of becoming a mother or not at a particular time and with a particular partner, but not to any choices that depend on the characteristics of the foetus. The reason often given for this conditional support of abortion rights is that selective termination of impaired foetuses expresses negative valuation of disabled people and/or discriminates against impaired foetuses. A common analogy (e.g. Asch and Geller, 1996) is that it is not ethically different to select against girl foetuses than to select against foetuses with genetic disorders. Many people have the intuition that selective termination of female foetuses is wrong, usually because it sends negative messages about the value of women. Opponents of selective termination of impaired foetuses use the same argument about the value of disabled people.

The problem for blanket anti-abortionists, as the late Ronald Dworkin (1984) has pointed out, is that few of them are totally consistent. For example, many anti-abortionists would permit abortion in cases where the pregnancy has arisen as a consequence of rape. Others would permit abortion in cases where the life of the mother is in danger. Equally, blanket anti-abortionists often do not oppose the taking of life in other circumstances, for example, in war or capital punishment. Dworkin concludes that anti-abortionists, although they say they are motivated by a belief that abortion is murder, must be mistaken. If abortion is murder, it remains murder even if the cause of the pregnancy was rape. After all, the foetus is not to blame for the circumstances of its conception. The mother may be very distressed, but it would be possible for her to have the child and give it up for adoption, which would be preferable to murder.

The problem for maximal feminists is that the idea of women having property rights in their bodies and hence the right to decide about their pregnancies ignores the fact that pregnancies affect third parties, not just women. After a certain point in pregnancy – certainly by the third trimester – the interests of the developing baby have to be balanced with those of the pregnant woman. Particularly in the later stages of pregnancy, it seems objectionable that a baby who may be able to survive independently outside the womb has no rights, and the mother is entitled to have it killed. The extreme feminist position has the merit of consistency, but leads to repugnant conclusions.

The problem for the disability rights selective objection to abortion is that it is inconsistent. It seems intuitively true that if it is permissible to terminate pregnancy at all, it is permissible to terminate in the case of disability. It does not make sense to me that it is acceptable to have an abortion for social reasons, for example, the timing of the pregnancy is inconvenient, or the woman does not want a baby with this particular man, or the prospective parents do not want another addition to their family, but not for the morally significant reason that the foetus is affected by an impairment. Moreover, it is only possible to speak of discrimination against impaired foetuses if they are humans entitled to full moral rights, and if this is the case, all abortion is wrong, not just abortion of impaired foetuses (Warren, 1997).

Two examples further erode the disability rights selective opposition to selecting on the basis of foetal characteristics. First, there are many cases of profound impairment, where the prospective life is very seriously affected, where disability rights critics often waive their objection: for example, metabolic disorders such as Tay-Sachs disease, where babies usually die by the age of 5 or Lesch-Nyhan syndrome, where the child may grow to young adulthood, but in a state of very severe physical and mental distress. If these are situations in which diagnosis can be taken into account, the general principle that it is wrong to choose on the basis of foetal characteristics is undermined. Second, a situation could be imagined when a young single woman becomes pregnant and is considering whether to have an abortion. For a woman of 16 or 17, the characteristics of the foetus could be very relevant to her decision. She might think that she could possibly cope with a child, knowing that support will be available, that childcare will be available, and that she has a chance of continuing her education and achieving a good quality of life for herself and her baby. Contrast this with her prospects if she has a baby with a serious impairment. There may not be enough support, there may not be appropriate childcare, and it may be almost impossible for her to achieve her aspirations. The future for both her and the child might be very bleak. To this young woman, the question of the characteristics of the foetus are not separable from, or irrelevant to, the question of whether she continues the pregnancy.

Unlike the blanket anti-abortionists, and many of the maximalist feminists, I hold the gradualist position (Gillon, 2001). This suggests that the developing foetus should be regarded as having increasing moral status as pregnancy progresses. The early embryo has potential, but it is not a full human being with all the status and protection which that implies (the analogy of the acorn versus the oak is sometimes used). The third trimester baby may still be in the womb, but has a good chance of viability, and is in most morally significant respects a person with human rights. Gradualism is a tenuous answer to the abortion question, because it is difficult to state exactly when the transition to human moral status occurs. Significance is often attached to biological milestones – such as the capacity for sentience or viability outside the womb, both of which occur at the earliest between 20–24 weeks, in high-income countries. Beyond these metaphysical and legal questions, it is important to add that abortion is neither a tragedy (as many anti-abortionists claim) nor an insignificant clinical procedure (as some pro-choice activists claim). All termination or loss of pregnancy, at any stage, may be sad and regrettable, because it involves the extinction of a growing human life, full of potential and promise. In particular, psychological evidence suggests that the termination of a wanted pregnancy after diagnosis of foetal abnormality at 18–20 weeks is associated with guilt and distress on the part of the parents who have to make that difficult choice, especially the prospective mother (Astbury-Ward, 2008). Later termination is associated with more symptoms of post-traumatic stress (Coleman *et al.*, 2010). The pain may continue for many years, perhaps even a lifetime (White-van Mourik, 1994).

While the gradualist position can be interpreted as supporting general access to first trimester termination, with second trimester termination in circumstances of foetal anomaly, third trimester termination is morally very contentious. It is at this point that a disability rights claim of unfair discrimination does have purchase. Current UK law on abortion states that it is prohibited after the 24th week of pregnancy, except in cases where there is a substantial risk that the child would be born 'seriously handicapped' (Shakespeare, 1998a; Sheldon and Wilkinson, 2001). In other words, third trimester foetuses are protected in law, unless they are at risk of impairment, in which case they are not protected until birth (and not always then). A simple charge of discrimination (Shakespeare, 1998a) fails, because here a distinction is being made on morally relevant grounds: a foetus with serious impairment is different from a healthy foetus, and to some, this relevant difference is a sufficient reason for overturning usual protections. Others resolve the inconsistency (or discrimination) by arguing in favour of permitting late termination for any pregnancy, not just pregnancies affected by impairment (Savulescu, 2001). I find this objectionable, because to me, a third trimester foetus has moral status.

In practice, late abortion necessitates foeticide. After 24 weeks, a baby is viable outside the womb, given medical care. At this point, if birth is induced, the baby would be born alive, and hence doctors would be compelled to attempt to keep it alive (although some utilitarians argue this is unnecessary). The differences between most impaired foetuses and non-impaired foetuses do not seem sufficient to justify such killing of an otherwise viable baby. The legal loophole permitting late abortions was intended to cover the very small number of cases where the foetus was non-viable (likely to die in pregnancy or soon after birth), but seems to have been exploited in other cases where the impairment was not incompatible with life (notoriously, in one instance, a case of cleft lip and palate, see Allison, 2003). For these reasons, it seems to me urgently important to tighten UK law so that late termination is only permissible where the life of the mother is in danger, or when it is inevitable that the foetus will die before birth or in the neonatal period.

Early non-invasive screening, using the new combined test (serum test plus nuchal translucency) in weeks 10–12, should reduce the numbers of women who find out that they are carrying a pregnancy affected by

Down syndrome after an amniocentesis around weeks 18–20, and who therefore may end up wanting an abortion near or after the legal limit. One study found that 71 per cent of abortions after the first trimester were because a woman had not realised she was pregnant, and only 2 per cent were associated with foetal abnormality (Coleman *et al.*, 2010), which suggests that better education and health provision might be the key to reducing the demand for later abortions.

While first and second trimester prenatal diagnosis and selective abortion are regrettable and distressing for prospective parents, it is hard to claim that it is morally wrong or should be further prohibited. We live in an age where scientific knowledge can provide information about the characteristics of the developing baby. Where there is evidence of a serious condition which may cause considerable suffering or restriction to the future child, and difficulties and restrictions for other family members, a utilitarian would argue that it is not wrong to enable pregnant women and their partners to exercise their right to access abortion: by doing so, they make their own lives easier, and reduce the amount of suffering in the world (Glover, 1977; Harris, 1992).

By contrast, virtue ethicists discuss selection abortion in terms of the moral character of the parents, and which decisions are compatible with good parenting (MacIntyre, 1999; Vehmas, 2002). Rather than discussing parental duties or foetal rights, virtue ethics emphasises parental responsibility, and the unconditional love of a parent for his child. For example, MacIntyre argues that the virtuous parent is orientated towards the child's needs, not their own needs, whatever those needs may turn out to be: 'Good parental care is defined in part by reference to the possibility of the affliction of their children by serious disability' (1999: 91). For him, parents of disabled children are the paradigms of good parenthood, 'who provide the model for and the key to the work of all parents' (ibid.: 91). To me, the virtue ethics position has more purchase after the birth of a disabled child, than in pregnancy when serious impairment is predicted. MacIntyre is perhaps over-idealistic about the virtues of good parenting. Because I cannot accept that abortion prior to 20 weeks is morally wrong, it seems to me that abortion on the grounds of serious impairment must also be justifiable.

Abortion is a moral harm, because it involves killing and the deprivation of a future of value to the foetus (Savulescu, 2002). This harm has to be compared with the moral harm of avoidable impairment (Glover, 1977). The equation will play out differently for different people, depending on the resources they have available to them, the seriousness of the impairment, their beliefs about their own capabilities, and their view of what makes a good life. These are difficult positions, which are the private responsibility and concern of individual women and men, and should be discussed with humility and caution by philosophers, activists and others who do not have to live with the consequences.

Will selective termination of impaired foetuses harm existing disabled people?

The expressivist argument could be interpreted in non-consequentialist and consequentialist ways (Michael Parker, pers. comm.): the former suggests that termination reflects or expresses a discriminatory attitude, and that this would be wrong even if no disabled person was negatively affected. In other words, some motivations for selective termination are wrong, even if selective termination is not always wrong. However, the latter and more powerful version of expressivism grounds the wrongness of selective termination in the harms that result as a consequence: the implications are that other people will have to live with the consequences of decisions to terminate pregnancies affected by impairment, not just the parents. It is claimed that there will be negative consequences for disabled people, if policies and practices that allow people to terminate pregnancy to avoid having disabled children are permitted.

Clearly, many disabled people and their supporters feel offended by prenatal diagnosis. But this does not mean that prenatal diagnosis is wrong: as Steve Edwards claims: 'One is obliged to take into account consequences of one's actions which might harm others, but it does not follow that those harms count for more than the suppression of one's free choice' (2004: 419). While there is evidence that some disabled people feel offended and discriminated against by prenatal diagnosis, there is no strong empirical evidence that material harms to disabled people result from selective abortion. For example, the increase in prenatal diagnosis and selective abortion does not seem to have resulted in a worsening of attitudes towards disabled people, or a reduction in standards of care, or quality of life. On the contrary, the irony is that the increasing availability of genetic knowledge has coincided with the increasing acceptance of disability rights and slowly improving provision for disabled people.

Disability rights activists assume that abortion on the basis of impairment suggests that it would be better to be dead than disabled. However, as Anne Maclean and many others have argued, there is a distinction to be made between abortion suggesting that disabled people's lives are not worth living, and a case where an individual person cannot cope with a disabled child (Maclean, 1993). For example, parents may feel that having a disabled child will damage their partnership, or impact negatively on their other children. They may fear economic hardship, particularly if one parent has to give up working to care for the disabled child. They may be prepared to sacrifice freedoms to parent children for the first twenty years of their lives, but not to continue in a parental role towards an adult disabled child who remains dependent. There are many extraordinary stories of the degree of selflessness and commitment that MacIntyre calls for, and such people should certainly be welcomed and applauded. But not all prospective parents will be prepared to make the sacrifices and endure the difficulties that disabled families sometimes face, and it is their right to forgo this future, which does not imply that they do not like, respect and accept disabled people.

It might even be argued that selective abortion can benefit existing disabled people. For example, some couples both carry a recessive genetic condition, which causes a risk of serious impairment – such as cystic fibrosis – in their children. They may only discover their risk as a result of having an affected child. Much as they love that child, they may decide that they cannot cope with another disabled child, and use prenatal diagnosis to avoid that possibility. The benefit to the existing child is that the parents can concentrate their attention and care on him, and do not have to try and support two children with high support needs. This example also shows that it is compatible to love and respect an existing disabled person, while taking steps to ensure that the impairment does not recur.

This claim should not be confused with an implicit reason that is sometimes given for selective termination. Advocates of screening – or indeed prospective parents – may believe it is in the interests of the potential disabled child not to be born, because life with impairment causes suffering or restriction (Glover, 1977). The question of whether a foetus has interests is complex and contested (Sheldon and Wilkinson, 2001: 89). However, it seems plausible that it is always in the interests of a potential person to be born, unless the life they would lead is worse than not existing at all (Harris, 2000). Very few forms of impairment involve so much suffering that non-existence would be preferable. In other words, prenatal diagnosis can be justified in terms of the effect on parents and other siblings, but cannot be justified in terms of the benefits to the life which is prevented from coming into existence as a result, except in the most severe cases of impairment. A child is not harmed by being born, which is why 'wrongful birth' litigation should not be permissible (Spriggs and Savulescu, 2002).

In contrast, opponents of screening argue that the person who is harmed by selective termination is the foetus with impairment. But if this is the basis on which disability rights advocates oppose selective termination, then the position has broader implications. For example, if they argue that impaired foetuses are persons, and thus that selective termination is discrimination towards, or harm to, disabled people, then their position is not just opposed to selective termination, but to all termination. If an impaired foetus is a person who is entitled to pro-tection, then any and each foetus is a person entitled to protection, and thus all abortion has to be murder (Gillon, 2001: 118).

Above, I have tried to demonstrate that preventing impairment is not wrong in principle. I have argued that the expressivist objection is not a strong reason for prohibiting screening. It is not incompatible to seek to prevent impaired children coming into the world, and also to support the rights of existing disabled people (Buchanan, 1996). I have further suggested that the expressivist objection has the implication that abortion in general is wrong. It appears to me inconsistent and illogical to support abortion rights in all circumstances except where the foetus is likely to grow into a disabled person. Abortion, on any grounds, is morally serious, but during the first and second trimester of pregnancy I believe that the choice should be a legal right, which is left to individual conscience to decide.

Is there a duty to diagnose and terminate pregnancies affected by impairment?

Some commentators have argued that prenatal diagnosis is not just permissible, but also obligatory. Others have suggested that prospective parents have a duty not just to test during pregnancy, but also to terminate pregnancy if the foetus is found to be affected by impairment. For example, the IVF pioneer Professor Robert Edwards has stated: 'In the future, it will be a sin to have a disabled child' (Rogers, 1999). It should be noted that pronouncements of this kind, though rare, are of exactly the same form as the pre-1945 eugenics which society more generally repudiates.

The range of spiritual and ethical views as to the acceptability of abortion suggests to me that neither society nor the state can prescribe the course of action an individual should take during pregnancy. The principle of reproductive autonomy suggests that prenatal diagnosis and termination should be available, within certain agreed moral limits, for those who wish freely to avail themselves of it. Society's role consists in providing information, counselling, support, and high quality professional services to help safely deliver the chosen outcomes.

What could be the basis of any duty to test or terminate pregnancy? It has already been established that a disabled child is not harmed by being brought into existence, where the only other alternative was not to exist at all, unless the impairment is so severe that it is worse than death. Prospective mothers do have a duty to take all reasonable steps (folate supplement, forgoing excess alcohol and drugs) to ensure that they do not damage a foetus during pregnancy (a future person), but this cannot extend to preventing the birth of an impaired child (a potential person). However, John Harris (1992) and others argue that there are wrongs which are not harms to individuals: creating disabled children, on this account, is wrong because it increases suffering or decreases utility.

Thus, it could be argued that the prospective parents have a duty to society or to the state not to have a disabled child. It is in the interests of society to have productive and healthy citizens, and therefore testing and termination of potentially impaired or unhealthy babies are required. This is classic eugenics, and contrary to justice, human rights, and the reproductive rights of parents. A more important objection draws on evidence that many disabled children grow into productive adults with good quality of life (and indeed, many non-disabled children grow up into unhappy adults with poor quality of life). The idea of disability as automatically equivalent to burden and suffering cannot be sustained empirically (Albrecht and Devlieger, 1999; Brouwer *et al.*, 2005). Although it could be conceded that there will be a small proportion of disabled people who may never be productive, and who may need care throughout their lives, how much of a problem is this in a prosperous Western society? Subordinating personal morality and individual human rights to collective interests can only be justified in extreme cases of emergency, which do not pertain in the prenatal diagnosis scenario. The social and economic burden of dependent disabled people in advanced economies is small, compared to expenditure on other items, for example, military spending.

Moreover, if parents have a duty to avoid disability or poor quality of life in their offspring, there are contentious implications. For example, there are other social groups whose offspring may be perceived to be a burden in society, for example, socially excluded communities in the inner cities. But to suggest that such social groups might have a duty not to have children would be regarded as outrageous and offensive by most people. The relevant point about socially excluded people – or about minority ethnic communities who experience racism and consequently a poor quality of life – is that the disadvantage is a consequence of social arrangements. Rather than preventing the birth of people who experience oppression, every energy should be devoted towards removing the source of the social exclusion. Exactly the same argument is made by disability rights advocates (e.g. Asch, 2003). A more supportive and inclusive environment will enable more people with impairment to be independent and productive. Therefore, rather than individual parents having a duty to avoid the birth of disabled children, should it not be society which has a duty to welcome and include disabled children and adults, so that the social problem of disability can be mitigated or eliminated?

My conclusion is that there can be no duty to diagnose or prevent impairment in pregnancy. My position is close to that of Matti Häyry's 'non-directive compromise': prenatal diagnosis is morally contested and there are good arguments for and against the practice (Häyry, 2009). It would be untrue to claim that people with impairments suffer while people without impairments do not suffer or become burdens. All lives involve suffering and dependency, and the only way to avoid suffering is to forgo reproduction entirely. All decisions about screening and termination are difficult, and can only be made by those people who have to live with the consequences – either the distress of abortion, or the potential stress of supporting a disabled child, or an additional child. Society should assist people to make good decisions, and support them with the consequences of their decisions. In particular, justice demands that the state should devote more resources to supporting families with disabled children, and to promoting the well-being of disabled adults, rather than acting as if prenatal diagnosis or other biomedical interventions will solve the problem of disability. As Abby Lippman argues:

> Social conditions are as enabling or disabling as biological conditions. Why are biological variations that create differences between individuals seen as preventable or avoidable while social conditions that create similar distinctions are likely to be seen as intractable givens?
>
> *(1994: 160)*

Is prenatal diagnosis a real choice?

In this chapter, I have articulated a liberal position on prenatal diagnosis, which runs counter to the oppositional rhetoric of some disability rights campaigners. However, this does not mean being naïve about choice, or about the context in which prospective parents make their choices. I do not believe that there is a coherent drive to eliminate disability from the population. But there are undoubtedly problems with how screening is offered and choices communicated (Shakespeare, 1998a; Hampton, 2005). In this final section, I will explore the contexts in which pregnant women and their partners make their decisions, in order to demonstrate that choices may not be as free and fully informed as clinical rhetoric suggests. These comprise the 'near patient context' and the 'broader cultural context'.

By the former, I refer to how women and men experience pregnancy services and the offer of screening (Rapp, 1997). There are three areas in which choice may be undermined. The first is information. A good decision depends on relevant and high quality information, which is communicated clearly and understood by the patient. Over many years, social and psychological research has cast doubt on the availability of adequate information in screening (Shakespeare, 1998a; McLaughlin, 2003). Since 2003, the UK National Screening Committee has a policy of all pregnant women being offered good quality antenatal screening for Down syndrome, regardless of postcode. Yet the attention to ensuring the technical quality of the triple test (hormones in blood serum) and combined test (serum test plus nuchal translucency measurement on ultrasound scan) has not yet been matched by consistency of good quality information provision.

In particular, screening information cannot simply be about the experience of having a test, the technical details of the test, and the reliability of the test. There is evidence of considerable ignorance about what screening tests can detect (Skirton and Barr, 2010). The most important question is what the test is for: in other words, information about the conditions which the screening programme is intended to enable women to avoid, if they so choose:

> If counselors, midwives and obstetricians are truly committed to patient decision-making and to informed reproductive choice, they should be providing enough information about life with a disabling condition so that prospective parents can imagine the ways in which life can be worthwhile as well as those in which it can be difficult.
> *(Asch, 2003: 335)*

Good quality, balanced information about Down syndrome, spina bifida and other conditions detectable through ultrasound scan, chorion villus sample or amniocentesis is rarely available (Williams *et al.*, 2002). Failure to offer this information carries the implication that it is obvious that someone would want to avoid these conditions, the only question being whether the test is effective in providing the diagnosis. Providing negative information, or information limited to a shallow clinical description of the features of the impairment, carries the implication that the condition is a medical problem which is best avoided (Alderson, 2001). Only if full information about the lives of people who have the condition and their families is provided, can prospective parents make an informed decision as to whether they wish to avoid this possibility in their own family. In 2002–5, I led a pilot project to provide life stories of people with Down syndrome, spina bifida, Turner's syndrome, Klinefelter's syndrome and cystic fibrosis, based on interviews and photographs of a range of people affected by each condition: although the resulting website was well evaluated (Ahmed *et al.*, 2008), we did not succeed in having it taken on as part of mainstream NHS information provision.

The second 'near patient' context which may undermine choice is the attitude and behaviour of medical professionals. If midwives, obstetricians and others working in maternity services imply that women have a duty to have tests or terminations, or if they are unsupportive to women who decline the screening offer, or if they are prejudiced about disability, then clearly, choice is undermined. There is evidence that professionals can be directive in this way, particularly from international surveys, but also sometimes from research in the UK (Wertz, 1998; Mao, 1998; Shakespeare, 1998a). The majority of professionals seem to have a strong sense of ethics (Hashiloni-Dolev and Weiner, 2008), and to be non-directive and pro-choice (Ahmed *et al.*, 2012). Occasionally, individual practitioners make it clear to pregnant women that they believe screening to be a great benefit which no sensible person could refuse. In other cases, patients ask the professional what they would do themselves, which puts the professional into a difficult position (Schwennesen and Koch, 2012): they do not want to be directive. Sometimes, the solution is to say 'the majority of women do x'. Offering the evidence is a way of shaping the individual's response: she will likely go with the crowd, or the majority will make her feel okay about her desired action.

Communication is particularly difficult with people whose first language is not English, or who are very young (Ahmed *et al.*, 2012). Midwives and healthcare assistants are the main points of contact with pregnant women, and they may have limited knowledge themselves (Skirton and Barr, 2007). They have a difficult task in both ensuring that the prospective parents understand that there is a slim chance that screening may force them to make difficult choices, and reassuring them that all is likely to be well. Thus, one study found that:

> [By] focusing on the present and the initial screening during the first trimester, and providing minimum or no information about possible options after a positive diagnosis, including living with a Down's child or terminating the pregnancy, midwives may have given the impression that innovative screening was unlikely to reveal an abnormal pregnancy.
>
> *(Tsouroufli, 2011: 433)*

This relates to the third element of the 'near patient context', the routinisation of maternity and screening services in UK and some other countries, what one research team refer to as 'screening creep', 'a subtle but rapid process of incorporation, routinisation and consequent consumer demand' (Williams *et al.*, 2005). As Tsouroufli puts it: 'Fast processing of women, promoting of screening as a safe test and staff's expectations routinized the offer of first trimester screening' (2011: 434).

While obstetrics has successfully minimised maternal and infant mortality, this has been at the cost of the autonomy of pregnant women. Screening becomes a conveyor belt, and choice is consequently undermined (Press and Brown, 1997). For example, the downside of the new first trimester combined screening test is that there is very short window for prospective parents to decide whether they want it. Research finds midwives getting over this problem by ticking the box for the combined test, but explaining to women that they can always decline later if they decide against it – replacing an 'opt in' with an 'opt out' system with consequent threat to patient autonomy (Ahmed *et al.*, 2012). Alison Pilnick's analysis of actual midwifery consultations suggest that rather than women making an informed choice to have nuchal screening, it is more of an 'assent' than a 'consent' model (Pilnick, 2008). In Denmark, the first country in the world to introduce free routine first trimester combined screening, overall take-up is at least 90 per cent (Schwennesen and Koch, 2012).

Obstetric ultrasound is a particularly ambiguous technology (Williams *et al.*, 2005). The purpose of costly scans during pregnancy is not just to reassure women, enable parents to bond with their babies, or provide pretty pictures for relatives. It is also to detect foetal anomalies, so that termination of pregnancy may be offered (Schwennesen and Koch, 2012). There is nothing necessarily wrong with that, as long as couples are clearly informed that they are having a diagnostic test, which in a tiny proportion of cases may lead to a heart-rending choice about ending a wanted pregnancy. Ironically, the new generation of high-quality three-dimensional and four-dimensional ultrasound machines gives a better image of the foetus, which promotes bonding and may make it harder for the small minority where serious abnormality is diagnosed (Williams *et al.*, 2005; Roberts, 2012). Danish evidence shows how sonographers try to communicate sensitively – for example, avoiding the language of 'high risk' or not enacting the image on screen as a living child, where they detect signs of abnormality (Schwennesen and Koch, 2012: 290).

By 'broader cultural context', I refer to cultural and social knowledge and attitudes to disability and parenthood. Prospective parents may be largely ignorant about disability. They may not know any disabled people: for example, only 50 per cent of respondents in a UK survey of prospective parents had had contact with a person with Down syndrome (Skirton and Barr, 2010). They may not be aware of the transformations in opportunities and rights which disabled people have experienced. They may have negative attitudes, for example, still thinking that disability is 'a fate worse than death', and they may fear their own loss of health and ability. They may not be able to imagine parenting a disabled child, and may fear that the life of a disabled child may be marked by suffering and restriction (Mackenzie and Scully, 2008). These fears may be reinforced by negative cultural stereotypes, and by messages about the benefits of genetic research and prenatal screening. A disabled person who cannot achieve qualifications, or look normal, or have a good career, or live independently may be regarded very negatively in contemporary society. All of these psychological and cultural factors may operate to undermine the possibility of a prospective parent choosing freely (Hampton, 2005). Moroever, as more and more people choose to test and terminate, it will become harder for others to resist and reject selection (Beck-Gernsheim, 1990). I do not suggest that individuals are brainwashed or coerced. However, they may often be fearful and ignorant and sometimes prejudiced. For these reasons, achieving true choice in screening depends on a more extensive debate about the rights and potential of disabled people, and about the duty of society to accept and support those who need help and cannot achieve full independence.

Conclusion

In this chapter, I have attempted to clarify complex arguments about a very emotive and painful issue in contemporary society. Ironically, both those who oppose and those who advocate prenatal diagnosis can make the mistake of exaggerating the potential of screening to detect and eliminate disabled children. Genetic intervention is not the solution to the disability problem, nor is it a significant threat to disabled people. Only about 10–20 per cent of disabled people have congenital conditions, most of which would not be detected through screening. Technological and economic constraints mean that very few potential conditions are currently diagnosable, although it is conceivable that the situation may change in future, with 'gene chip' techniques which allow testing for hundreds of alleles (Check, 2005).

While pre-implantation genetic diagnosis (PGD or embryo selection, sometimes labelled 'designer baby technology') enables detection of more conditions, only a handful of couples each year have PGD in the UK, because it is costly, complex and unreliable. PGD technology is closely regulated by the Human Fertilisation and Embryology Authority. The only people who are likely to have access to the service are those with a history of severe genetic disease – for example, recessive conditions such as cystic fibrosis and muscular dystrophy – or who have chromosomal anomalies which make it unlikely that they carry a pregnancy to term. Therefore, while interesting dilemmas are raised (Zeiler, 2005), in terms of disability rights, this option seems less problematic than existing prenatal diagnosis (contra King, 1999). In the more than twenty years since PGD began, it has not expanded beyond a tiny niche of high-risk families. For this reason, the analysis in this chapter has concentrated on ubiquitous screening in pregnancy, where the problems of informed consent and emergent eugenics may potentially arise.

I conclude that prenatal diagnosis is not straightforwardly eugenic or discriminatory. While the *practice* of prenatal diagnosis certainly requires careful monitoring in the UK, and probably urgent attention in certain other jurisdictions, the *principle* should not be objectionable or contrary to disability rights. Central to the issue of prenatal diagnosis is the difficult question of abortion. Avoiding impairment is not necessarily problematic, but ending developing life in the womb usually is. As a gradualist, I argue that termination is permissible in the early stage of pregnancy, and believe that diagnosis of significant impairment is one of the grounds that justifies the moral seriousness of abortion. Testing should preferably be limited to serious conditions that undermine quality of life (Henn, 2000). However, the privacy of those faced with these difficult decisions should be respected, and their autonomy supported. Everyone has an interest in helping prospective parents make better decisions, which they are less likely to regret at a future date. We should be on hand to offer counselling, good quality information, and support, but we should not venture to dictate where the duties of prospective parents may lie. Nor should we interpret a decision to have a test or a termination as expressing disrespect or discrimination towards disabled people. Choices in pregnancy are painful and may be experienced as burdensome (Kelly, 2009) but they are not incompatible with disability rights.

7

JUST AROUND THE CORNER

The quest for a cure

While issues at the beginning of life and end of life are most controversial in the bioethics of disability, there is another relevant class of questions which concerns the acceptability or otherwise of attempts to prevent or cure impairment. The imagery of miracle cures is central to cultural representations of disability and medical research, and recent decades have seen an expansion of such coverage with the Human Genome Project, gene therapy and stem cell research. Disability activists and disability studies writers have challenged the obsession with cure, arguing that:

1 Disability is about social barriers and social oppression, not impairment.
2 The priority is structural change, not altering individuals to conform to social norms.
3 Cure discourse individualises and pathologises impairment, which should be understood in terms of difference, not deficit.

In this chapter, I interrogate the debate around cure, challenging both the mainstream approach to medical research, and the disability rights response to it. After outlining some mainstream disability studies response to medical research, I explore the principle of cure, and show how the diversity of impairment experiences makes it dangerous to generalise about disabled people's views. Next, I look at some of the practical issues which make the rhetoric and practice of cure problematic, focusing on stem cell research and the role of Christopher Reeve. Then I discuss some difficult cases, before concluding by placing the cure debate within the broader context of bioethics and disability rights.

Three arguments from Part I of the book are relevant to this chapter. First, I argued that a progressive response to disability should devote attention to the problem of impairment, which plays an important part in the lives of many disabled people. Second, I argued that a multi-level approach is required to the disability problem, one that recognises that medical interventions to treat or minimise impairment are valuable, alongside (and not as replacements for) interventions at the social and structural levels. Third, I criticised the reliance on an ethnic conception of disability identity. This is relevant here because some disability rights activists challenge attempts to prevent or cure impairment because they see it as a threat to their own existence, or as expressing the view that their lives are not valid.

The disability movement on cure

Disability rights organisations and activists sceptical about or opposed to gene therapy or stem cell research have sometimes found themselves in uneasy alliance with anti-abortion voices concerned about embryo research. However, most disability activists are not anti-abortion, and their concern arises from the broader opposition to cure (Beresford and Wilson, 2002; Leipoldt, 2005). This scepticism is usually not couched in explicitly anti-research terms. For example, the official statement of the British Council of Disabled People argued that social model approaches are not incompatible with medical research:

> Only on the crudest reading of the social model could it be argued that this model is about rejecting medical treatment or research. The medical model itself is not about medical intervention, but rather the medicalisation of disabled people. This is what we reject ... We are also not making a case against medical research, but rather one for a more equitable distribution of effort and resources in order that a real difference can be made now in the lives of disabled people.
>
> (BCODP, n.d.)

Goggin and Newell (2004: 51) have discussed what they call the 'mythical structure' of the stem cell debate, in the Australian context. They argue that stem cell therapy is seen as deliverance from catastrophe. The underlying assumptions of this mythic structure are:

- Disability is individualised, not created by society.
- People with disabilities are to be acted upon.

- Technology as both value neutral and beneficent.
- Magnification of voices supportive of the technology.
- Heroic delivery of us from disability as moral trump card.
- Technology deals with disability: political issues not needed.

Neither of these accounts seems to be based on an intrinsic objection to stem cell research, unlike the faith-based opponents who are concerned about embryos. Instead, there is resentment about the prioritisation of medical approaches to the disability problem, and what is seen as a neglect of contextual approaches to the disability problem. These critiques often rightly highlight the unbalanced coverage of disability, claiming that media fascination with unproven research leads to a neglect of political issues. Medical therapies are unproven, perhaps impossible, and in any case inappropriate, given the everyday problems of disabled people. Neither account acknowledges that a successful medical therapy would be a good outcome: both bracket the issue of potential clinical benefit, either by saying that cure is impossible, or by ignoring the possibility in favour of more political questions.

Underlying these critiques is the prevailing disability rights unwillingness to engage with the question of impairment. Whereas the narrative of cure sees disabled people as people with impairments, the social model approach sees disabled people as victims of social oppression and exclusion. To focus on curing impairment is to challenge the whole basis of the social model story about disability, and therefore it becomes unacceptable (Oliver, 1989). It often appears that what is at stake in these bitterly fought arguments about medical cures are competing identity narratives.

Many disability rights accounts of medical research focus on hype, and claim to be opposed not to cure itself, but to irresponsible promises and raised expectations. For example, the newsletter *Disability Awareness in Action* special report on biotechnology says:

> Few of us would be opposed to research that holds the promise of finding cures for humankind's killer diseases – although we should be aware of the difficulty in separating what can be achieved from what scientists hope will be achieved.
>
> *(http://www.daa.org.uk/biotech_special.htm)*

Michael Oliver's inaugural professorial lecture 'What's so wonderful about walking?' (republished in *Understanding Disability*, 1996) gives a more sustained analysis and critique of the hyping of medical research. At the outset of his lecture, Oliver quotes from his first published sociological paper: 'the aim of research should not be to make the legless normal, whatever that might mean, but to create a social environment where to be legless is irrelevant' (Oliver, 1978: 137). He goes on to describe medical research charities as forms of millenarian movement, which he defines as 'a collective this-worldly movement promising total social change by miraculous means' (1996: 100). He is deeply sceptical of the track record of medical research:

> The problem is of course, that throughout the history of human-kind, the number of cures that have been found to these 'chronic and crippling diseases' could be counted on the fingers of one hand and still leave some over to eat your dinner with.
>
> *(ibid.: 101)*

In particular, he criticises the International Spinal Research Trust, which in 1986 was promising cures for spinal cord injury within five years. In other publications, Oliver (1989) has compared conductive education, a therapy for children with cerebral palsy, to Nazism and child abuse. However, these criticisms prompted a backlash from people directly involved, arguing that some of the Peto interventions can generate significant outcomes for people with these impairments (Beardshaw, 1989; Read, 1998).

It is not clear whether these challenges reflect the attitudes of disabled people in general. The only survey of disability activists, conducted on behalf of RADAR by Agnes Fletcher (1999), found considerable support for genetic research which might result in cures for impairment and illness: 73 per cent of respondents believed it would be great if new genetic treatments could be developed for conditions like cystic fibrosis or muscular dystrophy. It is clear that there is a range of views on the principle of cure, and on specific therapies. While it is important that disabled voices are heard in the debate, it is misleading to assume that disabled people will speak with one voice (Hughes, 2009).

The principle of cure

One reason for the diversity of views in the disability community is the diversity of impairment experiences among disabled people. The particular experience of impairment will influence an individual's attitudes to disability and to medicine. This is not to claim that two people with the same impairment will have the same views, but to make the broad generalisation that the complexity of impairment effects contributes to disagreement among disabled people.

For example, people with congenital impairments that are largely static in nature tend to be well adjusted to their situation, partly because they have known no other state. Impairment is their normality, and people may be very well adapted to their situation. Other family members may have their condition, due to genetic factors, and they may associate with other people with the same condition. In this context, impairment becomes a part of personal identity, to the point that the individual cannot conceive of themselves without their impairment (Edwards, 2005). Development of a positive sense of self may depend on a positive reading of impairment, which is re-valued in a community based on difference. The classic examples of such impairments include restricted growth, blindness and Deafness. However, many people with cerebral palsy and other conditions present from birth may also value their difference as part of their identity.

In this situation, there may be little enthusiasm for cures, and indeed complete cures for these conditions are unlikely. Corrective surgery in childhood may have been experienced very negatively. Cure may be seen as irrelevant or even threatening and, in the case of an activist, politically offensive. While there is often a worsening of health states due to age, the conditions are not associated with premature mortality or major health complications. People may be different, for example, people with Down syndrome, and even restricted in their choices and abilities, but they generally accommodate well to their situation, and minimise the role of impairment in their lives.

Compare this with those who have acute degenerative conditions. Some of these may have been present at birth due to genetic inheritance, but often they only become problematic during childhood, or else they are acquired in midlife. The individual may have known normal functioning, or at least better functioning: they may have appeared normal, rather than different and disabled. People subsequently experience health problems and degeneration of physical and sometimes mental state. Impairment may not be seen as part of personal identity: it may be seen as an external threat, or as an illness for which cure is hoped for (Novas, 2006; Hughes, 2009). The classic examples of this group of impairments are multiple sclerosis, muscular dystrophy, Friedreich's ataxia and similar rare genetic conditions. HIV/AIDS has many similarities. In these situations, there may be considerable interest, even a desperation, for cures (see, for example, patient views expressed in the journal, *Euroataxia*, at www.euro-ataxia.org). Often these groups are organised and run by parents of children with the condition, who may campaign, fund-raise, and even commission research that contributes to therapies (Novas, 2006).

A third group are those who develop impairments as a result of the ageing process. This may be the largest section of the disabled population, covering conditions such as arthritis and rheumatism, heart disease, strokes and Parkinsonism. Many people with these conditions may see impairment and restriction as a normal part of ageing. They are less likely to identify as disabled or as part of the disability community, retaining their lifelong sense of themselves as normal. Impairment will be regarded as a pathology. They are likely to want rid of their impairment or illness – particularly if it has been of rapid onset – but many will be resigned to their situation and have low expectations of cure.

Finally, there is the group of those who have acquired static impairment in midlife, for example, people with spinal cord injury. Like the late-life acquirers, this group have lived normal lives, and sudden impairment may be unfamiliar and devastating. They may be able to separate their identity from impairment for a time, which may make the process of adaptation more difficult. Once rehabilitation is complete, they do not identify as ill, because they have a static state. The main limiting factors may be experienced as social barriers and social attitudes. However, there may be subsequent physical degeneration as the ageing process sets in (as with post-polio syndrome). People in this group vary in their identity. Some deny their difference, seeking normality; others take the radical disability identity route; others feel defined by their impairment, which they continue to see as pathology and hence seek cure. For example, Michael Oliver is a famous case of a tetraplegic claiming that his injury had a positive impact on his life, and that he would not want a cure, while Smith and Sparkes (2004) discuss a group of men with spinal cord injury, the majority of whom were very definitely 'waiting for the cure'.

This brief sketch of four experiences of impairment/disability shows that individuals will differ in the extent to which they normalise impairment, and the extent to which it becomes part of their identity. The complexity of this debate increases further when different types of cure or therapy are considered. Complete elimination of impairment or disease state is very improbable for most disabled people (although medical successes with childhood leukaemia and other illnesses should not be ignored). However, there is a range of interventions that have changed the experience of impairment over the past century. For example, immunisation has reduced the incidence of infectious diseases such as smallpox and polio. Understandings of disease processes have minimised other conditions through prenatal interventions, for example, phenylketoneuria is a genetic condition which leads to severe learning difficulties, but a simple blood test after birth identifies vulnerable infants, who are placed on an exclusion diet and therefore can attain normal functioning. Administering folate before conception and in the early stages of pregnancy reduces the incidence of spina bifida. Against these successes are the scandals of pharmaceuticals that have actually generated impairment, most notoriously Thalidomide, but also other teratogens such as anti-epilepsy drugs.

Another class of interventions enables the affected individual to gain better life expectancy, although they do not cure the impairment. In public health terms, a reduction in mortality is associated with a gain in morbidity. For the individuals concerned, this is obviously a major benefit, and is evidence that the cure rhetoric has some validity. For example, new understandings of diabetes and insulin in the 1920s led to the survival of those who developed Type one diabetes. Spinal cord injury (SCI) was associated with premature mortality, until better management after World War II enabled people with SCI to achieve normal life expectancy: in much of the developing world, SCI is still a terminal condition. Similarly, heart/lung transplants have increased life expectancy for many people with cystic fibrosis, and the simple technique of nocturnal ventilation has enabled longer survival of young men with Duchenne muscular dystrophy (Eagle *et al.*, 2002). The use of combination therapies has converted HIV/AIDS from an acute terminal illness into a chronic condition.

Many of these beneficial interventions enable people with illness or impairment to move from one disease state to another. For example, spinal stabilisation enables some people with spinal cord injury to have a partial rather than total break of spinal nerves. Gene therapy has successfully cured Severe Combined Immune Deficiency in some children, although they have subsequently developed leukaemia. Current gene therapy research aims to convert Duchenne muscular dystrophy into a less severe variant of the disease. Some interventions for people with sensory deficits cannot cure deafness or blindness, but can achieve gains in sensory function that are experienced as improvements.

Another class of intervention is targeted at improving functioning or quality of life. For example, pacemakers, cochlear implants, and joint replacements have all been experienced positively by people who were previously limited by their physical condition. Surgical interventions such as limb-straightening have enabled restricted growth people with bow legs or malformed joints to be more mobile and avoid worsening of their conditions. People with cerebral palsy have taken muscle-relaxing drugs which reduce spasm. Prozac and other SSRI drugs have enabled people at risk of depression to function more effectively each day.

Finally, there are those interventions that seem more designed to normalise or provide cosmetic improvements than to tackle an underlying functional problem. For example, cosmetic surgery for people with Down syndrome, or limb-lengthening for people with restricted growth, or other aesthetic surgery or orthopaedic interventions. Here an individual – or their family members – facing negative social reaction can seek medical help to minimise difference and fit in. From a disability rights perspective, these interventions may be seen as 'blaming the victim'. Rather than solving the disability problem by removing social barriers, the individual is corrected to fit in with the norm. However, often interventions have both social and functional benefits. Sometimes it is unrealistic to expect major social or cultural change, and in the meantime seemingly cosmetic interventions can improve quality of life. Negative social judgements may also be based on the dangerous assumption that psychological problems are not as serious as physical problems.

This sketch of different impairment states, and different aspects of cure and therapy, is not intended to offer a systematic analysis of the field. However, it suffices to demonstrate that there is a considerable variety of experiences, reactions and interventions, and to challenge simplistic generalisations or blanket political opposition. People have different reasons for turning to medicine, and will have different reactions to their own impairment. Moreover, some cultures will be more supportive of difference than others.

Nor is medical cure or therapy incompatible with social change and civil rights: rather than seeing these as alternative strategies, it is possible to see them as complementary. For example, De Wolfe, who experiences ME, has called for recognition of the importance of cure, and the expansion of the social model to include illness:

> Most people who feel continuously weak, tired, giddy, in pain, will inevitably construe themselves as potential clients of curative medicine. By contrast with certain impairments discussed by disability activists, illness often does constitute tragedy, both for its victims and for those close to them.
>
> *(De Wolfe, 2002: 261)*

Yet this is not to deny that social arrangements also make a big difference.

Almost all disabled people, even where they are happy with the way they are, are unwilling to lose further function; while they may not want a cure, they do not want to lose the abilities they have currently, or have their health state worsen. For this reason, it seems to me that it is misguided to oppose cures and therapies in principle: each should be taken on its merits.

Cures in practice

While cure may be acceptable in theory, there might be problems in practice. For example, cures may be inappropriate responses to the challenge of disability, either because the person is not experiencing their difference negatively, or because barrier removal or social change would be a more effective response to their problems. In other cases, the side effects or other costs of cure may be more problematic than the illness or impairment itself. For example, people with mental illness have long documented the negative impacts of pharmaceuticals that reduce psychotic symptoms or mood swings, but lead to lethargy and other negative symptoms. Cochlear implants sometimes cause complications including potentially lethal infections such as meningitis, and in some cases they fail to achieve useable hearing. Limb-lengthening is a very stressful procedure causing considerable pain, frequent infections around the sites where pins are inserted to bones, and confinement to wheelchair for many months. Even preventative medicine such as immunisation, while benefiting the vast majority, causes major impairment in a tiny proportion of those to whom it is administered.

However, the major practical problem with the cure agenda is the way that new medical research findings are associated with hyperbole and raised expectations, which then do not translate into benefits. This is a common theme in disability studies and disability activist reactions to medical research and media reports of cures. Sociologists of science and medicine have also drawn attention to the cycles of hype and disappointment around the new genetics (Smart, 2003) and other pioneering research such as xenotransplantation (Brown and Michael, 2003) and gene therapy (Martin, 1999; Stockdale, 1999). For example, in the early 1990s, there was considerable scientific excitement about gene therapy (Orkin and Motulsky, 1995; Stockdale, 1999: 82). The discovery of the CFTR gene which causes cystic fibrosis led the medical director of the US Cystic Fibrosis Foundation to say 'We're not talking decades, we're talking years, a few years.' But still there are no cures in prospect – while there have been therapies and treatments which have alleviated the condition (Littlewood, 2004), it is still incurable: 'These representations have consequences for people living with CF. They can give a false sense of hope, distress parents, and alienate adults with the disease' (Stockdale, 1999: 87).

The pursuit of cure has a long history, long pre-dating genetic or stem cell research. For example, the spinal cord injury community have been discussing the prospects for cure since the 1950s, as Nicholas Watson has noted, such as this example of optimism:

In the past twelve months paraplegia has been dealt some serious blows. Paraplegia has been attacked from all four sides this year. The four attackers: PVE, NPF, PN and the medical researchers … Medical science has come up with some advances too. Researchers have been able to repair damaged cords in animals and get nerve impulses past the break … A new substance to grow spinal nerves has been developed by Walter Reed scientists.

However, this extract comes from an editorial entitled 'Kick Him While He's Down' from *Paraplegia News* in 1959. Writing in *Paraplegia News* five years later, James Smittkamp is more realistic about the prospects:

Twenty years ago the medical profession was almost unanimous in its belief that a cure was impossible. While this is still the majority view, some doubt of the old dogma has crept in and a few doctors now believe a cure can be found. But it will require considerable investment of talent, energy, money and time … From this reasoning two specific goals emerge: the elimination of paraplegia by finding a cure, and the alleviation of paraplegia until a cure can be found. Taking first the search for a cure, our problem is to determine the most promising approach … the obvious answer is specific research. Since most doctors still consider a cure impossible, we must go to those few believers who still believe that 'all things are possible'.

(Smittkamp, 1964: 6)

This quotation shows that the impetus behind cure rhetoric often comes from people with the conditions and their families, not just from the scientific or medical community. These historical quotations also suggest that contemporary headlines such as 'Human stem cells allow paralysed mice to walk again' (Sample, 2005) should be treated very cautiously.

Representing people living with genetic conditions or other impairments as desperate for the cure can be a powerful way of drawing public attention to the condition, and levering charitable or governmental funding, as Nik Brown argues: 'The telling of sickness narratives in the context of technological promotion is a powerful means of creating research space, attracting investment and justifying morally challenging research' (2003: 8). Brown talks about hope as part of the 'dynamics of expectation' and discusses patient group participation in lobbying and funding research – 'a simultaneously moral and corporeal form of engagement' – although his own research found that patient organisations are now more ambivalent or sceptical, having had hopes dashed: 'the welding together of painful pathological biography and the fate of a biotechno-logical promise takes place at enormous cost to those who, for however long, are persuaded to share in the hope' (ibid.: 8).

Yet, while those who hype medical research should be criticised, there is also a danger of those in the disability rights community – or indeed deconstructive social scientists in general – if they appear to relish the failure of medical research. Often, disability activists and social commentators take on the role of realists and cynics. Yet surely it would be wonderful if gene therapy or stem cell therapy did turn out to be effective in curing impairments and illnesses. While it is too soon to talk of cure, it is also too early to dismiss the possible potential of these frontier sciences. The difficulty for non-scientist commentators is how to form a judgement as to when the hype is justified. For example, early 1990s hype on gene therapy did not translate into benefits. Is the current debate about stem cell research to be judged as similarly misguided? Is stem cell research more promising than gene therapy was, or will it be another busted flush in five years time? Nik Brown argues: 'Communities of promise are constantly presented with the difficulty of judging the veracity of future claims. And we engage with these pro-cesses of judging whilst knowing that things rarely turn out as expected' (ibid.: 17). This uncertainty makes it hard to explain to patients who are asked to donate tissue – or even surplus embryos – what will happen in future, and who might benefit from – or profit from – the research. Much depends on trust (Ehrich *et al.*, 2012). Anthropologist Sarah Franklin claims that

> It is a mistake to think we can somehow factor out the hype, the media, or the work of the imagination in assessing the promises or the risks of new technology. This is not going to be possible, now or in the future, because it is precisely the importance of imagining new possibilities that fundamentally defines the whole issue of the new genetics and society.
>
> *(Franklin, 2003: 123)*

Cultural representation of cure

To look a little closer at the cultural representation of cure, I will focus on the example of stem cell research, and in particular the death of the actor Christopher Reeve in 2004. Reeve, who had suffered a very sev-eral spinal cord injury after a fall from a horse, had been a leading international figurehead in the quest to cure spinal cord injury. Through his profile and contacts, he was able to raise large amounts of money, which was used to fund The Reeve-Irvine Research Center, the strapline for which is 'Finding the cure'. Reeve and his medical allies always argued that regenerating the spinal cord was an achievable goal. He was quoted as saying: 'The time is at hand for breakthroughs in one of mankind's most heartbreaking problems, one that until now has resisted solution' (www.reeve.uci.edu/infodev.html). Many disability rights activists disliked what Reeve stood for. He was seen as being unrealistic, as giving false hope, and as unrepresentative of disabled people. For example, he reportedly spent £270,000 on treatment and therapy each year, had eleven attendants, and benefited from donated equipment. He thus had privileges and opportunities unavailable to any other disabled person. Moreover, Reeve almost exclusively campaigned for medical research, rather than for disability rights. He could be dismissive of disabled people who didn't share his obsession with cure, and believed it was wrong to accommodate or come to terms with impairment. For these reasons, while some disabled people derived hope and inspiration from him, others rejected his work, the way he was represented, and even saw him as a traitor.

I examined coverage of Christopher Reeve's death in *The Times*, *The Independent*, the *Guardian*, the *Daily Telegraph*, and the *Daily Mail*. Across the five newspapers sampled, there were 24 separate news stories, features, leading articles, op-ed pieces and obituaries. Coverage was dominated by words such as inspirational, indomitable, heroic, inspiring. *The Times'* treatment was typical: the front page news item was headlined: 'The all-American hero whose battle with disability gave hope to millions'. The obituary described him as 'tirelessly campaigning for the disabled and their rights', a far from accurate description. A leading article saw Reeve as 'a source of inspiration for many who have been confronted by disability'. The *Guardian* leader writer reported that '[Reeve] subsequently became a role model for disabled people in the way he refused to allow the condition to conquer his spirit as well as his body, and for the tireless way he campaigned on disability issues.' As I argue in this chapter, the actual response of disabled people was more complex than this suggests.

Perhaps it is unreasonable to expect balance after someone has died? Yet critical or balanced statements were conspicuous by their absence. For example, *The Times'* leader mentioned that Reeve 'was criticised by some for encouraging expectations beyond science's ability to deliver', and there were brief references to pro-life opposition to embryonic stem cell work (as well as an opinion piece by Michael Gove expressing anxiety about embryo research). *The Times* was typical in quoting actors, scientists and one representative of a spinal research charity, who were all positive about Reeve's role and message. A more critical scientist, Colin Blakemore, was quoted in *The Independent* and also wrote a more balanced piece for the *Daily Mail*:

> It is absolutely wrong to raise false expectations about the speed with which medical research progresses, but it takes people like Reeve, with their commitment and their certainty that they will be cured, to carry it forward.

Blakemore highlighted the difficulties with stem cell research, and pointed out the simple fact that it was never going to have been possible for Reeve to have walked again. Jeremy Laurance in *The Independent* ('The truth about Superman's achievements') and Ian Sample in the *Guardian* ('Is this the future of medicine?') stressed the uncertainty around stem cell research, and the time it would take to achieve clinical applications.

It is very rare for disabled people themselves, particularly critical voices, to be quoted in stories about cure research (Shakespeare, 1999a). Goggin and Newell (2004) analysed 300 news and features items on stem cells from Australian print media between May–June 2002. Disabled people were very rarely quoted as authorities, with the exception of several first-hand testimonial to the desire for salvation from people such as Christopher Reeve himself. Even a critical social analysis of different voices in the stem cell debate neglects disability rights perspectives (Ganchoff, 2004).

In the aftermath of Reeve's death, only two identified disabled people were quoted in the newspapers that I looked at. The *Guardian* quoted *Washington Post* columnist Charles Krauthammer (a wheelchair user) who called Reeve's public pronouncements 'disgracefully misleading', but in the context of a piece which concluded with a hope message and was entitled 'Life and death of a hero'. In the same newspaper, there was a piece by a spinal cord injured man explaining opposition from people with SCI and spinal injury units:

> Reeve was a controversial figure among people with spinal injuries and particularly with the more traditional medical establishments of spinal injury units. His message of hope for a cure was regarded as irresponsible and misleading. Whenever his name was mentioned it was either with frustration or a sneer, and I have often heard it said: 'His name is a dirty word in this house.'

However, the author's own views were very positive about Reeve and cure.

While the mainstream media were very positive about Reeve, the same cannot be said for the disability press. For example, activist Tara Flood was quoted in *Disability Now* as saying that Reeve 'Clearly surrounded himself with people who made him believe a cure was just around the corner' when it was 'potentially generations away ... He was in a position where he could have done huge amounts for disabled people but chose a different route.'

Bill Albert argued that the problem was that Reeve saw his disability as a medical issue. However, *Disability Now* did include one dissenting voice from the Spinal Injuries Association who was more positive about Reeve's work. Online, the BBC website, recorded many testimonies from disabled people and others who were very positive about Reeve, with phrases such as 'Reeve was an inspirational figure' and 'Reeve changed how I look at life.' No quotations from disabled people who opposed Reeve were featured, although it's impossible to know whether this was because they were not sent in, or because they were censored. Certainly, disability rights contributors to online discussion groups such as the international disability research list were largely negative about Reeve, and when I wrote a more balanced column on the BBC Disability website, I received very negative feedback from the radical community.

Studying media coverage of embryonic stem cell research in 2000, Clare Williams *et al.* (2003) found that there were five TV news bulletins which featured patients or patient support groups speaking in favour of stem cell research, and no examples of them speaking against (out of a total of eight bulletins). Only Labour MPs featured as often in bulletins. They also found that 22 newspaper articles featured supportive scientists and doctors, while four featured supportive patients or patient groups, and none featured critical patients or patient support groups. The views of both disability rights groups and women's voices were marginalised in the coverage. As I have shown, the same is true of coverage of Reeve's death.

Yet it would be wrong to assume that the disability community has a single or coherent view of people like Christopher Reeve, or stem cell research more generally. While the mainstream media may have been dominated by non-disabled pro-research voices, ordinary disabled people did write in to support Reeve's work. Other research finds patient activists in favour of stem cell and other medical advances (Ganchoff, 2004). Moreover, disability activist and disability studies debates are skewed towards anti-cure, anti-Reeve voices.

Difficult cases

Examination of media coverage and lay voices shows the importance of capturing the complexity and variation in disability responses. Looking more closely at a few case studies of cures and therapies shows the need for nuance in judgement. The Hastings Center volume, *Surgically Shaping Children* (Parens, 2006), provides just such a pluralist and carefully argued account of three sorts of therapy decisions: (1) correction of cleft lip and palate; (2) gender reassignment surgery; and (3) limb-lengthening in children with restricted growth. As the authors show, such cases are complex, because the patients involved are often too young to choose freely for themselves: parents have to make difficult decisions in what they believe to be the best interests of the child. This brings into conflict two values at the heart of parenting: to support the well-being of our children, and to let them develop in their own way. The contributors to the Hastings Center volume broadly agreed with parents deciding on early surgery to repair cleft lip and palate; opposed parents deciding on behalf of their children when it comes to intersex surgery; and believed that children themselves should be supported to make decisions about limb-lengthening.

One problem of the Hastings Center's approach (and of previous research in this area by Priscilla Alderson, 1993) is that there is a risk of individualising the treatment decision. In other words, while I support the involvement of children in decisions about their treatment, there is a risk of both children and adults being influenced by a wider cultural climate in the direction of accepting normalisation. For example, I think it is possible that children who consent to limb-lengthening may be implicitly influenced by their non-disabled parents' desires, as well as by the broader cultural messages in wider society. Limb-lengthening decisions are taken in the early teenage years, a period of the life course when pressure towards, and desire for, social conformity are at their height. Evidence that those who have undertaken the surgery are glad that they have done so is also problematic: after so great an investment of time and endurance of pain, and with a changed body shape, it is hard for any individual then to admit it may have been a mistake, or to say that they are not happy with the result.

One of the more controversial forms of cure is use of cochlear implants to correct hearing impairment. This has been opposed by Deaf people, who challenge the impairment-based definition of deafness. To Deaf activists, being Deaf is about being a cultural minority, not being disabled (Kermit, 2009). Deafness becomes a cultural identity based on a shared language, like a minority ethnic community. For this reason, Deaf people often refuse to identify with disabled people, whom they regard as having impairments. Deaf people usually welcome the birth of deaf children, who can then be enculturated into Deaf culture, through the use of sign language. Recently, there was also the controversial case of a Deaf lesbian couple who took active steps to maximise the chances of their child being deaf by choosing a Deaf sperm donor (Scully, 2012).

There seem to be internal contradictions in the Deaf approach to cochlear implants. First, if Deafness is really nothing to do with impairment, then logically there would be no reason for Deaf people to oppose impairment reduction. Second, if Deafness is about being a member of a sign language community, there is nothing to stop hearing children of Deaf adults being members of that community too: indeed, there is a thriving Children of Deaf Adults (CODA) movement which enjoys membership in both Deaf and hearing worlds.

Third, the vast majority of deaf children are born to hearing adults. Because their parents are not native signers, it would not be easy for these children to become native sign language users. For them, the best option may be to maximise speech and hearing through cochlear implants, so that they can have a chance of communicating with their parents and joining the hearing world. The dilemma for Deaf children of Deaf adults is that the maximum benefit of a cochlear implant comes when the child forgoes sign language and concentrates entirely on learning to speak and hear and lip read (Kermit, 2009). Therefore, if Deaf parents implant their Deaf child, they are sacrificing their best hope of communicating effectively with their own child, who will additionally suffer from having parents whose speech is probably limited. For this reason, the opposition of Deaf parents to implanting their own children is understandable, but should not prevent hearing parents using this technology to improve the life chances of their Deaf child.

A difficult case is presented by autism and other forms of 'neuro-diversity' (Happé, 1994; Hodge, 2005). In recent years, partly due to the development of internet-based forms of communication, a community of people with autism, Asperger's syndrome and related conditions have challenged the devaluing and pathologisation of these experiences. From a 'neuro-diverse' perspective, different ways of thinking and relating are not impairments, but just differences (Moloney, 2010; Wheeler, 2011). A more flexible society would be able to accommodate neuro-diverse people, and value their strengths and aptitudes, rather than seeking to prevent or cure these conditions.

While not dismissing this approach, it should be noted that the majority of people on the autistic spectrum do have significant problems arising from their cognitive differences. They may have severe learning difficulties; they may have extreme difficulties relating to other people or participating in society; unlike dominant media representations, they may have no compensating skills or aptitudes. In other words, those people with high functioning autism or Asperger's syndrome who talk of autism as an alternative style may not always be representative of others with the condition. While it is always valuable to promote acceptance and an understanding of difference, many families would welcome prevention, therapy or cure of autism (Kelly, 2005). The case of autistic spectrum conditions is a reminder of two important features of impairment high-lighted in previous chapters. First, there is a hierarchy of impairment: different impairments have different impacts, and the same impairment can have different effects. Second, mild to moderate impairment may not be a difficulty for anyone, given supportive and flexible environments prepared to respect and value difference. However, severe forms of impairment will often cause considerable problems and limitations and sometimes suffering and distress for the individual and their families. The importance of promoting cultural respect and social acceptance for people with impairment should not blind us to the importance of mitigating or preventing impairment via individual medical or psychological therapies.

Conclusion

In this chapter, I have argued for a more balanced approach to cure and therapy within disability studies. From a critical realist perspective, committed to understanding the operation of disability on different ontological levels, biomedical and psychological intervention has an important role. It would be foolish to hope for quick results from stem cell or gene therapy research. It would be dangerous to rely on medical research as an alternative to barrier removal. However, if safe, effective treatments eventually materialise, then disabled people will benefit and quality of life will improve. Resort to medicine is not contrary to other objectives of disability rights, and activists and scholars should be critical supporters of the endeavour to mitigate or prevent impairment.

However, a wise approach to the issue would also recognise the ubiquity of impairment. Medicine will never banish the problems and limitations of embodiment. As argued previously, impairment is a predicament that faces everyone, in some form and at some time. The ambition to minimise illness and impairment should be balanced with the need to accept limitations, and find ways of living with them. Denigrating or misrepresenting the lives of existing disabled people in the search for cures, even with the noble aim of raising funds for research, cannot be justified. Obsession with normality and perfection, ultimately unattainable or false goals, is harmful to well-being and self-esteem (Martz, 2001).

Biomedical research is not the only way to enhance the lives of disabled people, either in Britain, or globally. In fact, an international perspective reveals that there are more pressing disabling conditions than the rare disorders or late onset conditions for which stem cell research and genetics may eventually bring benefits (Shakespeare, 2005b). The majority of the world's citizens are still impaired by preventable diseases such as malaria or TB, or other socially caused conditions arising from accidents, malnutrition, poverty and war. Some 90 per cent of the world's pharmaceutical research is conducted on diseases which affect 10 per cent of the world's population (Flory and Kitcher, 2004). As Philip Kitcher argues: 'When millions of children die every year from malaria, how can we justify our expenditures on research into Lesch–Nyhan syndrome, cystic fibrosis, even the common forms of cancer?' (1997: 324).

Another interesting feature of contemporary biomedical research is that while most projects are directed at ameliorating impairment and illness, new products and techniques find wider application in non-disabled populations (Juengst, 1998). Examples such as Viagra, Human Growth Hormone (Conrad and Potter, 2004); and Prozac (Elliot, 1999) show how difficult it is to police the line between therapies and enhancement (Buchanan *et al.*, 2000: 118). Jackie Scully and Christoph Rehmann-Sutter (2001) argue that the use of the therapy/enhancement distinction further reinforces the pathologisation of impaired and people with impairment. They argue that attention should be paid to the consequences of concrete intervention, rather than reliance on a simplistic distinction to validate/invalidate therapeutic approaches. While the therapy/enhancement debate is beyond the scope of this chapter, it is important because it suggests that rather than equalising the natural lottery – creating greater equality by compensating and correcting impairments which render people disadvantaged – some biotechnologies may ultimately increase inequality, because they enable those who are non-disabled to further enhance their capabilities, leaving the impaired at a greater comparative disadvantage.

While these points, cautions and concerns are important – and have been well made by many bioethicists and some disability studies commentators – they do not provide intrinsic objections to pursuing medical research, alongside other strategies. But they do suggest that there are pressing questions for wider social regulation and debate, in order that the coming applications of biomedicine should be exploited to benefit the many, rather than the few, and to enhance, rather than to exploit and divide. We require what Flory and Kitcher (2004: 59) define as 'well-ordered science', where the voices of those directly affected are heard, where research is directed towards those questions which are most significant, and where scientists take their moral obligations seriously.

8

AUTONOMY AT THE END OF LIFE

Disability issues in bioethics are highly contested because they bring up powerful emotional issues: questions about the permissibility of technological intervention; the vulnerability of disabled people; the widespread non-disabled perception that impairment is a fate worse than death; the historical backdrop of abuse, oppression and murder. These factors are common to debates at both the beginning of life, and the end of life. Fears about eugenics and about euthanasia form the substrate of the disability rights response to bioethical arguments about autonomy and the value of life (Asch, 2001).

End-of-life questions are poignant, first, because they seem to threaten the very existence of disabled people, even more personally and directly than questions about prenatal diagnosis. Second, if individuals are permitted to end their life on the grounds of suffering and restriction, this potentially sends a message that impairment is so awful that no one would want to go on living in such a state. Third, a narrow focus on impairment and suffering again risks obscuring the social contexts which often determine the quality of disabled people's lives, in particular, the availability of independent living and civil rights protections from exclusion and discrimination.

In recent years, the end-of-life debate has assumed a high profile in many Western countries. The US state of Oregon legalised assisted dying for terminally ill mentally competent adults in 1997 and the neighbouring state of Washington followed; the Netherlands legalised voluntary euthanasia in 2002, after a thirty-year period of non-prosecution of such cases; Belgium legalised voluntary euthanasia in 2002 (Finlay et al., 2005); assisted suicide for chronically ill and disabled people is permitted in Switzerland.

In Britain, there have been a string of high profile legal cases such as those of Miss B, a disabled woman who wanted her ventilator to be turned off so that she could die, rather than live in an impaired state; Diane Pretty, a woman terminally ill with motor neurone disease, who petitioned for her partner to be able to assist her to commit suicide; and Reginald Crewe and other terminally ill individuals who have sought to travel to Switzerland where the voluntary organisation Dignitas offers an assisted suicide service. Partly in response to such cases, Lord Joffe has introduced several bills into the House of Lords to permit assisted suicide in Britain, supported by the Voluntary Euthanasia Society, now called Dignity in Dying (Epstein, 2005). In the United States, there was huge public interest in the case of Terry Schiavo, a brain-damaged woman whose former husband petitioned for her life-support system to be switched off, against the wishes of her parents and 'Pro-Life' campaigners.

Assisted suicide or mercy killing have also been the subject of the high profile and award-winning films *The Sea Inside* (Dir. Amenabar, 2004), *Million Dollar Baby* (Dir. Eastwood, 2004), and *Amour* (Dir. Michael Haneke, 2012). This unprecedented coverage of end-of-life issues perhaps contributes to the perception and fear among disabled people that their lives are in danger.

Notwithstanding the validity of these concerns, it is important to note that the passionate debate about disability rights at the end of life also bolsters an identity politics approach. Organisations such as Not Dead Yet, high profile battles against euthanasia enthusiasts such as Dr Jack Kevorkian, and emotive comparisons with Nazi euthanasia all fuel a plot narrative which variously suggests that other family members, doctors, or society desire the death of disabled people. Such a victim position is potent in raising the profile of the disability rights movement, and bolstering disability identity (e.g. Darke, 2004). The potent image of vulnerable disabled people is also encouraged by the vociferous 'Pro-Life' movement that uses an alliance with disabled campaigners to back its 'sanctity of life' position in opposition to choice, both at the beginning and end of life.

Typically, the discourse of disability rights opposition operates at the level of generality, rather than specifics: interventions are usually emotive and rhetorical, rather than rational and analytical; individuals are denounced; diverse issues are conflated; there is a lack of evidence for claims. This simplistic disability rights critique obscures the range of issues at the end of life. These include decisions about resuscitation (cardio-pulmonary resuscitation, or CPR); advance directives and living wills; withdrawal of treatment; assisted suicide; voluntary euthanasia; non-voluntary euthanasia. Each raises different questions, and a careful response should differentiate between them, even though they all raise questions about the death of people who may be defined as disabled.

In particular, it is important to distinguish situations where the autonomy of disabled people is undermined (abuse of Do Not Resuscitate Notices, non-voluntary euthanasia) from situations where disabled or terminally-ill people themselves are exercising their autonomy by requesting assistance with death, or withdrawal of treatment (advance directives, assisted suicide). The failure to draw relevant distinctions and the failure to engage with the clinical realities undermine many disability rights critiques. As an example of the complexities of what appears to be a straightforward end-of-life issue, I will turn briefly to the DNR ('Do Not Resuscitate') controversy.

The background to this controversy are instances when disabled or elderly people have gone into hospital, often for minor operations, and discovered that a clinician has scribbled 'DNR' on their chart, without consultation. To the patient, this can be very distressing. It appears that a judgement has been made that the patient's life is not worth preserving, and that clinicians are unfairly discriminating between disabled and non-disabled people. Emotive claims such as 'The NHS is killing disabled people' express the outrage of the disability movement, and spread fear among disabled people who have to go to hospital.

Sometimes, fears of discrimination and prejudice may be justified. There are also fears that patients who are given DNR orders receive less good treatment (Mohammed *et al.*, 2005). And it is certainly the case that decisions about cardio-pulmonary resuscitation (CPR) should always involve discussion with the patient and their relatives, which is a central element in the good practice statement agreed by the UK Resuscitation Council and doctors' and nurses' organisations (Resuscitation Council, 2001). However, while there have certainly been abuses, claims such as 'the NHS is killing disabled people' appear to be exaggerated.

Furthermore, CPR may not always be the straightforward benefit that it appears. It is likely that the general public have an exaggerated view of the efficacy of attempts at resuscitation. Even professionals regularly over-estimate the possibilities of CPR being successful (Wagg *et al.*, 1995). Most lay people's experience of CPR comes via medical soap operas such as *ER*. On television, CPR has a very high success rate. One study of television representation showed short-term survival (one hour) after resuscitation in 75 per cent of cases (Diem *et al.*, 1996). By contrast, 40 per cent short-term success is accepted to be the upper limit in practice, and most sources give a figure of 25 per cent of patients being successfully resuscitated in the short term. The same TV study found 67 per cent of CPR cases survived until discharge from hospital.

By contrast, a range of studies of long-term survival have produced figures of 2–30 per cent for those experiencing cardiac arrest outside a hospital, and 6.5–15 per cent for those experiencing arrest while in hospital. For elderly patients, it is suggested a figure of 5 per cent long-term survival after CPR would be more realistic. Unrealistic media portrayal, therefore, reinforces the perception that CPR is a miraculous intervention with a high chance of success. For this reason, many clinicians prefer the acronym 'DNAR' to clarify that the decision is 'Do Not Attempt Resuscitation'.

Not only does CPR not succeed, in the majority of cases, but it can also cause harm to patients. CPR involves: checking that airways are clear, and sometimes inserting a tube into the mouth and airway; air or oxygen being pumped into the lungs; vigorous repeated pressure on the chest to pump blood to brain and other vital organs until normal heartbeat is restored; it may include the use of an electric shock (defibrillation) to restart the heart. CPR is often a distressing experience for patients, relatives and staff. There are some disabled or elderly people for whom CPR could be hugely traumatic or sometimes even lethal. For example, people with osteoporosis or osteogenesis imperfecta have frail bones, which could be damaged if clinicians attempted to restart their heart, resulting in a fractured sternum or ribcage and possibly lacerated lungs. The outcome would either be a much more painful death at the time, or temporary survival in a state of extreme discomfort. For the rest of the minority who survive CPR, research shows that 20–50 per cent suffer neurological impairment, ranging from slight brain damage to persistent vegetative state (Mohr and Kettler, 1997). In other words, choosing to decline CPR may be a rational choice, given the realities:

> If CPR were a benign, risk-free procedure that offered a good hope of long-term survival in the face of otherwise certain death, few people would ever choose to have medical personnel withhold resuscitation. But controversy surrounds the use of CPR precisely because the procedure can lead to prolonged suffering, severe neurologic damage, or an undignified death.
>
> *(Diem et al., 1996: 1581)*

For the same reasons, doctors may think CPR is contra-indicated in such cases and suggest DNAR.

The evidence shows that if the CPR procedure and outcome evidence are properly explained to patients, they are more likely to decline resuscitation and to request DNAR notices. For example, in one study,

41 per cent of acute patients initially opted for CPR. When informed of the evidence about efficacy and outcome, 22 per cent opted for CPR. In a group of people with chronic illness whose life expectancy was less than a year, only 11 per cent initially opted for CPR. After being informed of the evidence, only 5 per cent opted for CPR (Cherniack, 2002: 303). Of course, an alternative way of interpreting these findings are that those who explain CPR and DNAR to patients are doing so in ways which encourage or even subtly coerce people into adopting an approach which clinicians themselves approve of.

Abuse of DNAR must be exposed and opposed. Moreover, DNAR should not trigger diminished quality of care (Mohammed *et al.*, 2005). Yet, properly used, DNAR notices have a place in medicine. There has been a transition from medical paternalism to a partnership model in DNAR guidelines. DNAR notices are used in a minority of cases, and the abuse of DNAR is rarer still. All medical decisions should be based on a consultation between professionals and patients, although doctors have to use their professional judgement as to whether a course of action will be clinically effective and in the patient's best interest. Equally, it may be rational for a patient to request a DNAR notice. Everyone, disabled or not, has an interest in having a good death, and CPR is often painful, undignified and futile. The conclusion I draw from the CPR/DNAR debate is that calm and evidence-based deliberation is usually more useful to disabled people than extreme rhetoric.

My position on end of life, as will become evident in this chapter, is based on consistent support for the choices and desires of disabled people themselves, not on disability rights ideology. For most of the time, the disability rights movement supports the autonomy of disabled people. The slogan 'choices and rights' has been an important rallying cry in many life domains. For example, autonomy is the basis of the independent living philosophy, which campaigns for disabled people to have control over their own lives. It seems to me to be inconsistent to support autonomy for disabled people in all matters except the moment and manner of their death. The remainder of this chapter will focus on the assisted suicide debate, in order to analyse these general issues within a particular and topical context.

Assisted suicide and disability rights opposition

The most famous disability rights group campaigning against assisted suicide is the US group, Not Dead Yet, founded in opposition to Dr Jack Kevorkian, the former physician who encouraged 130 ill or disabled people to die by offering his services. Their strapline is 'the resistance' and their website argues 'Though often described as compassionate, legalized medical killing is really about a deadly double standard for people with severe disabilities, including both conditions that are labeled terminal and those that are not.' Not Dead Yet sees assisted suicide as giving medical professionals immunity from killing disabled people. Founder Diane Coleman argues that economic pressures within the private healthcare system, together with lack of protection within the courts, will threaten disabled people if assisted suicide were legalised in the United States.

Most US disability rights activists and disability studies academics appear to support the position taken by Not Dead Yet (e.g. Gill, 1992, 2000; Silvers, 1998). For example, the historian Paul Longmore (2003) wrote eloquently on the Elizabeth Bouvia case, and argued that assisted suicide activists have a much broader agenda than the right to die in terminal illness, seeking to extend coverage to all disabled people. Adrienne Asch takes a position in support of Not Dead Yet in her account of bioethics and disability (2001). However, a few writers on disability, for example, Batavia (1997), have adopted positions in support of autonomy.

In the UK, disability rights opposition to assisted suicide was prompted by the House of Lords Bill to legalise assisted suicide, introduced by Lord Joffe in 2004 and 2005. Joffe would have mandated physician–assisted suicide in a very narrow set of cases. An individual would only be able to take advantage of the provision if

1 She was terminally ill, and expected to die naturally within a short period and
2 She was suffering unbearably.

The Bill thus extended to disabled people the power to end their lives – which non-disabled people are able to do through a decision to commit suicide – as well as ensuring that doctors would be able to give assistance and advice to terminally ill people so that the appropriate drugs to ensure successful and painfree suicide were made available and used effectively.

Organisations in the UK disability movement have been almost unanimous in their opposition to all attempts to promote legal reform in the direction of assisted dying, as were the majority of disability rights academics and activists. The phrase 'Not Dead Yet' is also used by British campaigners (www.notdeadyetuk.org), in particular, by high-profile Independent Living activist Baroness (Jane) Campbell. In 2004, I submitted evidence and appeared as a witness in favour of the Joffe Bill, but to my knowledge was the only prominent voice from the disability movement who spoke out in favour of assisted suicide. Due to the 2005 election, this version of the Bill failed. When Lord Joffe reintroduced his Assisted Dying Bill in November 2005, the *Disability Now* newspaper again printed a selection of prominent disabled people's views: 13 argued against the Bill, four argued in favour. Meanwhile, the majority of respondents to the *Disability Now* November 2005 poll argued in favour. Given that the Joffe Bill appeared to promote the autonomy of disabled people, ensuring the right to a good death, and not undermining the possibility of a good life, why did the leaders of the disability movement, almost without exception, oppose it?

One class of fears centres on the environment in which people make decisions. Disabled people may be vulnerable to different pressures, which in practice undermine the possibility of them making an autonomous decision. For example, in the immediate context, direct pressure may be exerted on disabled people to end their lives against their will. Healthcare systems and relatives may want to save the costs of supporting a dying person for many months. There are historical and contemporary precedents for so-called 'mercy killing'. There are fears that disabled people will be pressured into requesting assisted suicide by relatives or professionals.

More generally, the wider cultural context may also influence disabled people. Decisions are always made in a social context. Campaigns for assisted suicide (AS) and voluntary euthanasia have sometimes emphasised the pain, humiliation, and difficulty of disability in ways that are derogatory to disabled people, and cause fear and alarm in non-disabled people (Hurst, n.d.). Similarly, most people are afraid of dying and of death: 'The phrase "death with dignity" is very often used to mean the deliberately procured death of an ill or disabled person, and strongly implies that vulnerable people are only "dignified" in death' (Davis, 2004: 1).

Exaggerating the difficulties and suffering of impairment-related death – and ignoring the success of palliative care – will distort people's reactions and perhaps stimulate demand for AS.

Making AS available might also send an implicit message that it is logical and desirable for disabled people to end their own lives, or that disabled people's lives are inferior to those of non-disabled people (Campbell, 2003). This cultural belief may influence the attitudes of people who live and work with disabled people. These messages and attitudes in turn might feed back into disabled people's own views about their actions and choices, making it more likely that they will choose AS, even if it is against their best interests and perhaps they would not freely have taken that step in the absence of influence.

Many disabled people feel vulnerable and depressed from time to time, particularly after the first diagnosis of impairment or chronic illness.

Living with both impairment and disability is not easy. Many disabled people have at different points wanted to end their lives. With support and over time, most disabled people have come to terms with their impairments and learned to accommodate to their restrictions, reporting a good quality of life and no longer wishing to end their own lives. Disabled opponents of AS, many of whom have gone through this trajectory themselves, fear that other disabled people may make irreversible decisions, soon after the onset of impairment, and deny themselves the possibility of living a better life as a disabled person in future.

There may also be an impact on people who are not currently disabled, but may be anxious about becoming impaired. Fear of impairment is widespread among non-disabled people who are unfamiliar with disabled people. Research has shown considerable cultural prejudice against disabled people and a commonly expressed belief that it would be better to be dead than disabled. These fears need to be challenged, and the positive aspects and contributions of disabled people need to be emphasised. Impairment and disability are part of the human condition, and society needs to come to terms with disability, not encourage people to think that disabled lives are not worth living.

Of course, the influences on a person's decisions to seek AS can be material, as well as cultural and attitudinal. If the full range of independent living options (housing, technology, assistance, etc.) is not available, then the lives of people with impairments and terminal illnesses will seem harder and they may be more likely to opt to end their lives. The disability movement has argued that a person must have had access to the full range of care and independent living possibilities, prior to being entitled to request AS. Equally, the hospice movement provides evidence that palliative care and pain relief can ease dying. The availability of palliative care and of hospice care is very important. A person must have had access to these facilities, prior to being entitled to request AS. In countries like the Netherlands, where voluntary euthanasia is an established practice, the hospice movement and palliative care have not developed to the same degree as in UK.

Second, there is a set of questions about those who may be entitled to have an AS request honoured. 'Unbearable suffering' has been presented as a qualification for AS. But how should this be defined? It is almost impossible to agree an objective measure of pain and suffering, and everyone reacts to impairment and illness differently. Not everyone finds a particular level of pain or restriction unbearably awful. Many disabled people are living with the pain and dependency, technological and physical, which is cited as evidence for the rationality of a decision by others to seek assisted suicide. For example, many disabled people are tube-fed throughout their lives, yet tube-feeding for some assisted suicide advocates marks a stage of terminal illness when death would be appropriate and desirable. For example, Ed Roberts, an influential US disability activist, said:

> I've been on a respirator for twenty-six years, and I watch these people's cases. They're just as dependent on a respirator as I am. The major difference is that they know they're going to be forced to live in a nursing home – or they're already there – and I'm leading a quality of life. That's the only difference. It's not the respirator. It's the money.
>
> *(quoted in Priestley, 2004: 174)*

Disabled people living with tube-feeding, or ventilation, or other forms of high dependency, fear that their own lives will be devalued, or may even be at risk, as a result of the decisions or attitudes of others who do not want to live in such conditions.

Another qualification often cited is 'terminal illness'. But again, it is not clear how to define this state. Many disabled people – such as Jane Campbell, cited earlier – live throughout their lives with conditions that are defined as terminal. For example, impairments such as cystic fibrosis, muscular dystrophy, multiple sclerosis, are all currently incurable, and generally result in premature death. Some people who are diagnosed with these conditions decide that life is no longer worth living, even though they are currently not severely impaired. Would people with such impairments be considered terminally ill, and hence candidates for AS? Moreover, many of these illnesses have an episodic and fluctuating presentation: individuals may develop complications, enter a critical phase and appear on the verge of death, but with appropriate medical care, recover to live on for many more years. Only in retrospect is it clear when the terminal phase of terminal illness has begun.

Even though the Joffe Bill was restricted to people with terminal illnesses who were likely to die within a short period, many disability campaigners feared that it would be easy to extend the rights or cultural expectation of assisted suicide to disabled people in general, not just people who are in the terminal stage of a terminal illness. The fear of a slippery slope underpins both the contextual and the categorical arguments. If limited and careful AS legislation – such as the Joffe Bill – were approved, disability rights campaigners fear that the process would not stop there. They suggest the following narrative might unfold: the safeguards to ensure autonomous decision-making would be weakened, as legalisation made it more acceptable, and people began to feel pressurised to opt for death. The category of people who had the right to AS could be extended, to include those who are not in the terminal stages of incurable illness and in unbearable suffering, but also many people who are currently living with impairment, restriction and discomfort. By degrees, policy might be broadened until assisted suicide turned into voluntary euthanasia, and then voluntary euthanasia became non-voluntary euthanasia. However, this slippery slope has not materialised after 15 years of regulated assisted suicide in Oregon.

The third objection suggests that assisted suicide legalisation would be a form of unfair discrimination. For example, central to the Not Dead Yet case is that assisted suicide provisions violate equal protection under the Americans with Disabilities Act, because while non-disabled people would be prevented or discouraged from committing suicide, people with terminal illness – who are disabled people – would be permitted or encouraged to do so: legalised assisted suicide, in this reading, would legitimise disability discrimination.

A final objection, made eloquently, for example, by Alison Davis (2004), is the claim that life is an inalienable right. This means that life is a right of which you cannot be deprived, not even by yourself. According to this perspective, even if the majority of the public, including a majority of disabled people, support assisted suicide, it would still be wrong. Even if there was no evidence of abuse or coercion whatsoever, it should remain prohibited. Yet the idea that life is inalienable seems to be an *a priori* assumption. It is usually rooted in religious prohibitions. There seems to be no clear reason why those who do not adopt a theological approach to morality should accept the concept.

The autonomy argument for assisted suicide

The most powerful argument for permitting assisted suicide arises from the principle of autonomy (Woods, 2002, 2005). In liberal democracies, people are usually entitled to make choices as to how to live their lives, even if these choices conflict with the values of others, so long as their actions do not harm others. In other words, although I may not want to end my own life, neither I nor the state should prevent others taking this step. Control over one's own body is one of the most important of rights, and restrictions on someone's ability to choose how and when to die are regarded by many as intrusive.

Choice is a very important principle for the disability movement. For example, disability rights campaigners have fought for independent living, meaning the right to choose where and how to live and be supported. Where a person cannot carry out physical tasks, the principles of independent living suggest that she should be able to employ others to carry out those tasks, under her control (Morris, 1993a). Similarly, disability rights campaigners have fought for choices freely to express sexuality, to form relationships and reproduce, with assistance where necessary (Shakespeare *et al.*, 1996; Earle, 1999). Autonomy in healthcare is an important dimension of the choices and rights at the centre of disability movement ideology. For example, people should be free from unwanted treatment, and should be consulted in decisions that affect them.

It is therefore paradoxical and appears inconsistent that the disability movement should support freedom of choice in every area of life except the desire of a disabled person to end their life. Moreover, providing assistance to commit suicide could be said to empower a disabled person to realise their desires, in the same way as assistance in other activities. In law, people who are dependent on life-sustaining treatment already have the right to request withdrawal of treatment (for example, having their ventilator switched off, as Miss B requested). But those who are not treatment-dependent have no such possibility of ending their life. A disabled person might be unable to commit suicide, due to their physical situation, whereas a non-disabled person could carry through their wishes and take steps to bring about their own death: attempting suicide is no longer illegal in Britain. For example, Diane Pretty complained that she was physically incapable of killing herself without assistance, and needed her partner to help her die. Supporting her claim, Liberty, the human rights group, argued that she should have the same rights to kill herself as anyone else (Priestley, 2004: 173). Giving disabled people assistance to die would therefore remove an inequality, putting them in the same position as a non-disabled person. Logically, this seems a reasonable extension of the principles of autonomy and independent living and non-discrimination.

Moreover, the arguments of disability rights campaigners who oppose assisted suicide are themselves framed in the language of autonomy: it is claimed that if some people were to exercise their choice to commit suicide, this would infringe or undermine the choices of others not to commit suicide (Campbell, 2003). Yet it is not clear, conceptually, how this follows. Different disabled people have different views and desires. The desires or decisions of one disabled person should not have direct implications for the desires or decisions of another disabled person. For example, if some disabled people want to use personal assistance services, this does not imply that everyone else should be forced to adopt the same approach to support and care.

Empirically, some disabled people want to exercise the right to die: the cases of Reginald Crew, Diane Pretty, Miss B and others are examples of this phenomenon. Moreover, survey evidence suggests that disability activists and advocates who oppose assisted suicide are in a minority among disabled people. When the Disability Rights Commission conducted an online survey in 2003, 63 per cent of respondents supported new laws on end-of-life choice. Polling conducted by MORI for the Voluntary Euthanasia Society in 2004 found that 80 per cent of disabled people supported the Joffe Bill to legalise assisted suicide in controlled circumstances. This data seems to suggest that not only is the disability movement opposition to assisted suicide contradicting the important disability rights principle of autonomy, but also that disability rights advocates and organisations are not representative of the population which they seek to represent.

For example, Michael Hanneke's Oscar-nominated film *Amour* is about an elderly couple, where the wife suffers a series of debilitating strokes. She asks her husband to promise that he will not let her be taken to hospital. Towards the end of the film, she declines fluid. He wants to force her to drink, and asks whether she wants to die of thirst, and in that case whether it would not be better for him simply to kill her. She is unable to reply. Finally, he suffocates her with a pillow. Like all of Hanneke's work, the film is ambiguous. Yet Margaret Morganroth Gullette (2013) interprets this film as an advert for euthanasia, ignoring the agency of the wife who appears to desire to die. Gullette seems to think that the problem is simply the lack of respite care and the social isolation of the couple and that the husband's actions are straightforward murder, non-consensual termination of life. She is correct in viewing this as a very negative portrayal of end of life, but the situation which Hanneke presents seems far from rare: many people want to die, rather than experience prolonged suffering and dependency.

In some cases, society restricts liberty in order to protect people from the consequences of their actions. For example, in Britain it is compulsory to wear a seatbelt in a car or a crash helmet on a motor-bicycle, even though the only person who might otherwise be put at risk is an individual capable of freely choosing to travel unprotected. Prohibition of drugs is another example of protecting vulnerable individuals from bad decisions in their own best interests. It may be argued that terminally ill people also need to be protected from the consequences of a mistaken choice. Yet the person who fails to wear a seatbelt or helmet or uses drugs has not decided that they want to die. They have been careless, or believed that the pleasurable sensations outweigh the medical risks, or taken a gamble that they will not be harmed. These are different cases to the situation of someone who has thought carefully about their predicament, and expressed a deliberate and continuing desire to end their life.

Alternatively, it could be said to be inconsistent to limit the right of disabled people to assistance to commit suicide to cases of terminal illness. A fully consistent equality argument suggests that disabled people should be free to choose suicide at any time or for any reason, because this is a power that non-disabled people can exercise. Yet, there is a general presumption that suicide is to be prevented where possible. Even though suicide has been decriminalised, it is a moral duty for third parties to try to dissuade a person to commit suicide. Therefore, it would not be right for society to help any disabled or non-disabled person to commit suicide on autonomy grounds. The only socially sanctioned case where suicide becomes a legitimate choice is in the case of end-stage terminal illness. This is because having an end-stage terminal illness is morally relevant to the decision to end life. The individual does not have the prospect of a continuing life or of recovery from illness. The person may be suffering pain and discomfort and restriction. While they are aware that they are dying, they do not know when death will come. Modern medical care can keep people alive, who previously would have died much sooner. Dying people may have to endure days or even weeks of suffering, and witness their relatives and friends watching this extended process. Assisted suicide hastens death by a matter of days or possibly weeks.

In other words, choosing death can be rational for people in an end-of-life situation. The palliative care community largely oppose legalisation of assisted suicide, because of a belief that good palliative care can ease all deaths (Finlay *et al.*, 2005). But even with palliative care, hospice facilities and support, some deaths are difficult and it is rational to fear them. Of course, assisted suicide is certainly not something that all terminally ill people will want. Some people cope better with restrictions, find value in enduring suffering, and find alternative sources of meaning and pleasure. They will want to extend their life as long as possible, because they want to spend time with loved ones, and experience every minute available to them. But others find the prospect of prolonged dying unendurable and consider their suffering futile and unnecessary. In an era of self-determination and choice, many patients want to control the circumstances of their death (Miller *et al.*, 2004). Views on end-of-life decisions are highly personal, depending on religious and moral values, and an individual's capacity to cope with pain or restriction. One person's judgement does not have implications for another person's right to life or dignity or respect

For the same reason, it is not discriminatory to distinguish between terminally ill people and non-disabled people. Justice demands treating like cases alike, and unlike cases differently. If all disabled people were given access to assisted suicide, just because they were disabled, this would be discrimination (Davis, 2004). In normal situations, having a different physical or mental state should not be relevant to the judgement of the legitimacy of ending life. But in the specific situation of an end-stage terminal illness, where the individual is suffering greatly, there are morally relevant reasons to waive the usual prohibitions on suicide, and to enable patients to die painlessly and at a time of their own choosing.

Pragmatic arguments about assisted suicide

As well as arguments about the legitimacy of choosing 'a good death', the importance of supporting autonomy, and the empirical evidence of disabled people's own wishes, there are also several pragmatic arguments for making assisted suicide legal.

As with abortion, if assisted suicide is illegal, it does not mean that it will not occur. Because many people have a strong desire to end their lives to avoid the suffering of a slow and painful death, people will take steps to bring this about. For example, individuals will attempt to travel to places where assisted suicide is permitted. This can lead to the complications, distress and difficulty of 'death tourism', for example, in the case of Reginald Crew and others. Alternatively, some people will attempt to end their lives without assistance. This 'underground assisted suicide 'may lead to the dangers of botched suicide, and the risks of prosecution of assisters, fears of which may make a terminally ill person's situation more difficult and anxious (Magnusson, 2002). The analogy with back-street abortion suggests that providing regulated and medically safe provision is better than driving the situation underground, putting people at further risk of harm, and criminalising those who, often for good motives, seek to help people in need.

The second pragmatic argument is based on the suggestion that though the majority of people want to have access to assisted suicide, only a minority will ever choose to exercise their right to end their life (as data from Oregon and the Netherlands suggests). Knowing that assisted suicide is available may often reduce the anxiety of dying people. Fears of pain and other symptoms may be mitigated by the knowledge that there is another way out, if it all gets too much. The possibility of controlling death can be life-enhancing.

A national survey by Clive Seale (2006) reveals that in some cases, British doctors already hasten the death of their patients in different ways. The data shows that physician-assisted deaths are very rare: none of his respondents had assisted the suicide of patients, and only 0.16 per cent had performed voluntary euthanasia and 0.33 per cent non-voluntary euthanasia. This suggests that disability rights suspicions of doctors are misplaced. However, nearly a third (32.8 per cent) of respondents had alleviated symptoms with possible life-shortening effects (the so-called doctrine of double effect, where doctors knowingly prescribe pain-relief drugs which have the side effect of hastening death), and a similar proportion (30.3 per cent) had made decisions not to treat end-stage conditions, knowing that this would hasten an inevitable death. Doctors did not think that a new law would make much difference to their palliative care philosophy. It is interesting to compare with recent data from Belgium, where physician-assisted suicide has been legal since 2002: 81.8 per cent of physicians in Flanders and 64.5 per cent of physicians in Wallonia agreed that 'Life-ending on request can be part of good end-of-life care' (Cohen et al., 2012: 849).

Safeguards in assisted suicide legislation

If assisted suicide were to be legalised, appropriate safeguards would be necessary to protect vulnerable people and prevent abuse. These would govern eligibility for assistance to die, the decision-making process around death, and the broader cultural and social context within which assisted suicide was made available.

First, disabled people and terminally ill people need to have access to independent living and the full range of support services. Choices about death should not be made because life has been made unbearable through lack of choices and control. Moreover, palliative care is not currently available in many parts of the country. Palliative medicine can reduce pain and suffering at the end of life: assisted suicide is not an alternative to palliative care, but an addition to it. Some countries where assisted suicide is permitted have not made a commitment to palliative care, which makes it more likely for dying people to choose to end their lives prematurely, from fear of preventable pain and suffering. The broader cultural context is also important, because assisted suicide should not be promoted via negative images of disability and dying. Some of the advocacy around assisted suicide has stigmatised dependency and disability, and encouraged people to think that disability is a fate worse than death. Assisted suicide should be viewed as a last resort for a minority of people with terminal illness, not the expected and preferred option when faced with difficulty and disability.

Second, promoting autonomy should be balanced with protection, even if this verges on paternalism. Questions of definition need close attention in developing regulation of assisted suicide. The distinction between 'people with terminal illness' and 'terminally ill people' is very important, and not easy to specify. It is an important principle that the qualification for assisted suicide is the end stage of incurable disease accompanied by unbearable suffering. Simply being a disabled person is not a reason to be permitted assisted suicide. To broaden the eligible class too widely might be to put disabled people at risk in the way that critics fear.

Moreover, it is normal to fear disability and death, and it is often traumatic to incur or be diagnosed with incurable impairment or terminal illness. For example, Disability Awareness in Action quote Dr Ian Basnett, a quadriplegic, as saying of the period after the accident which left him quadriplegic: 'I was ventilator dependent for a while and at times said to people "I wish I was dead!". I am now extraordinarily glad no one acted on that and assisted suicide was not legal' (Hurst, n.d.). Experience shows that the initial anger and profound distress at onset of paralysis almost always give way to a more balanced and accepting attitude over time. Therefore, people who have recently developed or been diagnosed with impairment or terminal illness should be prevented from exercising the choice of assisted suicide. There should be a short-term infringement of autonomy for newly disabled people, until they come to terms with their situation. Understanding the complex fears and yearnings of those who desire euthanasia is important (Wood Mak and Elwyn, 2005).

Moreover, even people in the eligible category may not always be able to make a rational decision to request death. For example, depression and other mental illness could cloud their judgement and may prevent a person with terminal illness making a competent decision to request death. The right to request assisted suicide should depend on the mental competence of the person with terminal illness. Disabled people may become depressed at their pain and restriction and express a desire to die. For example, Alison Davis (2004) discusses a phase in her life when this was the case for her. She fears that had it been legal, she would have requested assistance, and suggests that most requests for death stem from depression.

Any request for assisted suicide should be subject to calm and careful scrutiny from both medical and legal professionals. Once a request has been made and approved, there should be a 'cooling-off period' for the person to consider their situation, at the end of which they should have to confirm once more that they understand the consequences of their decision and want to go ahead with assisted suicide.

Assisted suicide should only ever be available in very restricted circumstances: the end stage of terminal, incurable illness, when suffering becomes unbearable. Legalisation and regulation should be carefully framed, to ensure that the 'slippery slope' which opponents fear cannot occur.

Conclusion

Listening to the voices of disabled people and those directly affected is an important principle in bioethics. It is dangerous for non-disabled people to project their own fears and misconceptions as to what it might be like to be impaired: as Iris Marion Young (1997) has argued, it is not easy to put yourself in another person's shoes and imagine what their quality of life is like. It is equally important to analyse and challenge the voices of disabled people. For example, much of the vocal opposition to assisted suicide does not engage closely with the arguments about assisted suicide in the particular situation of end-stage terminal illness, which is the only situation where Lord Joffe – or I in this chapter – have advocated assisted suicide. The majority of people eligible for this measure would be people suffering from cancer or Motor Neurone Disease. The vast majority of disabled people would not be covered by the measure. For example, it would not permit people like Elizabeth Bouvia, who was disabled but not terminally ill, to have assistance to end their lives. For me, support for assisted suicide in end-stage terminal illness is not the same as support for voluntary euthanasia for disabled people, which I oppose for many of the reasons given by other disability rights commentators. There is an important difference between encouraging disabled people to die, and enabling dying people to die better.

Alison Davis (2004) argues that the legalisation of assisted suicide would lead to medical science being less concerned to cure illness or alleviate pain: rather than trying to do something about end-of-life situations and prolong life, doctors would prefer to sit by and allow people to die. This seems to be implausible. The whole of modern medicine is directed at trying to cure illness and keep people alive. The problem for many patients at the end of life is not so much that their doctors are eager for them to die, but that doctors find it very difficult to stop trying to help, to enable them to die naturally and have a good death. The reality is that people have to die of something.

Moreover, the vocal opposition of many disability rights groups and commentators to assisted suicide is not the whole picture. Many people who are in end-of-life situations request and desire assistance to achieve a good death. Surveys have found that the majority of disabled people and of the general population are in favour of assisted suicide. Even some disabled people's organisations – for example, Jerome Bickenbach (1998) cites the Coalition of Provincial Organisations of the Handicapped in Canada – have supported assisted suicide. In the UK, the National Union of Students disabled students campaign has supported law reform, and most recently a veteran UK disability rights campaigner, Anne Rae, has come out cautiously in favour of assisted suicide: 'This is not about disabled people saying they want to die because they are disabled; it is about any individual who finds themselves in an unbearable situation, a situation where they can no longer act for themselves' (Rae, 2012: 12).

Allowing people to kill themselves with medical assistance would be a major step. Fears about the vulnerability of disabled and terminally ill people are not without foundation, even though they appear to me to be over-exaggerated. The question becomes an empirical one: does the benefit to those who may choose to use assisted suicide, or who may be comforted by its availability, outweigh the threat to other people who may theoretically be pressurised into requesting the measure? Evidence from jurisdictions where assisted suicide or voluntary euthanasia is permitted – the Netherlands and Oregon – is not conclusive. However, in both countries, the vast majority of dying people do not opt for assisted suicide. Nor is there clear evidence of abuse of the law. After 30 years of assisted suicide in the Netherlands, there has not been an erosion of moral constraints nor extension to a wider class of disabled people. Since the Oregon Death with Dignity Act was enacted in 1997, only a few hundred individuals have died as a result of lethal drugs prescribed by their physician (Miller *et al.*, 2004).

It is tempting to interpret some of the disability rights opposition to assisted suicide as arising from the dominance of social model perspectives. For those who claim that disability has nothing to do with impairment, or that disability should not be medicalised, it is simply inappropriate to talk in terms of disease, suffering and death, because the solution to the disability problem is the removal of social barriers, independent living and social inclusion and respect, not attention to impairment. The power of social model approaches may have made it harder for the disability rights community to engage with debates about illness, impairment and end of life. Perhaps the social model ideology enables some to disengage from troubling questions about bodies and mortality.

Whether or not this is true, it seems to me that disability rights-based objections to disabled people's exercise of autonomy at the end of life are procedural, not substantial. Given that the disability movement supports disabled people to make choices in every other area of their lives, it seems inconsistent that disabled people should not be able to take control over the manner of their death. I believe that well-informed, well-supported, competent adults in end-stage terminal illness should be able to exercise this choice. With suitable safeguards and regulation, I support the introduction of assisted suicide legislation.

9

PERSONAL ASSISTANCE AS A RELATIONSHIP

> In many ways we are still discovering how this new form of social relationship works in practice. It feels to me that each family, each person's situation is very different, and each working relationship can be very different. Two types of people ... a PA that might work well with one type of disabled person might not work well with another, equally, someone who works well with one impairment might not work well with someone with a different impairment. I don't think there's any right or wrong way of doing things.
>
> (S, British PA user with physical impairment)

Personal assistance (PA) refers to the new ways of delivering personal support in daily living, which were devised by disabled people's movements in Britain, North America and Northern European countries from the 1970s onwards, as an alternative to traditional models of care (Morris, 1993a). Personal assistance was a key element in the empowerment of people with significant impairments, who had previously depended on residential care. Rather than living in institutions, or being supported in the community by paid carers supplied by the state, or being reliant on family and friends, disabled people began to receive payments directly to manage their own staff through arrangements such as the Independent Living Fund. As pioneer Simon Brisenden wrote: 'The point is that independent people have control over their lives, not that they perform every task themselves' (1989: 9). Being in control of how help was delivered meant having freedom and self-respect, rather than feeling dependent on the whims of family or workers employed by local authorities or charities. For this reason, Mladenov claims that: 'Personal assistance is a major condition for the possibility of disability equality just like rational debate is a major condition for the possibility of deliberative democracy' (2012: 4).

The PA model has since spread (Carmichael and Brown, 2002; Priestley *et al.*, 2010) beyond the core constituency of adults with physical impairments, to people with intellectual disabilities (Williams *et al.*, 2009; Manthorpe *et al.*, 2011), to older people and to children. Variations of the PA model can be found in all the Nordic countries, in the Netherlands, in North America, as the personalisation of welfare has developed in many high-income countries. It is important to note how heterogenous the PA model has become. In the UK, the diversity of approaches in different local authority areas, with multiple approaches and intermediate organisations, further contributes to the heterogeneity of the PA relationship on the ground.

Extensive research has already been conducted on the PA model and the wider personalisation of welfare (Pearson, 2012). Disability studies researchers have explored the benefits of independent living and the best infrastructure organisations to deliver the promise of empowerment (Morris, 1993a). Systematic reviews have explored whether the PA approach is cost-effective and results in greater user satisfaction for different client groups (Stainton and Boyce, 2004; Mayo-Wilson *et al.*, 2008). Social policy analysts have explored the market for care (Scourfield, 2005), and particularly transnational care migration, and questioned the reliance on low-paid migrant workers, usually women (Williams, 2001; Ungerson, 2005). From social policy and social work there have also been challenges to the personalisation agenda and the commodification of care (Leece, 2004; Spandler, 2004).

In this chapter, I want to bracket the social policy and health economy questions, and explore personal assistance as a social relationship. The chapter draws on the smaller body of research which has looked at the meaning and nature of the PA relationship, and how this is experienced by both PA workers and PA user (Yamaki and Yamazaki, 2004; Ungerson, 2005; Woodin, 2006; Kelly, 2010; Leece and Peace, 2010; Christensen, 2010; Mladenov, 2012), as well as by conversations with, and observations of, personal assistance relationships and my own occasional experiences of being a personal assistance user since I became paralysed in 2008. I will open by exploring the ideology of independent living and exploring why I think it fails to capture the reality of the relationship. Then I will consider in turn the situation of the PA worker and the PA user, before looking at some of the positive and negative emotions involved in this innovative form of support.

Personal assistance and independent living ideology

As expressed by the European Network of Independent Living (ENIL), PA does not mean the same consumerism or individualism which marks out the North American approach: 'Independent living does not mean that disabled people want to do everything themselves or live in isolation because we know that all people whether they are disabled or non-disabled are interdependent' (ENIL, n.d.). However, it does mean control by the disabled person. Mladenov (2012: 247) quotes Swedish pioneer Adolf Razka's idea of personal assistance as expressed in the European Centre for Excellence in Personal Assistance model, namely, that the disabled person chooses who works, with which tasks, at which times, where and how. One aspect of this is a preference for employing unskilled individuals, who can be trained and shaped by the disabled person, to deliver tasks in the way in which they prefer. An unskilled person will not have their own ideas or professional assumptions, unlike a nurse or another healthcare worker who might challenge the disabled person or seek to impose their own views.

Another important aspect, particularly in the British variant of this model, is that personal assistance departs from the tradition of care, by separating out tasks from emotions. The goal is for PA to be a cash service, controlled by the disabled person, where workers perform the tasks which the disabled person cannot do, without the need for emotions such as gratitude, resulting in independence, choice and freedom (Morris, 1993a) and avoiding the stigma of dependency. In a sense, the worker becomes a robot, the arms and legs of the individual who has impairments.

I want to question this independent living ideology, because I consider that any service between one individual and one or more assistants inevitably becomes a relationship (Marfisi, 2002; Woodin, 2006). A relationship involves feelings. These may be positive – gratitude, affection, respect – or they may be negative – frustration, resentment, dislike. A personal assistant usually works with a disabled person in their home and personal space, and witnesses their family and social life. In practice, I suggest, it is hard, if not impossible, to remove emotions from the equation. Therefore, I would agree with Clare Ungerson: 'A relationship between two adults involving touch (often extremely intimate touch), conversation, shared activities and sometimes shared living space, is hardly likely to remain a purely physiological analogy between brain and body parts for long' (Ungerson, 1999: 586).

The disabled person is likely to develop feelings of some kind for the person who assists them. The personal assistant is also an individual human being, with feelings and interests. They are likely to develop some sort of emotional bond with their employer. Moreover, they are not robots or body parts, they are workers, and consequently have rights. It is not enough to consider that as long as they are paid an acceptable hourly rate, there are no further responsibilities.

Who are PA users?

Looking more closely at the disabled people who use personal assistance schemes further complicates the straightforward model. Disabled people are extremely heterogeneous, encompassing people with either congenital or acquired impairments; people whose impairments are either physical, sensory, intellectual or related to mental health problems; as well as people who are becoming disabled as they age.

There is some research on which people with impairments end up as personal assistance users, which highlights the differences between younger disabled people, and older people who become disabled. For example, in Sweden, there has been a tension between younger disabled people, who are awarded personal assistance prior to their 65th birthday and continue the service into old age, and people who become disabled and have supports needs in old age, and who are then not entitled to personal assistance. In the UK, Leece and Leece (2006) researched the differences between people who used direct payments to employ personal assistants, and those who were users of traditional social care. The former tended to be younger than users of traditional social care. While the former had higher weekly income, this probably reflected higher levels of disability. The latter were more likely to have savings, reflecting their age. Overall, they did not find a social class difference between users of different forms of support. However, Leece (2004) highlights how the personal assistance model may be most attractive to middle-class people who are used to taking on employer roles and have the cultural capital to manage these relationships (see also Clarke *et al.*, 2005).

The personal assistance model began with people with physical impairments, and has since been extended to people with other impairments. If you have a physical impairment, you may literally lack the use of limbs, and require someone to drive your car, cook your meals, wash you or similar. You are physically limited but cognitively intact, which means you can decide what you want and dictate what happens. The robot analogy has some relevance. However, other disabled people have different needs, and this can complicate the model. For example, when we made *The Unusual Suspects* (Jackie Waldock, 2000), a documentary film for the BBC and the Open University, we included K, a woman with visual impairment, who spoke about wanting her personal assistant to be more like a companion, a paid friend, who would help her socialise and go out in town. Around the house and at work, K was independent and needed no help. But she wanted someone to do things with, because she lacked confidence or felt lonely in social situations.

The same may be the case for someone with learning difficulties. It is often not that the people cannot feed themselves or get around town. However, they may find it harder to decide what to do, they may need some support and advice in everyday interactions, and they may even need to be protected from their own impulses. For example, Reynolds and Walmsley report on the type of support that is often provided by family members and which PA schemes may need to replace:

> The type of care offered by relatives of people with learning difficulties or mental health problems is usually quite diffuse, involving being available and responsible when they are needed, offering company, emotional support and often fighting for services.
>
> *(1998: 68)*

It is important to note the heterogeneity of the intellectual disabled population (Carnaby and Cambridge, 2002). The majority of people with learning difficulties are individuals with mild intellectual disability, but the category includes others with more profound limitations of communication and cognition, as well as people who may have autistic spectrum conditions which impair interaction and social skills, but not necessarily intelligence. There are consequently a variety of models that apply in personal assistance with people with learning difficulties. For example, the Swedish JAG programme, which develops personal assistance for everyone, including people with intellectual disability, highlights the individuality of the different solutions in the report, *Ten Years with Personal Assistance* (JAG, n.d.).

Research in the intellectual disability field has shown how PA relationships with these PA users are more relational and involve more emotion than the independent living ideology suggests (Williams *et al.*, 2009; Kelly, 2010). Williams *et al.* (2009) analysed conversations between people with learning difficulties and their PAs which show that, while these are relationships of equality and respect, they are also different not just to traditional caring relationships, but also to PA relationships with people with physical impairments. More emotional work is going on, particularly emotional work by the PA to encourage, support, and sometimes guide the person with the ID. The researchers discuss the 'fine line between over-familiarity and professionalism' as well as the difference between traditional 'learning disability talk' and 'employer–employee talk' (ibid.: 826).

Who are personal assistants?

The question of who seeks employment as a personal assistant and why they do so, and what they get out of this work, is a very under-researched area. Generally, low-skill work that requires no qualifications is low paid and marginal to the economy, and attracts migrant workers, students, and women with caring responsibilities who wish to work part-time. Personal assistance work is predominantly done by women, who make up 87 per cent of these workers in the UK, 85 per cent in Norway (Christensen, 2012). Because assistance work is low paid and attractive to migrants, it often takes the form of a live-in situation in the UK, although this situation is apparently almost non-existent in Norway. The demographics of personal assistance highlight how it may often be the case that the worker will be vulnerable and in a less powerful role than the employer – for example, female, minority ethnic – even though the latter is disabled and the former is not.

Clare Ungerson (2004) describes the cash for care literature as being 'insouciant' about impacts on workers, because the emphasis is on the empowerment of users through direct employment. Analysing data across five European Union countries, she fears for the well-being of those working in this sector:

> These schemes are likely to foster the development of a care-labour market that is 'grey', marginalizing the workers and locking them into peripheral, low-paid and transient employment, while at the same time denying them social rights such as employment-related benefits, and excusing them social responsibilities such as the payment of employment-related taxes.
>
> *(Ungerson, 2004: 191)*

However, at least in the UK and the Nordic countries, there are strict regulations on hourly rate and tax and National Insurance contributions, so this assessment does not seem entirely relevant. Leece and Leece (2006) propose the development of support systems to protect PA interests – unions, networks, peer support, helplines, training.

From her research in Norway and the UK, Christensen (2010) highlights the different reasons why individuals choose personal assistance work. She distinguishes three ideal types. The 'continuing carer' is the caring person who wants to work one-to-one with someone who needs help; her category of 'search for new horizons' refers to the migrant worker who travels abroad to earn money and have new experiences; the 'pragmatist' is earning money as a student or while preparing for another job. Each of these types will have different motivations and approaches to the work. However, Christensen argues that the split between emotions and tasks does not necessarily make sense for any of these types of worker, each of whom are likely to get emotionally involved with their clients.

Independent living ideology and empirical evidence stress that disabled people usually prefer to employ untrained staff, whom they can train and ensure that assistance is delivered in ways they prefer. Yet this might make the worker vulnerable to harm, for example, through lifting or carrying in ways which cause back problems (Spandler, 2004: 191). Arguably, this also makes the PA worker more vulnerable, and locks them into an unskilled sector of the labour market. This may not be a problem for the person for whom PA work is a transient experience – the 'pragmatist' – but for the woman who chooses PA work as a career, it undermines the possibilities for progression. After many years of working for one employer, a worker may not be able to demonstrate transferable skills – their experience is in relating to one person – which is why PA work has been described as a career cul-de-sac.

Yet PA workers do find satisfaction from being able to empower their employer (Fisher and Byrne, 2012). They may also welcome the informality and lack of supervision of the one-to-one relationship, as opposed to the rules and procedures of working in larger and more organised care contexts (Glendinning *et al.,* 2000). As S, a disabled man who had had over 100 different workers over his adult life, said to me:

> There are people who come into the work, maybe care or personal assistance, it's like a refuge, because maybe they've had difficulty of getting work elsewhere, they could be anti-authority, don't operate well in social organizations.

He also stated:

> I've had plenty of workers who've worked with us, particularly through agencies, who've also worked in residential homes and they make absolutely fine workers, and they're very aware that when they work in a [residential] home environment it's very different approach than this environment ... so it's [about] adaptability as well.

Some forms of PA work do require training, such as support staff who work for people with learning difficulties (Carnaby and Cambridge, 2002; Fisher and Byrne, 2012). In Sweden, PA workers employed by municipalities are required to have some nursing competence (Clevnert and Johansson, 2007), although as in the UK, those disabled people who could express their own views tended to prefer untrained assistants.

Another debate is about employing relatives. For the classic PA user – the younger adult with physical impairments – the PA model has been chosen as an alternative to being reliant on family members, so it is rare for people to pay their relatives. However, it is not unheard of: I encountered one woman who consistently employed nephews and nieces to perform her support tasks. Clare Ungerson (2004) discusses how the wider 'cash for care' field encompasses many examples of remunerated carers or recognised carers across Europe, who are paid welfare benefits or other transfers in order to subsidise their work supporting older family members who become disabled. Thinking of the relationship aspects, if the PA worker is a family member, this could lessen the potential role conflicts of being in the family home or being a stranger delivering support (Clevnert and Johansson, 2007). However, given the sometimes strained relations between relatives, it could also create alternative conflicts by complicating interactions further.

Role issues in personal assistance

The PA model is new, and there is a lack of clarity over what type of relationship is appropriate between the user and the worker. Looking at the wider spectrum of 'cash for care', Ungerson (2004) in her studies across Europe found that 'cash for care' schemes did not change the relationship of informal carers to their relatives. But this is different from the classic independent living situation where two people encounter each other for the first time as PA user and PA worker. PA work involves the delivery of intimate care by a stranger, in the personal space of the PA user, and this unusual closeness needs to be managed somehow. It may be a long-term relationship over many years, or it may only last a few months. Boundaries need to be drawn, and some distance upheld.

Leece and Peace (2010) compared eight disabled adults and their homecare workers with eight disabled adults and their personal assistants. Perhaps unsurprisingly, PA users were more likely to use independence in the sense of decisional autonomy – as in independent living thinking – whereas homecare users were more likely to use it in terms of executive autonomy (doing things for yourself) – the traditional care model. However, it should be noted that not only had the PA users on average been disabled for twice as long as the homecare users, they were also generally of higher social class. All but one homecare worker said they controlled the relationship, and they were more likely to use infantilising language. Most PA workers said their employer was in control, and talked about trying to be unobtrusive, and keep out of the way when there were visitors. However, they also had closer relationship with their employers than homecare workers, perhaps because the latter had multiple clients whom they spent less time with. The conclusion from this research was that personal assistance was empowering for both parties.

There are a variety of ways that different individuals relate to their workers, and this varies in terms of the personality of the individual, their disability, as well as between countries. Theorists have distinguished two dimensions in their analysis: hierarchy versus equality, and emotions versus formality. For example, Ungerson (2005) talks about 'hot' and 'cold' relationships. A 'cold' relationship can easily be brought to an end without feelings of guilt, because it is simply the contractual relationship between two strangers. A 'hot' relationship is a long-term arrangement which survives despite tensions – perhaps with a paid relative, or when a person cannot easily recruit an alternative worker, or when a worker cannot easily leave and find an alternative form of work. Perhaps the ideal is a 'cool' relationship, marked by acceptance and respect on both sides, clear boundaries and tasks. A distinction has also been drawn between control and closeness in support relationships. These 'hybrid' forms of support work combine user control with closeness, which is unusual in the wider context of paid work.

In Britain, with a very distinctive class tradition, reinforced in literary and cinematic representations, a powerful model is of master and servant. The latter exercises deference, does not challenge their employer, comes when they are called, and does not speak unless spoken to. They do not eat or socialise with their employer, and hover in the background. I have experienced some PA users who operate exactly this type of relationship with their 'staff', albeit tempered with humour and informality as well. Sometimes, it is to protect their own privacy, and to ensure that the PA worker does not take over their social life or adopt their friends, or interfere with their parenting of their children. Christensen (2012) records some more negative experiences that can arise, for example, where the PA worker is abused and exploited and treated with disrespect. For these reasons, some authors have argued that the individualised relationship is a threat to socialised welfare, and risks a return to the pre-war era of the servant class (Graham, 1991; Williams, 2001).

But it has been suggested that the modern PA relationship is very different from the historical master–servant model: 'The disabled employers are not supported by social distance and deference as nineteenth-century country house ladies and gentlemen were: indeed, the social construction of impairment in itself demeans disabled people' (Ungerson, 1999: 594).

Not all PA users in the UK adopt the master–servant model. As S, who comes from a Northern working-class family, said to me:

> We've got a very strict rule that workers always eat with us. Me mam comes on a Sunday, she cooks for everyone. If we go out, then workers sit with us, their meals are paid for. We're having no truck with that kind of servant thing.

Moreover, the PA worker today has more freedom to leave and seek alternative employment if they do not like it. However, their vulnerable position in the labour market as low-paid, low-skilled workers means that they do not have complete freedom to exit, particularly if they are migrant workers.

Another model is more like the historical idea of the companion, the paid friend who sometimes accompanied the wealthy lady. Here there is more equality, although still an element of deference. The employer sets the agenda, it is a cash relationship, but socialising together is part of the expectation, much like with K to whom I referred earlier.

In Norway, with less of a class tradition and more instinctive equality than Britain, the dominant independent living idea is of professional friendship, which is reinforced by the training and information provided by ULOBA, the disability movement intermediate body that promotes and organises personal assistance. Professional friendship sets limits to the relationship. The disabled person – who may well be lonely – can enjoy the company of their assistant and have a dialogue. However, 'Although it is important to have PAs emotionally involved, it is important too to keep some distance in order to maintain control. And viewing them as paid friends helps because it makes them more equal' (Christensen, 2009: 128). Christensen concludes that the term 'interdependence' is more relevant than independence. From British research with professionals who work with people with learning difficulties, Fisher and Byrne (2012) conclude that maintaining boundaries and stressing the professionalism of the role are important.

In Norway, the disabled person manages the PA worker but usually the worker is employed by ULOBA or another infrastructure body: only 11 per cent employ the worker directly (Christensen, 2012). In the UK, the disabled person receives funds under a direct payment, and is therefore the employer of the worker. According to one survey (UK IFF), 42 per cent of PA users receive help with employment aspects, 26 per cent of whom use a support organisation as an intermediary. S, the British long-term PA user I interviewed, said:

> To have a personal assistant, you don't have to be employing that person directly, and we've got into this culture in this country of thinking that personal assistance means direct employment ... To think that control equals being an employer is fine for a few hundred severely disabled people where it works really well, but for the vast majority of disabled people, for the vast majority of home-carers, that's dragging them into major difficulties potentially.

In the UK, the dominance of the individualised direct employment model influences the roles and relationship, as well as who is likely to be able to benefit from the model – not everyone wants the stress of recruiting or managing staff (Carmichael and Brown, 2002; Scourfield, 2005). Moreover, in Norway, PA users are more likely to have a formal contract and job description, whereas only 34 per cent of UK PA users were using a formal job description with all their personal assistants. Analysing these differences, Christensen concludes: 'The encouragement of a self-selected and strongly individualized employer role creates the possibility of developing the extremes of either master/servant types of relationship or strong solidaristic/emotional-based relationships' (2012: 410).

The model and relationship may be different again when the PA user is a person with learning difficulties. For example, under the JAG programme that operates in Sweden, a service guarantor helps recruit and supervise workers for the person with intellectual disability, and ensures quality of assistance. The personal assistant works within a framework established by the service guarantor. Therefore, the person with learning difficulties is in a very different role from the classic person with physical impairment who directs their own assistance.

Emotional dimensions

Although the PA model appears revolutionary, it still comes down to relationships. Asked to describe the nature of the relationship between a PA user and their workers, S replied:

> Delicate, I think that's the best word I can think of to describe it, it's delicate and it can go wrong at any time, and you always have to act delicately ... it's like any relationship, that trust can go overnight and you never get that back.

The attitudes of PA workers to the disabled people they work for remain critical, as research regularly demonstrates:

Respect, dignity, being treated equally, trust and reliability were all identified as critical factors in how service users felt about the service they received. At their best, relationships with staff maximised choice and control, reinforced self-esteem and dignity, and made users feel genuinely valued and cared for; at their worst, they could enforce dependency and passivity, erode self-esteem and be intrusive.

(Vernon and Qureshi, 2000: 272)

Different traditions, cultures and roles have implications for the emotional connections between PA user and their workers. As Christensen (2012) says, the less regulated and more individualised situations contribute to powerful feelings and bonds, both positive and sometimes negative. Leece (2004: 7) argues that 'warm, friendly relationships' of 'affection, loyalty and friendship' develop between PAs and their employers: her research in Staffordshire revealed PAs regard their employers as their friends or family members, and often worked more than contracted hours, but also benefitted from the convenience, the cash and the comfort. This hints at the complications when a PA worker becomes a friend, and boundaries become muddied: 'In these employer/employee relationships of one-to-one intimacy, it seems to be imperative that boundaries be set, but it is not clear where' (Ungerson, 1999: 595).

For example, feelings of guilt or obligation might trap workers into working beyond their contracted hours, or the employer may ring them up at all hours to request emergency help. Sarah Woodin (2006) found that because they did not have enough allocated hours, PA users sometimes had to make informal arrangements with PA workers for favours outside of working time.

Personal assistance relationships can become very close, and involve intimate personal care. As Ungerson also says: 'Friendship, though, is more permeable: once feelings of affection arise, then the consequences of crossing boundaries can range from the minor pain of social embarrassment to the personal risk of a broken heart' (1999: 597).

The negative aspects also arise when things go wrong. It may be very difficult to end such a close relationship if bad feelings arise, or if the worker is exploiting the employer, for example, through theft or becoming unreliable (Manthorpe *et al.*, 2011). As well as examples of disabled people being rude and demanding to their workers, Christensen (2012) also found an example of a disabled person being abused by a personal assistant who moved into the house with her children and exploited the situation for her own ends. Swedish research highlights the ambivalence and complications in cases when young people have personal assistants, where power was often unequal and the relationship not mutual (Skär and Tam, 2001).

The individualised, privatised nature of personal assistance, and increasingly the personal budgets, mean that when things go wrong, it may be harder for abuse to be detected and restorative action taken. Flexibility and informality are wonderful when things go well, but dangerous when they go bad. Ungerson suggests it is down to the luck of finding a good employer – or worker:

> For these workers, it was often a matter of luck whether they had a 'good' employer or not. The fact that they were frequently working alone with no colleagues, and operating in a segment of the labour market which credentialism has barely touched, meant that they were vulnerable to exploitation based on emotional blackmail.
>
> *(2004: 204)*

Unlike in Britain, in some countries of Southern Europe and elsewhere, with under-regulated care sectors and many migrant workers, the PA user has absolute control and gets good value for money, but the workers have little choice, little personal time and no rights (ibid.).

Concluding thoughts

Paying for care is a very widespread phenomenon in developed societies. Ungerson's work shows the very many different cash for care models across Europe. She is particularly interested in arrangements for delivering support to older people, whereas the independent living literature is almost exclusively concerned with younger disabled people. The wider context is that many people in Britain pay for some form of assistance or support – the figure of 670,000 people in 2001 has been quoted (Leece, 2004) – comprising older people in residential homes, nannies and childminders, cleaners and gardeners and/or entirely private support arrangements. While personal assistance needs to be understood within the wider context of cash for care arrangements, the particular history and culture of independent living mean that it is distinctively different in comparison to the arrangements increasingly being made for older people who become frail or confused (Ungerson, 2005).

In this chapter, I have tried to draw on the emerging research literature about the personal assistance model to demonstrate two points: first, assistance and support are more complex and diverse than the simple independent living ideology generally suggests; second, that personal assistance always entails relationships and emotions, never simply the delivery of tasks. Debate on assistance and support should be based on the recognition that people are different in their support needs, in their aspirations, and in their values. Different forms of assistance and support are needed which support individuals in appropriate ways which enable them to flourish and achieve their projects. One size will not fit all – either the historic form of residential care, or the current ideal of independent living (Fisher and Byrne, 2012). Whatever form of care and support is adopted needs to be based on respect for both parties – those who deliver care and support and those who receive it. None of this is to undermine the value and benefit of the PA model, which seems, in almost all cases, to be much better for both worker and user than relying on municipal homecare or family support, let alone residential care.

I agree with the quotation from S that opens this chapter, when he emphasises the novelty and diversity of the PA relationship. However, I do not believe that there is 'no wrong way of doing things'. I and other theorists have begun to bring in the feminist ethic of care as a model for understanding care relationships in the disability sector (Williams, 2001; Shakespeare, 2000; Watson *et al.*, 2004). I think that personal assistance should be explored using the ethic of care, not just the ethic of rights that has hitherto predominated. The British approach to personal assistance is problematic, as even sympathetic commentators have begun to suggest: 'In developing a masculinist approach to care, the disabled people's movement seeks to promote autonomy for disabled people but eliminates emotion from the caring process by transforming it into a formal, contractual, exchange relationship' (Hughes *et al.*, 2005a: 271).

All support and care systems need to balance individualism and mutuality, as Selma Sevenhuijsen argues:

> The feminist ethic of care points to forms of solidarity in which there is room for difference, and in which we find out what people in particular situations need in order for them to live with dignity. People must be able to count on solidarity, because vulnerability and dependency, as we know, are a part of human existence: we need each other's disinterested support at expected and unexpected moments.
>
> *(1998: 147)*

So rather than taking an individualised approach, we should recognise the importance of the relationship between each side of the PA equation: worker and user. It would be wrong for the liberation of disabled people to be achieved on the back of the exploitation of their support staff. The feminist ethic of care theorist Jean Tronto denies that the individual employment of a support work necessarily means that care is being commodified or the worker is being exploited:

> But to strip care out of such a relationship, to see it as a source of practical assistance embodying neither emotional nor ethical sensitivities and sensibilities to the personal and interpersonal conflcts that come from needs associated with ageing, illness or disability, cannot provide a basis on which to embody well-being for those cared for or satisfaction for those paid to care.
>
> *(1993: 72)*

The ways in which personal assistance is conceptualised and set up will have a huge influence on the types of relationships that develop, as the comparison of Norway and Britain indicates (Christensen, 2012). Carol Thomas (2007) calls for more funding and higher rates of pay, which would certainly help, but this does not seem the complete solution. It is possible for a low-paid worker to be treated with respect and find satisfaction in their work, and conversely, for someone to be well paid but treated like dirt and feel resentful. Ungerson's conclusion about cash for care in general probably also applies to personal assistance in particular:

> These policies or systems do not create unqualified benefits or utility. It is important to understand how their initial construction impacts on the empowerment and independence of both users and carers, and also to recognise that the location of care-users and the type of labour market they are able to access will influence the ways in which the care relationship develops and its quality.
>
> *(2004: 210)*

To use Nancy Fraser's terminology, the need is for recognition, not just for redistribution. However, this is not to deny the importance of properly funding personal assistance schemes. But the real way forward, as Kröger (2009: 409) argues, would be for personal assistance 'to find a balance where the needs and interests of both parties are respected'.

10

FRIENDSHIP

Introduction

Back in 1996, when my colleagues and I wrote *The Sexual Politics of Disability* in 1996, I think we made an error. By making sexuality our primary concern, we failed to understand that intimacy is perhaps a greater priority for disabled people. Sexuality is an important form of intimacy, and modern Western societies are fascinated with sexual acts and sexualised bodies. But friendship and acceptance are more fundamental than sex. Despite the implication given by much of the media and popular culture, sex may be comparatively unimportant to a wide section of the population. From a life course perspective, sexual desire appears to play a major part in life between the age of puberty and until midlife: perhaps three decades out of a possible 70 or 80 years. Of course, children are in many ways sexual beings, and it is offensive and inaccurate to see older people as asexual. Yet sexuality is undoubtedly different at different stages of the life course. Moreover, even during the peak period of sexuality, many individuals and relationships are not dominated by sex. Leonore Tiefer (1995) cites a historic study in *New England Journal of Medicine*. A survey of 100 self-defined 'happy' couples found that there was some sort of arousal or orgasm dysfunction in the majority of cases but that the couples considered themselves happy both sexually and non-sexually nonetheless (Frank *et al.*, 1978). It has been well observed that frequency and importance of sexual activity decline as a relationship continues and matures, and other ways of relating become more important. But whereas sex is not always a priority, for almost all human beings, the need for intimacy, companionship, and acceptance remains central from birth to death. People can survive, even flourish, without sex, but the majority of individuals would be desolate without friendship.

The importance of friendship

Humans are social animals. There are some rare people who seek solitude and shun company. Some people have different ways of relating, for example, those on the autistic spectrum. But most human beings seek company, recognition and acceptance, and without it, life can be bleak, tedious and lonely. Friendship is important for emotional, practical and even medical reasons. Ray Pahl, the sociologist who pioneered the study of friendship, talks about the importance of the 'social convoy', referring to the group of linked individuals who make their way through life:

> The accumulation of supporting experiences of various forms eventually leads individuals to feel securely that they are capable and competent people and that they can be confident in knowing that there are significant others who believe in them, who love them and who can be counted on in a crisis. Having this social support empowers people to live more effectively and, indeed, more healthily and for longer.
>
> *(Pahl, 2000: 149)*

Communities and networks are not just important because they make people feel happy and connected. Networks play a number of other functions as well as emotional support: instrumental aid (lifts, childcare, loans, finding work); appraisal (helping evaluate a problem or solution); and monitoring (Pescosolido, 2001: 472).

Research has linked lack of social support to adverse medical conditions. There is evidence that more diverse social networks are associated with resistance to illness. Separated and divorced people have higher mortality from certain diseases than married people (Pahl, 2000: 145). Socially isolated people die at two or three times the rate of people with a network of social relationships and sources of emotional support (Brunner, 1997). It is not clear how these mechanisms operate, but possibly psychological distress causes immunological changes which cause vulnerability to disease. It is known that cortisol, the hormone released in situations of stress, has bad effects on the heart and brain.

Friendship is not a simple matter. There are different sorts of friendship, and the social meaning and form of friendship have probably been different at different historical times and in different places. Moreover, different people do friendship differently, for example, male friendships typically are based on shared activities, whereas women's friendships typically are based on communication. In general, women seem to be better at friendship and interaction than men (Traustadóttir, 1993). In terms of the benefits provided, it has been suggested that there are two types of friends. First, there is the intimate friend, with whom one shares private experience and emotions. This type of friendship can be a deep and caring bond, based on trust, liking, and probably a history of shared experiences. Intimate friends may not see each other frequently, but are there when needed. People may not have very many intimate friends, perhaps only two or three. Second, there are friends who are there for company and sociability. This is what is meant by a social life – friends who are available to do things with. Someone may need a large number of such friends, to maximise the chance that a friend is on hand at the time they're looking to socialise. Both types of friendship might characteristically provide practical help from time to time, for example, assistance or advice. And reciprocality is a necessary feature of friendship – each serves a function for the other, and there is give and take in the relationship. Marion Barnes, talking about how each seeks the best interests of the other, states:

> The mutuality and reciprocity of friendship reflect the significance of equality as a defining characteristic. The openness and trust that exist among friends are not inflected by the status or power differences that operate in many other social and familial relationships.
>
> *(2012: 86)*

She also points out that friends also provide support and assistance, alongside families, something I became aware of when I became spinal cord injured, and friends visited regularly during the ten weeks that I was in rehabilitation, providing support as well as food parcels so that I could better endure hospital. In the twenty-first century, friends play a greater role than in previous periods in human history. A century ago, we would have been socially and culturally determined by our family. Fifty years ago, this role would have been played by our work and career. Now it is the people we do things with that count. Developing rich and varied social connections and having friends is a hidden but vital dimension of society: 'In order for a citizen to be fully engaged in a good society, access to material resources is not enough: access to psychological resources is also necessary' (Pahl, 2000: 164).

Disabled people and isolation

If friendship offers benefits that are medical and practical as well as emotional and social, then this is another reason why friendship should be particularly important to disabled people. Disabled people often have more difficulties than non-disabled people in dealing with both their bodies and health, and the environments and systems which they have to negotiate. They rely more on others to provide assistance on a day-to-day basis, and they may be more vulnerable to medical complications.

Yet while disabled people may have greater needs of friends, they are less likely to be well integrated into networks and friendship circles. Disabled people differ from most other disadvantaged groups because they experience significantly greater isolation and loneliness. For working-class and minority ethnic people, their neighourhood will usually provide community. Moreover, the family may be a haven in a heartless world, where there are others who share the experience and who can provide role models. Women will also often be able to find role models, friends and supporters among female family and friends. Lesbian and gay people may find families and neighbourhoods threatening and isolating. Yet, for many, networks and subcultures can provide alternatives, particularly in urban areas. Some gay and lesbian people find their identity and their community in the commercial gay scene. Others turn to alternative communities or create 'families of choice' (Weeks *et al.*, 2001) as an alternative to their local neighbourhoods or biological families.

By contrast, disabled people may not know any other disabled people in their family, neighbourhood or wider community. They may find it difficult to identify as disabled. They may be excluded from social settings. Prejudice, ignorance and hostility may create barriers which prevent connecting to strangers or make entering public spaces an ordeal (Watson, 2003). Disabled people may lack the energy or skills or resources to socialise. Community care has ensured that most people with impairments live in local neighbourhoods, not in segregated institutions, but many disabled people remain effective prisoners in their own homes. This may be because of environmental barriers, lack of money, feelings of vulnerability, or problems with mobility. It is known that older people are at risk of losing social contact and intimacy, but disabled people may also experience these difficulties. Reviewing two decades of literature on community-based services, Traustadóttir (1993) concludes that most disabled people continue to be isolated, lonely and have few friends. This disconnection may be more likely at particular times of the life course (Priestley, 2004) or for certain groups of disabled people.

For example, families which have a disabled member tend to be socially isolated. Parents may be struggling to survive on low incomes without sufficient services, and may not have time to support their disabled child to develop friendships. Evidence from social research with disabled children suggests that isolation from the peer group is a major issue for many young people with impairments (Priestley *et al.*, 1999; Skär, 2003). Some children may travel long distances to schools which can provide facilities for them, whether segregated or mainstream. The consequence is that they may lack friends in their own neighbourhoods. Many disabled children spend most of their time with adults. These may be their own parents, or special needs assistants in school, or other carers and therapists and support workers. Because they are always accompanied by adults, they are denied access to the social world of children, and they may be unable to take part in age-appropriate activities and express the typical resistance of children and young people. Research shows that many disabled children have few or no friends. They may have 'Hi, friends', but not genuine intimates. For example, Huurre and Aro's (1998) study of adolescents with visual impairment found that they often had fewer friends than their peers and were more likely to report loneliness and low self-esteem. Karl Atkin and Yasmin Hussain (2003) found that young Asian disabled people were isolated and lacked networks. For example, when asked about leisure, Shakeel replied: 'Spare time? I think every day is spare time for me' (ibid.: 169), and Nasira told them: 'I don't have any friends because I don't go anywhere ... They don't want me to come round because I'm disabled, you see, they don't want to know me' (ibid.: 169).

Aitchison (2003) found that the young disabled people he researched with spent more of their leisure time in solitary and home-based pursuits such as watching television, listening to music, or playing computer games. On average, his 15 respondents had only one visit with a friend in the study fortnight. McMaugh (2011) found that while a third of the Australian children with disability who participated in her research had very positive and happy relationships with their friends, another third did not have a single friend. Pippa Murray's (2002) survey of 100 disabled teenagers found that most described lives as tainted by isolation, loneliness and exclusion. Lack of appropriate support – transport and personal assistance – was the major barrier to participation. Whereas professionals thought leisure opportunities were valuable ways of developing life skills and independence, young people's goal was friendship.

People with mental illness are another group of disabled people who are particularly likely to be isolated. For many people with mental illness, the community may be seen as frightening and lonely (Lester and

Tritter, 2005). It may be difficult for people to sustain relationships, both because of the prejudice and fear associated with mental illness, and also because of the impact of mental illness on behaviour. People with psychosis are three times more likely to be divorced than the general population (Meltzer *et al.*, 2002). A survey of 3000 people with severe mental illness found that even among those who had contact with support organisations, a quarter had no or very little involvement with community activities (Pinfold, 2004). In four out of ten cases, the social networks of people with mental illness were limited to other people using or working in the mental health services; 84 per cent of people with mental illness felt isolated, as opposed to 29 per cent of the general population.

People with learning difficulties also face problems with friendship (McVilly *et al.*, 2006). After de-institutionalisation, they may be present in the community, but not participating in it. Often, people with learning difficulties are isolated in subgroups of professional workers, and peers with learning difficulties. Bernert's US study found that the lives of women respondents with learning difficulties were centred on the disability agencies which provided their accommodation and sheltered employment. A minority associated with people outside their agencies: 'The women could not choose their social groups or the activities but they could choose whether or not they wanted to participate in the activities. Socializing with individuals outside of their social groups was not necessarily assisted, so the women had to assume responsibility for these interactions' (Bernert, 2011: 132).

One study found that only one in three people using learning disability services had even one non-disabled friend (Robertson *et al.*, 2001). In their study of people living in supported accommodation in Northern England, Emerson and McVilly (2004) found that 81 per cent of people with learning difficulties wanted to have more friends, and 65 per cent wanted a 'best friend' relationship. While 65 per cent had engaged in friendship activities with another person with learning difficulties, and 25 per cent with a friend who did not have learning difficulties, the median number of friendship activities over a four-week period was two. The researchers concluded that it was the setting, not the characteristics of the individual which determined the level of social activity. Research on the accommodation goals of people with learning difficulties indicates that access to social networks of family and friends are vital aspects of living arrangements (Barr *et al.*, 2003). Respondents prioritised having privacy in their homes, but also feared being alone.

Other groups within the disabled population may not experience this degree of social exclusion. For example, people with restricted growth usually do not experience cognitive limitations, are able to work or participate in society, and often resist identification as disabled. Yet my team's research with people with restricted growth in the North of England found a different social profile to the general population: out of 81 respondents, 47 per cent were single, compared to 30 per cent of the general population. Only 39 per cent were or had been married, compared to 69 per cent of the general population. While 12 per cent of the general population live alone, 33 per cent of our respondents lived alone. It would be wrong to conclude that all restricted growth adults are therefore lonely and isolated, but the data is suggestive of a group who may have less social contact than their non-disabled peers.

Even where disabled people do have friends and companions, they may find it harder to experience everyday intimacies which non-disabled people take for granted. This is not just a matter of having children or having a family life, important though these issues are. Many experience frustrations and difficulties with communication, which cannot be simply attributed to oppression, but also arises from the very real problems of understanding some people with speech impediments. Some disabled adults experience little physical contact with others. Their body may usually be experienced in terms of pain, restriction and lack of control. The main occasion when others touch their body is when carers or personal assistants or professionals lift and handle them in daily living situations, or for medical interventions.

How can the isolation and loneliness of some disabled people be explained? It would be misleading to conclude that this was an inevitable outcome of having an impairment. However, neither is it simply a matter of social oppression. Wider societal trends, the particular barriers faced by disabled people, and the social predicament of impairment all contribute to the problem. So far, the widespread acceptance of disability rights approaches has not made a big difference to the social lives of disabled people: 'Despite the success they have found in strengthening their status in the public sphere, people with disabilities – particularly intellectual disabilities – experience loneliness and isolation in the sphere of their personal lives' (Reinders, 2008: 6).

The decline of community and struggle for connection

Western societies became increasingly individualised and atomised during the twentieth century, as traditional ties of family, religion and community declined. A range of social, economic and demographic factors reduces the strength of networks of kin, friends and community. For example:

1 Families are smaller and more dispersed.
2 Organised religion is a minority experience: social networks built around religion are less common.
3 People are more mobile, leaving their community of origin to attend higher education, and often relocating several times during their lives to find work.
4 Pressure of careers means that working-age people are less likely to have time to dedicate to community activities. Because more women work, fewer people are exclusively home-makers.
5 Non-face-to-face interaction – through telephones and the internet – and passive forms of leisure – television and other multimedia – may have taken over from unmediated social engagement for many people. Rather than using the same local shops and services, and developing relationships with staff, people may drive to out-of-town shopping centres, where transactions are usually anonymous.

These factors, to varying degrees, erode continuity and interconnection. None of these changes make friendship impossible, and of course friendship in many ways has never been more important in contemporary society. These factors may contribute to changes in the form of friendship as much as to the decline of friendship. People may make friends quickly, for example, through work, or parenting networks, but move on equally quickly. People may not know their geographical neighbours, or take the time to make friends in their local communities, because they are connected to networks of interest. By contrast, in the past, communities were based on long-term and stable familiarity and shared activities within localities. The anthropologist Mary Douglas differentiates between strong ties and weak ties:

> Strong ties are best for certain dependent categories of the population such as infants, elderly people, the handicapped and the chronically infirm. But strong ties broken are hard to mend: it is not easy to foster them at the right phase in the life cycle and to loosen them at other times. Weak ties, on the other hand, appeal to our cultural bias in favour of an open society.
>
> *(quoted in Pahl, 2000: 159)*

All of these wider social factors make isolation and disconnection a problem for many people, not just non-disabled people. But they particularly impact on disabled people. Community care has meant that most disabled people are living in the community, just as the concept of community has been eroded.

Disability, friendship and social barriers

Developing friendships depends on having opportunities to meet people, and having the skills to develop and sustain friendships. If we are to avoid falling into the traditional mistake of viewing disabled lives as inevitably sad and tragic, it is also important to understand the role of social factors. This means seeking explanations for disabled people's isolation in terms of environmental and social barriers, including educational segregation, employment discrimination and inaccessible transport and social environments.

In *The Sexual Politics of Disability*, we argued that while the social model has been used to highlight the failures of contemporary social organisation – the badly designed transport, the prejudiced attitudes (Keith, 1996), and the discriminatory employers who disable people – it needs also to be used to show that the problem of disability and sexuality is not an inevitable outcome of our bodily differences. It is not because people cannot walk, or cannot see, or because they lack feeling in this or that part of the body that disabled people have sexual problems. As we argued, the problem of disabled sexuality is not how to do it, but who to do it with. The barriers to the sexual expression of disabled people are primarily to do with the society in which they live, not the bodies with which they are endowed. For example, many people find friends among the people with whom they study at school, college or university, and the people alongside whom they work. If disabled people are segregated in school, or excluded from further and higher education, and if they are twice as likely to be unemployed, then they will not only lack skills, opportunities and income, but they will also lack the social networks and self-esteem which successful participation in education and employment offers. If people lack money, they will be unable to buy drinks and meals, or tickets to films and other cultural events, even assuming that the venues for these activities are physically accessible.

Social and educational interventions to overcome social exclusion may well have paradoxical impacts on the inclusion and friendship opportunities of disabled people. For example, it has been suggested above that the presence of special needs assistants and other non-disabled helpers may lead to disabled children being excluded from peer groups, or finding it harder to reach out and make friends. Paradoxically, residential institutions and special schools were often places of security and friendship for disabled people, despite the problems of segregation, disempowerment and abuse in many settings. Edgerton (1984) showed how hidden sub-cultures in institutions emphasise sociability, harmony and self-esteem.

Having the right to live independently in the community is a good principle, but in practice often translates into being isolated in a private home in the middle of a neighbourhood where there are few opportunities for networking or friendship. For many disabled or elderly people, attending a day centre or living in a group home may be preferable to being bored all day or living alone. Many disabled people are in the community, but not part of the community.

Disability services may always not recognise the problem. Promoting friendship opportunities might not be on their agenda. Workers may not see it as their job to help their clients with making friends. Disability services may focus on group activities, setting their clients apart from the mainstream, rather than on promoting opportunities on an individual basis. Many services are preoccupied with risk and protection, and may be concerned at exposing their clients to unstructured contact with the rest of the world. If people with learning difficulties start exploring their sexuality, for example, they may become vulnerable to abuse or exploitation.

The development of a disability rights movement may have benefits for disabled people in overcoming isolation and loneliness, as well as in other areas. For example, anti-discrimination legislation, removal of social and environmental barriers, accessible transport, more opportunities to participate in mainstream education and employment, and more economic resources all improve the quality of life of disabled people. As a result, people may have more social contacts, more opportunities, and more access to the mainstream world, all generating more inclusion. Second, disability rights approaches improve self-esteem, by relocating the problems of disabled people from the person themselves, to the oppressive society. Also, by showing how disabled people are oppressed, not simply unfortunate, perhaps the social model creates a moral imperative for non-disabled people to reach out to disabled people to try and overcome oppression and isolation. Third, the disability rights movement creates and sustains social networks, primarily between disabled people themselves (Campbell and Oliver, 1996). Coalitions, direct action protests and disability arts cabarets all offer opportunities for disabled people to link up with others. Subcultures, whether based on disability rights, or on shared impairment, can provide contexts for oppressed individuals to make friends and gain confidence.

While these outcomes should be valued, it could be argued that there may paradoxically be negative effects of the emergence of disability rights. For example, the disability movement may not be welcoming or inclusive to all disabled people, and there have been claims that minorities or those with particular impairments are not always equally represented or supported. Moreover, the rights discourse may encourage a political identity which is rejecting of non-disabled people, and promotes hostile and self-segregating responses. Gaining more disabled friends may sometimes be at the cost of abandoning those non-disabled acquaintances or family members who are seen as patronising and inappropriate in their response to disability. Of course, this may not be a negative outcome: fewer, better friends who contribute to self-esteem rather than putting you down might be preferable.

A social model analysis of the lack of friendship and intimacy in the lives of disabled people cannot fully account for this persistent and neglected problem. By definition, it is a social not a biological phenomenon. But it is not simply a matter of discrimination. It is partly about the predicament of impairment. Broader social changes have created a world in which disabled people are particularly disadvantaged, and the problems of being impaired are exacerbated. It is not just that disabled people and older people are disempowered and devalued. The social ecology of contemporary living has less space for those who may be able to contribute little to reciprocal relationships. The dominance of secularism, individualism and consumerism may accord little priority to helping those who are isolated and excluded.

Achieving social interaction

Interaction between disabled and non-disabled people can be difficult for a range of reasons. Some of these are to do with the disabled person themselves. Some impairments make social relations more difficult. For example, people with speech impairments may be hard to understand (Paterson and Hughes, 1999). Deaf people may rely on sign language for communication, which many hearing people are unfamiliar with, or may have limited confidence with. Deafened or hard of hearing people may become very isolated as a result of difficulties of communicating with others. Most non-disabled people may not know how to go about communicating with a deaf-blind person. Some people with learning difficulties may also have little spoken language, sometimes relying on Makaton. In all these cases, relying on an interpreter may create a strained interaction. With familiarity and goodwill and patience, communication may become easier. But it may always be an effort for both parties to maintain a conversation.

In other cases, there may be no overt communication barrier, but interaction is still difficult. For example, people with learning difficulties may not behave conventionally or understand the subtleties of body language and ironic banter. People with mental health issues or cognitive

impairment may lack insight, become anxious or suspicious, or otherwise interact in unusual ways. They may forget previous conversations
or social contact. In the case of people with visual impairment, it may be
difficult to initiate contact, or to communicate non-verbal cues. The
lack of eye contact may be disconcerting for people unfamiliar with
visually impaired people. In other cases, physical difference or deformity
may be very distracting. As Erving Goffman (1968a) described, the effect
of stigma is to undermine the possibilities of interaction, at least at
the outset. It is difficult always to attribute these impairment effects to
oppression or discrimination, rather than to social embarrassment and
unfamiliarity. As Lenney and Sercombe (2002: 16) observe, 'The
dynamics at work when people with disabilities interact with others are
complex and contradictory.'

Impairment does not need to determine the outcome of interactions.
After all, many people with highly visible impairments or communication
difficulties manage social interactions very successfully. But, on average,
such impairments do contribute to the social isolation of many disabled
people. Those who achieve interaction do so by what Fred Davis (1964)
called 'normalizing': going more than halfway, by enabling the non-
disabled person to go beyond their preoccupation with the impairment,
and finding what they both have in common (Fisher and Galler, 1988:
173). Skill and confidence are required if disabled people are to manage
this move. Those who overcome social barriers often do so because
their impairments are compensated by other factors. For example, they
may enjoy cultural advantages of race, gender or status, or have resilient
or gregarious personalities.

However, more often, because of the experience of both impairment
and discrimination, and perhaps also because of the past experience of
difficult communication, disabled people may lack confidence and self-
esteem. For example, people with acquired brain injury may feel that
their sense of identity has been taken away by their impairment (Sherry,
2002). People who have been institutionalised all their lives may not
have a strong sense of individuality or autonomy. In general, disabled
people may have internalised negative messages from significant others,
or from society in general, and believe themselves to be incompetent or
invalid or undesirable. Alternatively, they may be angry and hostile
about their situation, resenting the way they are treated, and unwilling
to overlook actual or perceived slights from others (Keith, 1996). Both
of these are understandable reactions to the diffculties of impairment and
disability, but neither is conducive to comfortable relations with others.

Of course, it is important to note that the attitudes and behaviour of
non-disabled people are a major factor in the extent to which disabled

people are isolated or integrated into networks and communities (Keith, 1996; Tregaskis, 2004a). For example, there are various reasons why non-disabled people may be unwilling to make the effort to communicate with or associate with disabled people. If disabled people are segregated from non-disabled people, then lack of familiarity may generate fear and prejudice. Ignorance and lack of social skills might make it difficult for non-disabled people to overcome communication barriers or cope with unusual behaviour. Cultural representation of disabled people as asexual and uncool is unlikely to encourage non-disabled people to reach out to include disabled people in leisure or social activities. Because of their own insecurity, many people want to be associated with successful and high achieving people: disabled people may be seen as incompetent, and as discrediting people to be around. If disabled people seem to be distressed or suffering, then this may be uncomfortable to non-disabled people who try to avoid the difficult aspects of life. Because a relationship with a disabled person may be perceived as asymmetrical, it may be assumed that the non-disabled person will not derive any personal benefit from the relationship. Finally, those who are willing to look past these issues and reach out to disabled people may not want to get into a caring role. This may particularly structure women's responses: 'Because women are assigned the roles of nurturer, helper, and healer, getting to know someone with a disability may seem to imply that the non-disabled woman must automatically become a caretaker' (Fisher and Galler, 1988: 76).

In his theological discussion of friendship and intellectual disability, Hans Reinders concedes that effort is required to reach out to people with learning difficulties: 'Friendship is a very rare experience in their lives. People without a disability seldom want to become involved, particularly when it takes a strong commitment to do so' (Reinders, 2008: 4).

At the extreme, there may be fear of fostering a relationship of dependency, where the disabled person makes excessive or continuing demands which the non-disabled person is unwilling or unable to fulfil (DisAbility Services, n.d.: 16).

However, these negative responses are not the whole picture. There are many individuals who are willing to associate with disabled people, reach out to them, and include them in their lives and communities. For example, school children with disabilities may have friends and peers who support them, when they experience bullying (Bourke and Burgman, 2010). When people become friends with disabled people, the salience of the impairment may diminish: the disabled person becomes 'delabelled' (Taylor and Bogdan, 1989: 32) and accepted as normal, and the relationship can become reciprocal. Often, disabled children do have friends in their peer group, who look beyond the impairment and see the person. Traustadóttir (1993) argues that women are over-represented in social networks of disabled people, and play an important role in providing social support. Women seem to be more accepting than men of disabled people. Men may find it difficult to provide assistance to disabled friends, or may be ill-at-ease with emotional intimacy.

Following Taylor and Bogdan's (1989) work on the sociology of acceptance, we can identify several reasons why non-disabled people put in the extra effort and reach out to disabled people. First, people are bonded by the family relationships they have with disabled people: 'The family would not be the same family without the disabled family member' (ibid.: 27). Parents and siblings of disabled people who contributed to the AnSWeR website (www.antenataltesting.info) show how their lives have been enriched by disabled family members, and the commitment they have to them. Second, because there are actually major benefits to associating with disabled people. People like and enjoy the company of disabled people, as this respondent indicated: 'I really like spending time with him. Why? Because we both have active imaginations, we're artistic, share the same sense of humour, love chocolate, and like good coffee on Sunday mornings' (ibid.: 32).

Disabled people may be enjoyable and amusing, and their company may form an alternative to the more competitive, status-oriented or stressful social relations in the mainstream world. For example, it is often suggested that people with learning difficulties are more open, generous, trusting and light-hearted than non-disabled people. They may have a sense of humour and a joy in life which is very valuable (Vanier, 1999).

Third, non-disabled people may be motivated by the benefits for their own sense of self which they derive from reaching out to less fortunate people. They may get a sense of purpose in life. They may feel that here they are doing something rewarding. They may feel that they are better people as a result. They may in fact be socially valued by their community or society because of their charitable work. As a result of their work with disabled people, their own self-esteem may be enhanced (Wuthnow, 1991).

Fourth, people may make the effort to include and support disabled people for ideological reasons: they may have a religious commitment, and therefore believe that the role of a Good Samaritan or good neighbour or charitable person is desirable, is part of their religious faith, or may be rewarded in the afterlife. Alternatively, they may have a sense of social solidarity for political or humanist reasons, and believe that it is their duty to include others and to overcome oppression: for example, the women's movement explicitly fostered friendships between women, and friendships between women from different backgrounds (Fisher and Galler, 1988). People who work professionally with disabled people may extend this into friendships with disabled people in their personal lives.

Reciprocity seems to be an important element in proper friendship. This may remain a problem, even when disabled people are skilled in reaching out, and non-disabled people are motivated to make and stay friends. While personal assistance and better services may make disabled people less reliant on their friends, there will always be situations in which help is required. Disabled people may minimise their needs, in order to avoid asking for help from a friend and skewing the relationship. Reciprocity may also apply to topics for conversation, for example, censoring of conversations about sexuality and childbearing and even disability itself has been reported by disabled women (ibid.: 183). Non-disabled people may feel guilt about not sharing the limitations or difficulties of their disabled friend. All this complicates interaction, and sometimes affects the possibility for emotional openness and exchange.

Sometimes, friendships between disabled and non-disabled people occupy an ambiguous space. In describing the friendship between Michelle, a non-disabled woman, and Susan, a woman with significant learning difficulties, Traustadóttir (2000) shows Michelle used the language of work as well as the language of love. Whereas the ideal was for their relationship to be a true and mutual friendship, in practice, the day-to-day reality was of Michelle having to work hard to establish and develop their companionship. Normal friendships are usually homogenous and balanced. But these types of worked-at friendships do not conform to the culturally dominant view of friendship. Here, the rewards are not reciprocation and mutual support, but the satisfaction of making someone else happier and more included, and playing a socially valued role.

Friendship between disabled people

For many disabled people, it is other people who share their experiences or outlook who make the best friends. This is particularly the case for people with learning difficulties, such as the respondents in McVilly *et al.*'s (2006) study. There was more equality, and hence it was more comfortable to be friends with other people with learning difficulties, particularly people who had been at school together. This approach is not limited to people with learning difficulties: it has been suggested already that the disabled people's movement offers a forum where people can fraternise and form friendships and relationships.

Those who feel isolated, and subject to prejudicial social reactions, within mainstream environments often would rather hang out with others with whom their difference is accepted. This was one of the roles of the community mental health centres in Norway that Elstad and Kristiansen (2009) studied: people with mental health conditions benefitted from recognition, support, fellowship, participation, from each other as well as from the support staff. Something similar is reported from Sierra Leone, where Dos Santos-Zingale and McColl (2006) found that newly disabled people whom they studied preferred to be with other disabled people, to feel a sense of acceptance and belonging. Again, Milner and Kelly's New Zealand study (2009) found that disabled people experienced mainstream settings as alienating and oppressive: for them, inclusion was about being known. They wanted a place to escape the public gaze and a respite from feeling different – which was often their home or their vocational centre. Other people with disabilities can be a haven from a heartless world. However, collective action can also reclaim public spaces. Respondents in this New Zealand study who associated with other people with disabilities were able to colonise bars and swimming pools and support each other to change the communities around them. Similarly, the newly injured people in Sierra Leone used their collective weight to lobby for better assistance from government.

Bridging the friendship gap

If isolation and loneliness cannot simply be attributed to oppression, it is difficult to see how barrier removal alone could entirely solve the problem. A society with strong anti-discrimination legislation and good access would certainly be one in which disabled people were more socially engaged, but not all disabled people would automatically be included. Particular groups may be at particular risk of isolation – for example, people with learning difficulties or mental health issues – and particular points in the life course may be difficult for disabled people, for example, adolescence. Social welfare agencies and social movements need to understand these issues, and make a positive contribution to fostering social networks and community for and with disabled people.

Staff can be pivotal in promoting inclusion and friendship. Taxi drivers, carers, nursing and medical professionals do emotional work, providing friendship and validation, not just the obvious practical tasks. Many disabled people rely on their personal assistants to provide companionship as well as practical help. A traditional stress on professionalism and distance needs to give way to what Traustadóttir calls 'commitment and involvement' (1993: 122). Some currents in disability rights discourse risk neglecting these aspects of the helping role. Non-disabled people, and professionals in particular, can be seen as potential exploiters or abusers, rather than potential allies. Sometimes, personal assistants are treated as servants, and the psycho-emotional aspects of the role are downplayed, as discussed elsewhere in this book.

Services could be audited to explore whether they increase or decrease the isolation of disabled people. Rather than solely focusing on inclusion, provision should also aim to build shelter and inter-connectedness. For example, special needs assistants in classrooms often tend to increase children's isolation, even if they succeed in meeting other needs. Imagination may be needed to deliver support in ways which do not single out the recipient, or exclude them from other valuable interactions. New initiatives should be assessed in terms of whether they impact on possibilities of friendship and intimacy, helping build connections. For example, relying on email or telephone rather than face-to-face communication may be efficient, but at the cost of reducing opportunities for social contact: 'While the screen may open the user to new worlds, it may also serve to deepen isolation and prevent acquisition of the skills and confidence required to conduct relationships in the everyday world' (Seymour and Lupton, 2004: 302).

For other groups, providing online discussion opportunities may build connections and promote mutual support. For example, people with rare conditions may find comradeship in national and international list-servs such as the Shortlist e-group for people with restricted growth. People with communication or social interaction issues may find online groups easier to negotiate than face-to-face gatherings.

There is potential for staff to do more to help friendship. This can be as simple as providing transport to ensure that people with learning difficulties can meet their friends, or as subtle as helping people make up after arguments (McVilly *et al.*, 2006), particularly when people do not have the social skills to overcome conflicts.

For example, people who work with and for disabled people should promote a community development model of service provision, looking for opportunities for their clients to make connections and engage in social activities. Rather than only group activities, staff could facilitate individualised social activities for clients. A pro-active and imaginative worker could stimulate ideas, facilitate oppportunities, and act as an entrepreneur, based on creating connections based on shared interests. The Metro Access workers in Victoria, Australia, seem to be playing exactly this role, looking at how mainstream community organisations and activities can accommodate participation by disabled people.

Voluntary groups in the disability community create possibilities of friendship and companionship, as well as having instrumental value in campaigning or providing services. Disability rights groups, self-advocacy groups and more traditional self-help groups bring isolated people together and make spaces for friendships to grow. Cultural projects also play a role. Examples include the network of Arts Studios where people with mental health issues can drop in and spend time. The staff are professional artists, rather than care workers, and provide company, as well as fostering creativity. Theatre groups for people with learning difficulties (such as Olla in Sweden and The Lawnmowers in Gateshead, UK) can enhance confidence, challenge negative attitudes, and provide meaningful social activity. Disability arts cabaret nights and nightclubs for people with learning difficulties (e.g. the Krocodile Klub and the Big Snapper in UK) offer spaces where disabled people can socialise with others on their own terms (Price and Barron, 1999).

Various initiatives have tried to provide a framework in which genuine friendship can develop. In the absence of spontaneous social networks and traditional communities, artificial ways of creating companionship and friendship for disabled people need to be explored (Abraham, 1989). These include friendship circles (Perske, 1988) and bridge building. For example, Circles of Support (Gold, 1999) are networks of non-disabled people which provide friendship opportunities for a disabled child or adult. Often these have been organised by the parents of young people with learning difficulties with the aim of promoting the inclusion of their child. However, sometimes these friendships do not outlast the duration of the group meetings. Moreover, there is a tension between the hope for 'true friendship' and the danger of creating a support service which stigmatises the disabled person at the centre: 'We must guard against merely creating another generation of "professionals" and "clients", with the former group seen as perpetually competent, and the latter, perpetually needy' (Van der Klift and Kunc, 1994: 3).

Providing too much help can itself be disempowering. Friendship is an elusive thing which cannot easily be engineered. It is interesting that the needs of people with learning difficulties around sexuality identified in the Living Safer Sexual Lives action research project were more easily met than their request for help around breaking down loneliness and isolation (Johnson et al., 2002).

It has been suggested that people with learning difficulties or other cognitive impairments may benefit from training so that they can learn how to make friends. For example, programmes can teach friendship skills to adolescents with high functioning autism and Asperger syndrome (Duffield, 2001). This approach may seem patronising. However, learning how to communicate, how to be sensitive to boundaries, how to overcome jealousy or possessiveness, are all complex skills which are gained through experience and through watching others. Arguably, people can be helped to develop and practise these skills through role play, which facilitates mutual understanding and appropriate behaviour, and helps with conflict resolution. The danger is that a focus on skills means that people spend the time learning, not getting out and making friends. When the DisAbility Services Branch of the Department of Human Services, Victoria, commissioned research to investigate social networks among people with a cognitive impairment, and how these could be enhanced, their report focused on social inclusion, not just skills development. A major emphasis was on accessing communities based on shared interests – for example, sports and pets – rather than geographical proximity. The conclusion of their research was that a focus on friendship could bring about a major shift in the provision of services for people with learning difficulties.

In order to become friends, non-disabled people need to be able to learn about disability, both in general, and in terms of the specific individual with whom they are engaging. Ignorance and fear – including fear of doing or saying the wrong thing – are barriers to social interaction (Lenney and Sercombe, 2002: 17). Inclusion of disabled people in schools establishes familiarity between disabled and non-disabled people. Education about impairment and disability, and by disabled people, may challenge myths and establish ways of being together. Ultimately, disabled people may still need to explain and to educate their non-disabled colleagues and friends about what their own impairment means, and where accommodation will have to be made. This requires patience and commitment and communication from both sides.

Conclusion

In the course of writing this chapter, I looked at the index of half a dozen recent disability studies texts (Campbell and Oliver, 1996; Barnes and Mercer, 2003; Swain *et al.*, 2003; Swain *et al.*, 2004; Barnes and Mercer, 2004; Barnes *et al.*, 2004). There was minimal discussion of friendship, sexuality, or loneliness. Most of the research which has been done on friendship and disability has been restricted to issues for people with learning difficulties. Equally, mainstream studies of intimacy and friendship do not usually attend to particular issues for disabled people (e.g. Jamieson, 1998). The British disabled feminist, Liz Crow, wrote:

> I've always assumed that the most urgent Disability civil rights campaigns are the ones we're currently fighting for – employment, education, housing, transport etc., etc., and that next to them a subject such as sexuality is almost dispensable. For the first time

> now I'm beginning to believe that sexuality, the one area above all others to have been ignored, is at the absolute core of what we're working for ... It's not that one area can ever be achieved alone – they're all interwoven, but you can't get closer to the essence of self or more 'people-living-alongside-people' than sexuality, can you?
>
> *(Crow, 1991: 9)*

While endorsing Crow's point, it seems to me to be a broader and deeper problem than that of sexuality alone. Prior to sexual expression is the problem of basic companionship, conversation, and togetherness. Steve Taylor and Robert Bogdan (1989: 34) call for a sociology of acceptance: research into what can foster connection, how relationships can be supported, and how both disabled and non-disabled people can be enabled to form relationships with each other. This agenda should be an important part of disability studies, and it should be part of the social response to the challenge of disability. Policies which took the intimacy and friendship needs of disabled people seriously would see support as more diverse than simple daily living tasks. People with learning difficulties want staff who appreciate the importance of friendship, and prioritise it (McVilly *et al.*, 2006). As Hans Reinders writes: 'Institutional space creates new opportunites that will become effective only because of the support of people. Without people who are disposed to be supportive, opportunities will turn to frustrations' (2008: 44).

Trying to support inclusion and friendship opportunities for disabled people is complex and difficult. Different solutions each involve tensions and compromises. For example, the Camphill or L'Arche communities seem to provide safe and sheltered environments, where people with learning difficulties are supported within family structures, engage in work, and can have freedom to live normally. Yet this is achieved by creating a rather segregated and unusual rural village situation, in which very motivated non-disabled people live with a high proportion of people who need support (Vanier, 1999; Rawles, 2004). Equally, artificial ways of fostering connection may seem patronising. The skeleton of contact and exchange which such structures provide may not seem genuine or worthwhile. But over time, such relationships can develop into important and mutually satisfying connections. Moreover, to many people who benefit from volunteering schemes – particularly older people and people with learning difficulties – their benefits outweigh any anxieties about charity or paternalism which disability rights activists have sometimes expressed.

Traustadóttir (2000) warns against the idealism found in many rosy and inspirational stories of friendship between non-disabled people and people with learning difficulties. She shows how these relationships are in practice harder and more complex than they first appear, and are usually rather different from conventional mutually supportive friendships. There is a danger of over-romanticising the difficulties of enabling disabled people, particularly those with significant cognitive problems, to form true relationships and achieve intimacy.

While there has been considerable attention to the friendship needs of particular groups of disabled people – people with learning difficulties and with mental health issues in particular – it seems to me that community and connection are an issue for many others who have physical impairments, particularly those which affect communication or hearing. Older people, with and without impairments, are clearly also at risk of isolation. Moreover, in an atomised contemporary world, the benefit of initiatives to support disabled people may be experienced by non-disabled people too (Bates and Davis, 2004). The social gathering which supports the disabled individual gives something meaningful to the non-disabled participants, who may also feel lonely at times. The benefit of volunteering, to give another example, is in the fulfilment and meaning it provides to those who volunteer, as well as to those who receive support. Just as the isolation of disabled people is about wider social changes, not just the predicament of impairment, so the solutions to that isolation may have wider impacts beyond the world of disability.

11

THINKING ABOUT DISABILITY, SEX AND LOVE

Introduction

In *The Sexual Politics of Disability*, Kath Gillespie-Sells, Dominic Davies and I argued for a social model of disabled sexuality, based on the insight that the problem was not 'how to do it' but 'who to do it with' (Shakespeare *et al.*, 1996). Ten years after our book, Article 23 of the Convention on the Rights of Persons with Disabilities stated that: 'States Parties shall take effective and appropriate measures to eliminate discrimination against persons with disabilities in all matters relating to marriage, family, parenthood and relationships, on an equal basis with others': this is now a legal obligation on the 127+ states which have ratified the Convention. Undoubtedly, attitudes towards disabled people's sexuality are slowly changing, perhaps more rapidly for people with physical and sensory impairments than for people with learning difficulties (Morales *et al.*, 2011). For example, there have been many TV documentaries and feature films that touch on the issue, or take it as a central theme, such as *The Sessions* (2012, director Lewin).

Yet still the words 'disability' and 'sexuality' are often coupled with the word 'taboo', and commonly there is shock among family members and service providers to find that a disabled person is partnered or sexually active. For example, an Australian colleague told me as I revised this book:

> I once had a doctor respond with unreserved shock when I told her I was sleeping with someone (she hadn't asked, I had to volunteer it because it was relevant). I was 23. When she referred

me to a specialist her referral said, 'S has severe Osteogenesis Imperfecta. Surprisingly, however, she is sexually active.'

Similarly, in her account of being partner of a man with MS, Sarah Smith Rainey (2011) talks about the common assumption that she was her husband's carer, not his lover. Further afield, a study of reproductive services for pregnant women with disability in Lusaka, Zambia, found that staff often reacted to these women with disbelief: 'When they see you they laugh … seeing your disability and the pregnancy on the other hand' (Smith *et al.*, 2005: 124). Experiences and attitudes like this cause commentators to talk about the myth of asexuality, or to refer to the disability sexuality taboo. Liz Emens goes so far as to claim that 'normative desexualization is about utter exclusion of disabled people from the intimate realm' (Emens, 2009: 1338).

While on the one hand, these attitudes and assumptions are undoubtedly very common, I think it is hard to say that disabled people are desexualised, when there is widespread evidence that disabled people are having sex in great numbers. For example, empirical studies show that young people with disabilities are sexually active in similar ways to people without disabilities (Brunnberg *et al.*, 2009). In fact, large Swedish studies report an earlier age of sexual debut for adolescents with disabilities than their nondisabled peers: 57 per cent of girls with disabilities, as opposed to 43 per cent of nondisabled girls had had sex, and 39 per cent of disabled boys, versus 37 per cent of nondisabled boys (2007 study of 15–16-year-old participants in mainstream education, N = 2839): it was even higher for girls (60 per cent) and boys (50 per cent) with two or more disabilities (ibid.). The researchers connect this early sexual debut to the young disabled person's battle to be included and accepted. It was also associated with the use of alcohol, tobacco, or truancy. For some people, early debut was a consequence of abuse, a factor also reported among Deaf people in the Philippines (Gomez, 2011). A study from Sierra Leone found that 71 per cent of people with mild to moderate and 58 per cent of people with severe disability had been sexually active in the previous year, as compared to 92 per cent of non-disabled adults (Trani *et al.*, 2010).

Disabled adults are less likely to be in partnerships, but the disparity is not huge. Emens highlights US data showing that around 50 per cent of people with severe disabilities, 60 per cent of people with non-severe disabilities and 68 per cent of nondisabled people are married (Emens, 2009: 1326). Many groups within the disability population are unlikely to face significant barriers to sexual activity and partnership; for example, Deaf people who associate through Deaf clubs and other Deaf sub-culture. Equally, disabled people are heterosexual, bisexual, lesbian and gay and transsexual, in much the same ways as nondisabled people (Bedard *et al.*, 2010), as we also found in our 1996 study.

Data on comparatively high rates of sexual activity may be misleading, however, insofar as they also include people who are already married who become disabled, for example, as they grow older. After spinal cord injury, for example, evidence suggests that the majority of women – three-quarters in a Swedish study by Kreuter *et al.* (2008) – have sex within six months post injury. A Malaysian study of women with spinal cord injury noted that 40 per cent of the women continued to have sexual activity after injury, although there was a decline in the frequency of sexual intercourse (Othman and Engkasan, 2011).

The situation may be different for those who are born with impairments. In the research my team conducted with people with restricted growth in Northern England, 47 per cent of respondents were single, compared to 30 per cent of the general population. 41 per cent were married or in a long-term relationship, compared to 60 per cent of the general population. The situation is likely to be comparable or worse for people with congenital impairments that substantially limit communication or independence.

The second group of people who face particular barriers around relationships are people with learning difficulties who either are prevented from exercising choices around intimacy, partnership and parenting, or who require additional supports in order to flourish in the realm of sexuality. For example, guardianship laws in various European countries (e.g. Austria, Greece) mean that people with learning difficulties or mental health conditions require permission from their guardian to get married (European Fundamental Rights). A large Spanish study with people with mild to moderate intellectual disability (N = 376) found that 72.9 per cent had a partner, but 91.61 per cent did not live with their partner, and 98 per cent were unmarried (Arias *et al.*, 2009): experiences and aspirations regarding love were similar to those of nondisabled people, and where there were positive experiences of relationships, this contributed to emotional well-being. Sheila Jeffreys draws attention to the fact that women with intellectual disabilities are more likely than most sections of the disabled population to be partnered, claiming that this is because men want docile and easily dominated women. Whatever the truth of that suggestion, while intimate partner violence is an issue for all women with disability, women with intellectual disabilities are at particular risk of sexual violence and exploitation (Jeffreys 2008; Hanass-Hancock, 2009).

In the remainder of this chapter, I want to contribute to three debates. First, in what terms can we theorise the intersection between disability and sexuality in the human rights era? Second, how can we create services and systems that are supportive of sexual intimacy for disabled people? Third, how can we negotiate issues of autonomy and protection for people with learning difficulties?

How can we theorise sexual rights for disabled people?

In citing the UN Convention on the Rights of Persons with Disabilities, we open the question of the role of government in enabling disabled people to achieve sexual intimacy and relationships. As one of the respondents to Russell Shuttleworth's research said, 'The ADA [Americans with Disabilities Act] isn't going to get me laid!' This issue is discussed by Liz Emens, who writes that:

> The complexities of intimate differentiation – including its benefits for some members of subordinated groups and, more widely, for its role in the pursuit of love, lust, and happiness for individual seekers of many stripes – argue against a conclusion that the associated harms could justify individual level regulation.
>
> *(Emens, 2009)*

In some Indian states, subsidies have been reportedly offered to men who marry disabled women. At least in the Western world, arranged marriage is rare. It is clearly the case that people fall in love – or lust – in a free market of emotions, rather than with a carefully calculated scrutiny of possibilities and obligations. I would be very surprised to find that anyone actually asked themselves 'What are the essential functions of the job of being my partner?' (ibid.: 1360). People generally do not make explicit rational calculations of that nature when it comes to sex and love, otherwise life would be a lot harder for disabled people than it seems to be. Yet what Emens describes as the accidents of sex and love – who meets who, and who has access to the social, cultural and economic capital to be appealing – are nevertheless structured by access to employment and education and public spaces: '[B]y deciding the form of our communities' institutional and physical infrastructure, the state has shaped who meets whom, who interacts with whom, who has the chance to fall for whom' (ibid.: 1380).

As we argued in 1996, and as I reiterated in the first edition of this book, the more that societies are inclusive of disabled people – in terms of physical and virtual space, but also in terms of access to education, employment and public space – the more that disabled people will have the cultural, social and economic capital to participate fully in the world of emotions, sex and relationships.

But liberation is more than simply access. Veteran sexual rights campaigner and researcher Ken Plummer describes 'intimate citizenship' as something which should run alongside civil, political and social rights: 'the control (or not) over one's body, feelings, relationships; access (or not) to representations, relationships, public spaces etc.; and socially grounded choices (or not) about identities, gender experiences, erotic experiences' (Plummer, 1995: 151). This is a wider concern which highlights that many disabled people do not feel in control of their bodies, do not see themselves represented as positive and sexual beings in everyday culture, and do feel excluded from spaces where relationships are on the agenda. People with learning difficulties in particular are excluded from this sense of intimate citizenship, as they are from other aspects of citizenship (Mirfin-Veitch, 2003). Loneliness and isolation are an issue for too many disabled people. Kathleen Lynch *et al.* (2009) talk about 'affective equality', bringing in a feminist ethic of care concern with who gives love, support and care, and who receives it. In this perspective, being deprived of supportive affective relations is a serious form of injustice.

Margrit Shildrick (2012: 38) criticises the call for sexual citizenship, pointing out, correctly, that the sexuality of disabled people is both highly regulated and silenced. She worries that sexual citizenship does not contest what she calls 'the current neo-liberal understandings of sexuality' and 'fails to break with the devaluation of difference'. I await further elucidation as to why this is necessarily the case. In *The Sexual Politics of Disability* (Shakespeare *et al.*, 1996), we shared the testimonies of men and women who were hetero, homo and bisexual, originated from different cultures, many of whom contested notions of masculinity and femininity. Without negating the power of dominant patriarchal and heterosexist assumptions, it appears to me that the concept of sexual citizenship contains the notion that sexual rights have to be addressed alongside other human rights, and that disabled people should be considered as sexual beings alongside their peers, without imposing a notion of what sexuality should entail.

More importantly, if supportive affective relations – and sex – are a key aspect of personhood, deprivation of which constitutes injustice, then what can states do about this? How can they fulfil their obligations under Article 23 of the UN Convention? Given the split between the public and private realms of life, this is not a straightforward matter. There are good reasons for not wanting the state to interfere in people's bedrooms: historically, this interference has generally been repressive more often than it has been protective.

Here, Isaiah Berlin's distinction between positive and negative freedom may be helpful. Restrictions on negative freedom arise when states legislate for who can get married and have children. Historically, laws have prevented the marriage of people with disabilities – those with epilepsy, learning difficulties, AIDS, mental health conditions, for example – and mandated the involuntary sterilisation of some of these groups. It is clear that human rights demand the abolition of such restrictions on negative freedom. But is this enough to ensure affective equality? What more can states do positively to enhance the opportunities for disabled people to access sex and relationships?

Liz Emens (2009) sketches out a programme of actions that go beyond the state lifting formal restrictions on who can have sex or marry. She argues that the state should eliminate penalties, for example, when a person with disability loses welfare benefits if he becomes partnered to someone who is employed. Further, the state can help level the playing field, for example, by ensuring that individuals get sex education or even support in developing friendship skills. Measures to remove access barriers and achieve what she describes as designing the 'architecture of intimacy' might go beyond the obvious to include audio description in cinemas and promoting visitability of private homes, thus facilitating social lives. Finally, Emens suggests that the state could fund positive expressions of imagery around disabled intimacy and sexuality, such as cultural activities, arts and diversity campaigns.

Notions of sexual citizenship, sexual access, affective equality and the architecture of intimacy are important aspects of what might be called the liberal rights model of disabled sexuality. But as well as gaining access to the mainstream, perhaps it is also important to open up the possibility of disabled sexuality challenging the ways in which everyone conceives of what sexuality is and can be. Tobin Siebers has talked about 'sexual culture', exploring how sexuality may be different for disabled people. Different parts of the body may become erogenous zones; assistance may be required for participation in sex; the boundary between the public and the private may be violated. It is presumably this disabled challenge to sexual norms which Rob McRuer is thinking of when he proposes crip theory.

Another example of what is meant by a disabled sexual culture arises from what Rainey (2011) discusses: her account contrasts cultural representations of disabled sexuality with personal narratives by disabled people and their partners, arguing that care can increase, rather than hinder intimacy. Care is a two-way reciprocal process, not merely something which the non-disabled partner performs for the disabled partner. Disabled sexuality can perhaps contribute insights about the erotics of care that non-disabled people may not (yet) have experienced.

Services which support intimacy

Armed with notions like sexual citizenship, sexual access, affective equality and sexual culture, and having debunked the notion of asexuality, we can turn to what services can do to support intimacy.

Immediately, the lacunae and active barriers are evident. Services and professionals tend to ignore or downplay the dimension of sexuality when thinking about or working with disabled people. This may partly be because disabled people are considered, actively or by default, to be asexual, or to have a child-like innocence. Family planning clinics may be inaccessible (Anderson and Kitchin, 2000) and advice and support may be lacking (Earle, 2001). A survey on staff experiences of the sexuality of their clients with learning difficulties in Northern Ireland found that only 22 per cent of staff had had training around the issue, although 65 per cent had experienced one of the sexuality scenarios listed, for example, public masturbation or unwanted sexual advances (McConkey and Ryan, 2001).

Alternatively, and in particular for people with learning difficulties, services may only consider sexuality in terms of a perceived vulnerability to abuse, or conversely, the worry that people may behave in sexually inappropriate ways or put themselves at risk of HIV (Cambridge and Mellan, 2000). Instead, services should think in terms of supporting knowledge and confidence around sex, positive self-image, negotiation and communication and assertiveness. In a now classic paper, Hilary Brown talked about how services could support people with learning difficulties to achieve intimacy and sexuality (1994), rather than regulating and segregating.

From Sweden, Julia Bahner's research gives examples of how services for disabled people are obstacles to sexual encounters (Bahner, 2012). As an example, she cites how special transport services could be booked to take a wheelchair user to a bar or a nightclub. However, if he then encountered a potential partner, they could not travel home with him because the regulations did not permit passengers, with the exception of personal assistants. The same barrier is encountered on accessible taxis, trams or trains where there is only room for one wheelchair user at a time, thus preventing two wheelchair users going out together.

In hospitals or rehabilitation centres, the need for intimacy is rarely valued. Bahner cites the example of E, an interviewee with around-the-clock assistance (including from her husband), who recounted how when she was in the hospital, after much battle with the personnel, she and her husband managed to get him a bed to be able to stay overnight: 'Not because we would be able to have sex there, but just the fact that he could lie there beside me, hold my hand, caress me … I was so happy!'

My experience of spinal cord injury rehabilitation in the UK, was that patients were allowed to have one night with their partners in the 'independent living flat' in the hospital, and had to fight to be able to spend a whole weekend together – despite the fact that there were rarely other patients clamouring to use the facility. Sexuality is an important aspect of rehabilitation, yet the relevant information was not offered automatically, and there was no space or privacy where the newly disabled person could explore their sexual possibilities.

The issue of privacy for people living in residential institutions is well known. For those living in the community and supported by personal assistants, there is more freedom, yet there remains a challenge in achieving privacy with a partner. Sarah Woodin's research found that while having a personal assistant was vital to meet partners and go on dates, the presence of a personal assistant could be intrusive and even put off new partners (Woodin, 2006). In a small flat, it could be off-putting to have the personal assistant sitting in the living room while a couple retire to bed to have sex in the middle of the day. Sending the assistant outside for a walk was not an option in the Swedish winter (Bahner, 2012). Often, the way services are delivered does not take into account the need for intimacy and prevents the spontaneity that is often a part of sex for non-disabled people.

Spaces need to be created where people with disabilities can meet and socialise. Over several decades, the UK Outsiders Club has offered a space for disabled and non-disabled people to meet in a sex-positive context. More recently, nightclubs for people with learning difficulties have been run for and by people with learning difficulties themselves, for example, the Krocodile Klub in Gateshead, Beautiful Octopus Club in Leeds and others (Garbutt, 2010). Dating services, such as Stars in the Sky, are the logical next step (Hollomotz, 2011).

Beyond these possibilities lies the question of sex work or sexual surrogacy, the topic of the recent film *The Sessions* (2012, director Lewin). In some countries – such as Denmark, the Netherlands, Australia – the cultural and legal climate is such that a support worker is allowed to help a disabled individual with masturbation, or take them to a sex worker, or sex surrogacy services exist to meet the sexual needs of men with disabilities, or there are even sex workers who specialise in disabled clients (Wotton and Isbister, 2010; Kulick and Rydström, forthcoming). Elsewhere – Sweden, for example – a zero tolerance approach to pros-titution means that not only is there no sex work possibility, but nor are support staff allowed to take any step which might be construed as facilitating sex by their clients (Kulick and Rydström, forthcoming). Traditional radical feminists (Jeffreys, 2008) applaud this, because they believe that facilitating disabled sexuality is just another version of the exploitation of women by men.

In countries like Britain, the role of personal assistants and nurses in supporting their clients to have sex is ambiguous (Earle, 1999, 2001). However, I think that projects such as the Australian Touching Base network of sex workers who enable disabled people to access sexual intimacy are a positive development, and hard to interpret in terms of trafficking or oppression of women (Wotton and Isbister, 2010). Services like sexual surrogacy or sex work have to be discussed, if we are serious about ensuring that all disabled people are to access sexuality.

Balancing autonomy and protection

Many people with ID live in supported accommodation or with their families, hence the issue of privacy is particularly relevant to them (Noonan and Taylor Gomez, 2011). Families exert tremendous influence of where and how people with learning difficulties live, who they associate with, and what possibilities they can explore in their lives (Mirfin-Veitch, 2003). Families often disapprove of the dating activities of young adults with learning difficulties (Bernert, 2011). These adults aspire to normal adult roles – including sex – but are treated like children by their guardians. In group homes or sheltered workshops, staff set rules for displays of affection, television viewing, and bed times, and generally supervise relations between people with learning difficulties (ibid.: 134). Families do not prioritise sexuality issues (Burton-Smith et al., 2009). They may encourage their adult children with learning difficulties to get sterilised (Desjardins, 2012) or go on long-term contraception (McCarthy, 2008). The Living Safer Sexual Lives project (Johnson et al., 2000, 2002), drawing on the life stories of 25 people with learning difficulties, highlighted four themes: (1) the attitudes of service providers and families which were obstacles to relationships and sexuality; (2) the lack of information about sexuality; (3) the lack of clear policies and guidelines for staff; and (4) the loneliness and isolation experienced by many respondents.

Service providers are often anxious about liabilities regarding sexual activity by service users (Bartlett, 2010; Bernert, 2011; Noonan and Taylor Gomez, 2011). At a basic level, this may arise because staff members are uncomfortable about older people or people with learning difficulties having sex, which may reflect the staff's own discomfort with sexuality. Alternatively, a service user may be sexually active, by her own free choice, yet her parents may be unhappy about it and complain to the agency. More importantly, a person may be at risk of abuse. For example, staff may want to protect women they perceive as vulnerable from men with learning difficulties who may be known to be violent or perceived to be exploiting them (Hamilton, 2010). Or finally, the person may be unable to consent to sex.

In the UK, under the 2003 Sexual Offences Act, if an individual has a 'mental disorder impeding choice' – in other words, cannot refuse, choose, agree, understand or communicate – then engaging in a sexual activity with them is a crime, resulting in a custodial sentence and inclusion in the sex offenders register. However, only a low level of knowledge is required to consent to sex: the judgment in one court case (Re MAB) stated 'Her knowledge and understanding need not be complete or sophisticated. It is enough that she has sufficient rudimentary knowledge or what the act comprises and of its sexual character to enable her to decide whether to give or withhold consent' (quoted in Bartlett, 2010: 8).

The old way of thinking about consent was in terms of status. All people with a particular condition were regarded as unable to consent. This was clearly inappropriate, given the range of individual capabilities and situations:

> The vast majority of adults who fulfil the criteria for an inherent vulnerability will be able to live full, meaningful and autonomous lives, and should not be judged to be *automatically* at heightened risk of being constrained, coerced, or unduly influenced, relative to other adults, regardless of their circumstances.
>
> *(Dunn et al., 2008: 244)*

A functional approach is superior to the status approach, because it focuses on what an individual is capable of in what situations, and where he can give adequate consent, and where he cannot. However, this approach has also been criticised for being unduly individualistic. Safety and vulnerability are contextual, and it has been argued that an ecological approach is needed, taking into account that risk arises in interactions, rather than vulnerability being seen as a feature of an individual's impairment (Hollomotz, 2011). Andrea Hollomotz says it is not enough to send an individual on a sex education course where they learn to say no, because:

> Once individuals return to a 'home' environment in which they are disabled from making choices, from being private and being in

control of their bodies, they may forget what they have learned or realise that self-determination is not relevant to their lives. Whether an individual is able to exercise self-determination is therefore very much dependent on environmental factors.

(ibid.: 43)

However, while I agree with this general line of argument, it seems to me that Hollomotz is so committed to a social model approach that she fails adequately to account for the inherent vulnerability of some people with learning difficulties. If someone is naïve and trusting and shares personal information with everyone on the bus, or if she cannot tell if a male friend is genuine and sincere or exploitative and potentially violent, then I think most would agree she is inherently vulnerable, and a measure of support and shelter is consequently required.

Hollomotz draws on a study she conducted with a small group of people with learning difficulties (N = 29). Half of the respondents had experienced consenting penetrative sex, a quarter had kissed and cuddled, and most knew the basics of heterosexual intercourse. However, only 15 respondents could distinguish between consenting activities and bad or violent activities. Only five knew about sexually transmitted infections and the use of condoms. Hollomotz compares this group to another study with non-disabled young people that showed that 56 per cent had accurate knowledge about STDs (as opposed to 15 per cent of her sample of people with learning difficulties). She concludes that both disabled and non-disabled people can be vulnerable and that her respondents were not out of the ordinary. I do not think the evidence supports the conclusions she draws.

Over-protection is problematic for at least three reasons. First, the ethical principle of autonomy, reinforced by Article 12 of the CRPD, implies that people should be able to decide for themselves what they do and with whom. My view is that restrictions of autonomy are acceptable where they are essential to protect the individual's safety. However, any such restrictions should be as minimal as possible, and this is evidently not the case in many settings. The idea of vulnerability is used to deny people with intellectual disabilities the right to make choices and take risks and live independently. Second, over-protection has been argued to remove the possibility of people with learning difficulties developing the skills and knowledge they need to protect themselves (Dunn *et al.*, 2008; Hollomotz, 2011): 'Undue protection from risks and opportunities associated with everyday life may disable individuals from becoming competent social and sexual actors and from accessing information and services that have the potential to reduce sexual "vulnerability"' (Hollomotz, 2011: 1).

Third, over-protection can be counter-productive because it can cause individuals to assert their independence in dangerous ways, for example, through rebellious behaviour, deception, etc. (Bernert, 2011: 138).

A balance must be struck between overprotection and control (ibid.), and risk and danger for adults who may lack the abilities to understand and protect themselves:

> [P]rior to intervention, every attempt should be made to support adults with autonomous risk management regardless of the circumstances within which that risk manifests itself. Only when autonomous risk management is deemed ineffective should an adult be considered 'at risk'.
>
> *(Dunn et al., 2008: 20)*

Dunn and Archer suggest that it is particularly important to engage with the person's subjective experience of his/her vulnerability by hearing their own perspectives and feelings. Yet people with learning difficulties sometimes lack insight into their situations and therefore may well reject the idea of themselves as vulnerable (Hollomotz, 2011).

People with learning difficulties should be able to make mistakes, like everyone else. However, there should also be provision of supportive and sheltering services and staff who can protect them from any potentially dangerous consequences of their choices. This is an extremely difficult balance to strike. I believe it would be wrong to go from one extreme – over-protection, exaggeration of vulnerability – to the other extreme – denial that there is any inherent vulnerability and complete exposure to risk. People with learning difficulties are both like everyone else, but also different in important ways.

Ways forward

Enabling people to feel positive about themselves, and enabling non-disabled people to feel positive about them, reflect wider processes of empowerment and cultural change. The more disabled people achieve their other civil and social rights, the more they will have the confidence, self-esteem and desirability that make relationships possible. All other Articles in the Convention on the Rights of Persons with Disabilities are therefore supportive of Article 23, Respect for Home and Family, achievement of which is therefore effectively one of the outcome measures for the whole endeavour of human rights.

Services and policies should be developed in ways that do not undermine the aspirations towards friendship, intimacy and sexuality.

This includes housing, transport and other practical matters. Disabled people should be able to live and socialise with friends and partners, and to meet potential friends and partners. Privacy should be available as well as the support required to explore the sexual aspects of life, where needed.

Better responses are needed to the sexual desires and rights of people with learning difficulties. Having learning difficulties should not be equated with dysfunction and therefore an automatic need for protection and control. Services providers should listen to their clients and treat them in an age-appropriate way.

In particular, lack of knowledge and experience makes people vulnerable. People with learning difficulties should be supported to learn about sex and relationships, and to develop friendships and connections with disabled and non-disabled people that go beyond their immediate agencies or services (Bernert, 2011). Three specific learning needs were identified in one study (Swango-Wilson, 2011): (1) how to develop friendships; (2) how to develop lasting relationships and marriage; and (3) how to achieve safe intimacy (protection from STDs, pregnancy, etc.). Visual and concrete examples are appropriate for delivery of sex education (Mirfin-Veitch, 2003). Group discussions about sexuality for people with intellectual disability (Noonan and Taylor Gomez, 2011) can provide safe and private spaces for men and women to share experiences, both separately and together. Education is required for some people with learning difficulties, so that they recognise that, for example, masturbation is normal and healthy, but should be something for private, not public spaces. EasyRead booklets and DVDs are increasingly available (Johnson *et al.*, 2002).

Sexuality information should be non-judgmental. People with learning difficulties may not have the language to express their sexuality, particularly if they are lesbian, gay, bisexual or transgender (Bedard *et al.*, 2010). Various projects have aimed to educate, train and support people with learning difficulties around LGBT issues (e.g. Noonan and Taylor Gomez, 2011).

Education is also required for service providers and families (Johnson *et al.*, 2002), so that they can understand, respect and support the sexual autonomy of people with intellectual disabilities. Successful workshop interventions have been delivered in Australia, New Zealand, Iceland and other countries.

Conclusion

Disabled people have the same needs as other people, which include needs for intimacy and sexual expression. As Liz Emens (2009) notes, being in relationships is good for mental and physical health and well-being.

Disability rights campaigns and disability studies research should therefore address sexuality, more than they have yet done. It seems to me long overdue to go beyond the twin fixations with either asexuality or dangerous sexuality, to establish ordinary sexuality as a realistic objective for disabled people.

How could this be done? Artists, educators and media producers could develop and promote positive images, to challenge the idea that disability is inevitably unsexy. Educationalists and health promotion workers should ensure that young disabled people always have access to appropriate sex education in schools, and receive any targeted and specific education needed to empower them to protect themselves and relate effectively to others. Family members should be encouraged to understand that people with learning difficulties have needs for intimacy and sexuality, among other aspects of life. While people with learning difficulties and older people with dementia may be in need of protection and support to avoid the risk of abuse and exploitation, they should not be regarded as inevitably vulnerable or unable to consent. Service providers should audit their services to ensure that they are not being delivered in ways that undermine the possibilities for intimacy. More research is needed on which groups of disabled people face particular barriers accessing sex and relationships, and what works best to overcome those barriers. Research should also open spaces for the voices and stories of disabled people, young and old, about relationships and sexuality, building on the work we did nearly twenty years ago.

12

UNDERSTANDING VIOLENCE AGAINST DISABLED PEOPLE

Introduction

What do we mean by violence? What does violence mean in the lives of disabled people? In this chapter, I want to sift through some of the recent debate about violence and hate crime, and clarify ways of speaking about and responding to this most disturbing aspect of disabling social relations. As in other areas, I am keen to establish the science – what we feel most sure of – rather than get pulled into areas of theory and speculation.

It is necessary to begin by defining terms, given that academic and activist discourse has a tendency to escalate descriptions and to deploy the word 'violence' to describe a wider range of discriminatory or exclusionary processes experienced by disabled people, such as human rights violations in general, rather than restricting use of the word to examples of coercion or physical force. For example, poverty has sometimes been regarded as a form of violence (e.g. Chouinard, 2012). However, in this case, the word 'violence' seems to be used in a metaphorical sense, equated with 'damage' or 'oppression'. Beyond the immediate attention-grabbing unfamiliarity of the word 'violence' applied to poverty, discrimination or other human rights violations (e.g. Goodley and Runswick-Cole, 2011), it does not seem to add to our understandings of those undoubtedly negative and damaging phenomena to call them violence. Violence has the important connotation that a person or group of people are very directly and intentionally exerting power over another person or group of people. Only if 'violence' is understood in a metaphorical way can the regimentation of pupils in a school be understood as a form of violence (ibid.: 610). The danger of using 'violence' as a synonym for disciplinary processes in general is that it dilutes the concept and makes it harder to identify the extreme forms of violence that are unacceptable and damaging.

In this chapter, I will draw on the public health approach to violence developed by the WHO and the Violence Prevention Alliance. Here, violence is conceptualised in terms of five different forms:

- physical
- sexual
- emotional
- financial
- neglect.

This schema is intuitive and not overly narrow. After all, a purist might reserve the term violence for the use of physical force. Sexual violence is a subcategory of violence, which entails coercion – being forced into sexual activity by being threatened or constrained or hurt. Terms like emotional violence and financial violence seem to be beginning to stray into the metaphorical uses of the term, but retain the sense of a person inflicting direct harm on another.

The public health approach also tends to classify violence into different types, each of which might involve any of the dimensions described above:

- child maltreatment
- intimate partner violence
- youth violence
- elder abuse.

It appears to me valuable to concentrate on the definitions and parameters established in the public health approach. However, in exploring the intersections of disability and violence, it may also be necessary to expand or revise some of these categories to reflect the specific experiences of disabled people. For example, rather than the narrowness of intimate partner violence, we might be interested in other forms of domestic violence, such as that of the mother-in-law against the disabled wife. We also need to consider the abuse or violence of a personal assistant against the disabled person they work for. The wider category of institutional violence against children and adults with disabilities seems to be so widespread that it requires explicit naming.

What do we know about violence against disabled people?

Thankfully, there is growing awareness of the issue of violence against disabled people, as well as disabled people's greater vulnerability to crime in general (McDermott, 2012) thanks to increased media interest as well as to important campaigning publications such as the book, *Scapegoat* (Quarmby, 2011). To take some recent examples: in 2007, Fiona Pilkington killed both her daughter and herself, after years of being harassed to the point of desperation. In 2010, David Askew, a 64-year-old man with intellectual disability from Greater Manchester, collapsed and died after years of bullying from local youths, who would prey on him for money and cigarettes (Carter, 2010). In 2012, an enquiry was set up to investigate the widespread and ongoing abuses of people with learning difficulties at Winterbourne View, after undercover reporting at the private 'care home' by the BBC *Panorama* programme. Six members of staff went to prison as a result of criminal proceedings. In court, the prosecutor said:

> It is the Crown's case that generally the offences were motivated by hostility towards victims based on their disabilities. The offenders were operating in groups; the offences involved an abuse of power; an abuse of trust; the victims were particularly vulnerable and on occasion the ill-treatment of a patient was sustained, with the consequences of serious psychological effects.

But while there have been a number of vicious and disturbing cases reported, it is not clear how widespread the problem is, particularly compared to general levels of violence. Recorded hate crimes against disabled people have certainly increased, but this likely reflects, in part, increased awareness, better police response, and more reporting of incidents. Moreover, there is a lack of good quality data on the topic.

Studies may have small sample sizes, or unclear definitions and measures, or lack suitable comparison populations, such as the vast majority of documents reviewed by Chih Hoong Sin *et al.* (2009) for the Equalities and Human Rights Commission. For example, widely reported research about hate crime for Disability Rights Commission and Capability Scotland (2004) relied on a self-selected sample (N = 158) who responded to a survey. This does not tell us anything about how prevalent violence is among disabled people as a whole, although it does tell us something about the nature of violence for those people who have experienced it. Another example is a much quoted study of violence against women with disabilities in Orissa, India (N = 729), which concluded that every disabled woman was beaten at home, although this was not explicitly stated by the respondents. There was no control group provided for comparison with non-disabled women (Mohapatra and Mohanty, 2005). Advocates and activists, in their laudable efforts to raise awareness and ensure better responses to the issue, sometimes rely on inaccurate or misleading research, or no research at all.

Mindful of this, when I was at WHO my unit commissioned systematic reviews of research on the prevalence of violence against disabled people, in order to establish a solid understanding of the magnitude of the problem and encourage the violence prevention community to take the issue more seriously. A team from Liverpool John Moores University examined all the academic literature, graded the evidence for quality, and together we published two papers reviewing this data, one on children (Jones *et al.*, 2012) and one on adults (Hughes *et al.*, 2012).

With data on adults, we immediately encounter the difficulty that it is often not clear whether the statistics cover people with disabilities who are also subjected to violence, or whether the violence was the cause of the disability. For example, in countries like Sierra Leone (Trani *et al.*, 2010) and Guyana (Chouinard, 2012), there is a strong association between disability and violence. Yet these statistics may feature non-disabled people who become injured – for example, lose limbs – as a result of civil war, landmines, or in the latter example, cutlass attacks. To avoid this problem, the John Moores systematic review included only those studies of people with disabilities who had experienced violence in the last year: we assume these studies are more likely to be of disabled people who experienced violence, rather than non-disabled people who became disabled through violence. The prevalence estimate therefore understates the overall lifetime risk of violence. However, given this proviso, we found that people with disabilities were 50 per cent more likely than non-disabled people to have experienced violence in the last year: this corresponds to 3 per cent of all disabled people. The raised risk was increased to four times more likely for people with mental health conditions, corresponding to nearly a quarter of people with mental health conditions experiencing violence in the last year (Hughes *et al.*, 2012).

For example, one of the included studies was a large Canadian study (Brownridge, 2006) that found that women with disabilities had 40 per cent higher risk of violence compared to non-disabled women in the preceding five years, and to be at particular risk of the more severe forms of violence. Perpetrator-related factors – particularly behaving in a patriarchal dominating manner, engaging in sexually proprietary behaviours – were predictors of violence. Secondary analysis of a large US dataset also found that women with disabilities were more than 50 per cent more likely to have experienced intimate partner violence (Barrett *et al.*, 2009).

Since a new law in 1998, the US Department of Justice has disaggregated statistics on disability violence in America. The 2008–11 figures show that the average annual age-adjusted rate of serious violent victimisation for persons with disabilities (22 per 1000) was more than three times higher than that for non-disabled people (6 per 1000). The age-adjusted rate of simple assault for persons with disabilities (26 per 1000) was twice that for non-disabled people (13 per 1000). Men with disabilities suffered more violence in 2011 (42 per 1000) than women without disabilities (17 per 1000), but women with disabilities suffered the highest rate (53 per 1000). People with cognitive disabilities had by far the highest rates of victimisation. Serious violent victimisation increased for all disability groups between 2009–11: the unadjusted rate nearly doubled in the case of people with cognitive limitations (difficulties concentrating, thinking or making decisions) and people with independent living limitations (difficulties doing errands alone), and tripled for the group with self-care limitations (difficulties dressing, bathing).

Monika Mitra has analysed violence against people with disabilities extensively. For example, she found that 13.6 per cent of Massachusetts women with disabilities had experienced abuse in the year before pregnancy, compared to 2.8 per cent of women without disabilities, and 8.1 per cent experienced abuse during pregnancy, compared to 2.3 per cent of women without disabilities (Mitra *et al.*, 2012). Her analysis of findings from the US Behavioral Risk Fact Surveillance System (Mitra and Mouradian, forthcoming) echoes the Department of Justice findings regarding the vulnerability of men with disabilities: 19 per cent of men with disabilities reported lifetime intimate partner violence, compared to 13.3 per cent of men without disabilities, 35.5 per cent of women with disabilities and 22.1 per cent of women without disabilities. Men with disabilities were as likely to report attempted intimate partner violence as women without disabilities. Men with disabilities who experienced violence were also more likely to report poorer physical and mental health effects than other men.

Eric Emerson and Alan Roulstone (in press) analysed the UK Life Opportunities Survey, which depends on self-report by disabled people. This suggested that people with a disability were 2.3 times more likely to have been a victim of violent crime and 2.6 times more likely to have been a victim of hate crime than nondisabled people. However, only about a third of disabled people reporting a hate crime attributed this to their disability. In this survey, it was people with mental health or behavioural difficulties who were most likely to experience violence, with a six-fold increased risk of violence and a ten times increased risk of hate crime. About 1 per cent of people with mobility impairments had experienced a disability-motivated hate crime in the previous year, rising to about 7 per cent of people with cognitive impairments.

When it comes to children, it is less likely that the violence was prior to the disability. The Liverpool John Moores team also conducted a systematic review of prevalence of violence against disabled children, and found that they were at 3.68 times the risk of non-disabled children, which corresponds to 26.7 per cent of disabled children having experienced violence in their lives (Jones et al., 2012). This risk was accentuated for children with intellectual disabilities or mental health conditions.

For example, an Illinois sample of 100,000 under-6 children from low-income families found that children with behavioural or mental health conditions were nearly twice as likely as other children to be victims of child abuse and neglect, while children with chronic physical health conditions only had a very slightly raised risk and children with developmental delay or intellectual impairment were at no greater risk of maltreatment (Jaudes and Mackey-Bilaver, 2008).

Some of the tentative conclusions I draw from this emerging data synthesis is that prevalence of violence is indeed raised for disabled people; different groups of disabled people have different risks of experiencing violence; men with disabilities are at risk of violence to a greater degree than men without disabilities, and sometimes at higher risk than women without disabilities. Family members are the commonest perpetrators of abuse and violence, although institutions are also places where abuse and violence are very common. All of these facts should influence how we consider and respond to the problem.

How should we talk about violence against disabled people?

In the UK and the USA in recent years, disability activists, advocates and researchers have adopted the term 'hate crime' to describe violence against disabled people (Sherry, 2010; Quarmby, 2011). The term 'hate crime' is taken from discussions of homophobic violence and violence motivated by racial hatred. In these latter instances, there is clearly hate involved. Some people find gay people or ethnic minorities to be threatening or abhorrent: they go out with the express purpose of locating and beating up an individual from these communities, or else if they encounter someone at random, they decide to attack them because of their underlying animus. Exponents of the term 'disability hate crime' consider the same to be the case for disability. Thus, Dan Goodley suggests that 'hate crime is the logical consequence of the animosity to be found in the psychical defence mechanisms of the wider community' (2011: 96). Bill Hughes speculates that 'perhaps the phenomenon of disability hate crime – both cyber and corporeal – can be explained – in socio-emotional terms – as a manifestation of fear of impairment, resentment and hatred actualised as virtual or viscera violence against disabled people' (Hughes *et al.*, 2012: 70), which may be connected to a disgust at the vulnerability of disabled people, a 'disavowal of the slimy self' (ibid.: 70). Lennard Davis (2002: 156) suggests that the general public cannot easily accept that there could be hatred against disabled people:

> [B]ut the 'hate' against people with disabilities is a much more subtle and ingrained hatred. It is a hatred of difference, of the fact that someone cannot see a clearly posted sign, cannot walk up unblocked stairs, needs special assistance above what other 'normal' citizens need. This kind of hatred is one that abhors the possibility that all bodies are not configured the same, that weakness and impairment are the legacy of a cult of perfection and able embodiment.

Although I suspect that these theorists are overstating their case, it would be entirely understandable, after reading about Winterbourne View or the Pilkington case or other nasty vicious abuse of disabled people, that the term 'hate crime' would come to mind. There has been increasing news coverage of a series of truly appalling crimes in Britain, where individuals or families have been harassed over a long period of time (Quarmby, 2011). There are many examples of people with intellectual disabilities who have been befriended and preyed on for their welfare benefits or for somewhere to stay – so-called 'mate crime' – before in some cases being tortured and murdered. Furthermore, most people with intellectual disabilities can describe acts of physical violence committed against them by non-disabled people, such as the individual who told me about being tied to a tree and urinated on by young people. Back in 2000, the Mencap *Living in Fear* report (Mencap, 2000) showed that bullying was ubiquitous in the lives of people with learning difficulties: 90 per cent said they had been bullied in the previous 12 months, and 23 per cent had been assaulted. More recently, 62 of the 67 people with intellectual disability interviewed by Carwyn Gravell (2012) had experienced some form of harassment, abuse or crime, many of which involved cruelty.

People with other impairments can commonly list dozens of instances when they have been called names, stared at or otherwise mocked or bullied by non-disabled people, and some have experienced physical violence. For example, the research that my team conducted with people with restricted growth in the North of England (Shakespeare *et al.*, 2009) found that

- 96 per cent had experienced staring or pointing;
- 77 per cent had been on the receiving-end of verbal abuse;
- 75 per cent felt they often attract unwanted attention;
- 63 per cent of respondents often felt unsafe when out;
- 33 per cent had been physically touched by people in public;
- 12 per cent had experienced physical violence.

Most children with disabilities have experienced being called names or picked on at school, as Nick Watson and I found in our research in the 1990s. More recently, in the UK research conducted by Connors and Stalker (2007) almost half their small sample of disabled children had experienced bullying at school, while Bourke and Burgman (2010) found that nearly all their small sample had experienced bullying in Australian schools. Some 62 per cent of British young people responding to a 2012 Muscular Dystrophy Campaign survey had been taunted or verbally abused because they were disabled (Cassidy, 2012).

Some, although not all, of these very unpleasant experiences should certainly be called hate crimes. However, not all of them could be defined as crimes and it is not clear that they are all motivated by hate. Some actions are hate-filled, but are not crimes, some actions are crimes, but are not motivated by hate, and some actions are neither criminal nor hate-fuelled, but are still deeply distressing to the victim. I remain very sceptical about the widespread use of hate crime as a blanket term, because I think it mislabels certain actions which I think are better conceptualised as bullying; because I think it distracts attention from the commonest forms of violence against disabled people; and because it promotes fear among disabled people.

There is a continuum of violence, abuse and bullying, with name calling and staring at one end, and gradations of nasty inter-personal behaviour up to and including actual violence at the other. If every incident that falls on the continuum of violence is labelled as a hate crime, there is a danger of language-inflation, and of escalating a dispropor-tionate reaction disproportionately. The child who stares at a disabled person in the street should be told by their parent or care-giver that this is rude and unacceptable, and should be made aware of disability and disabled people, and supported so that they feel neither fearful nor hostile. The playground bully should be reprimanded, and if necessary punished, by teachers, but to call their actions a hate crime seems inappropriate. While no doubt those who commit criminal acts against disabled people may have started out as playground bullies, the vast majority of children who stare at or laugh at a disabled person do not go on to become abusers in later life. That is to say, there is a continuum, but there may not be a trajectory of escalating actions, in most cases. However, there are certainly times where bullying does become criminal. This seems usually to be when it is very persistent; where it is very extreme; or where it includes dimensions of gender, race, sexuality, disability, etc. In 2009, a 15-year-old boy who bullied a girl to the point of suicide was found guilty of aggravated racial harassment in Lincoln, which suggests that even playground bullying can be considered a crime in certain circumstances (http://news.bbc.co.uk/2/hi/uk_news/england/lincolnshire/8164081.stm).

Another problem is that the 'hate crime' discourse concentrates on one form of violence – predominantly youth violence – and obscures the much more significant and common forms of violence to which disabled people are subjected, namely, violence and abuse within the family or within institutions (see, for example, Conroy, 2012). Unless 'hate crime' becomes the synonym for all forms of violence and abuse, we need to have an awareness of the overall balance of risks involved. Violence from strangers or disaffected youth may be more newsworthy, but it is much less common than violence and abuse from known people and family members.

Above all, the thinking behind the hate crime label – and the increase in the sentencing for hate crimes mandated by Section 146 of the 2003 Criminal Justice Act – are that these acts are particularly bad, and worse than exactly the same acts when perpetrated without such a motivation. But why would it be worse to have 'short arse' shouted out after you than 'fat boy'? Would it be any compensation, if you were mugged for your purse, to know that at least the perpetrator was not harbouring discriminatory thoughts about you? If someone is beaten up because they are a Sunderland fan, that is not a hate crime, but if they are beaten up because they have a stutter, it probably is, which does not make sense to me.

In practice, there seems little difference: violence is violence. The creation of a specific and separate category of 'bias crime' or 'hate crime' only leads to semantic disputes and worries and confusions or disagreements about how a particular incident should be classified (Sin, 2013). Alan Roulstone *et al.* (2011) are concerned with the distinction between crimes committed because disabled people are vulnerable, as opposed to hate crimes. They conclude that the term 'hate' 'proves too high a legal and linguistic threshold to afford disabled people an equitable and responsive criminal justice system' (ibid.: 362) and prefer a phrase like 'disablist hostility and harassment' as an alternative. To me, this sounds like scant improvement.

Are disabled people 'vulnerable'?

As discussed in the earlier chapter about sexuality, there is a deep resistance in the disability studies field to seeing disabled people as vulnerable. On the positive side, this thinking reflects the assumption that rather than individualising problems, they should be seen as arising in particular contexts, which create vulnerability. On the negative side, there is a resistance to giving due weight to impairment, or to recognising the real differences between, for example, people with learning difficulties and non-disabled people.

Disabled people may have vulnerabilities arising from impairment. The person with mobility impairment cannot run away; the blind or deaf person can less easily perceive danger; someone with a speech or language impairment cannot communicate what has happened to them; the physically frail person cannot defend themselves; a person with learning difficulties may be naïve and trusting or too open with information. For example, Gravell reports the following anecdote from a person with learning difficulties: 'I was walking by the canal, and this man said he knew me from school. We went to the café and he took my phone and money' (2012: 17). For these reasons, people with these impairments may be particularly targeted by abusers or thieves.

However, other forms of vulnerability arise from the social context in which many disabled people are located. For example, in developing countries, disabled children often do not attend school. With siblings out at school and parents working, they may be at risk of sexual abuse from other family members (Save the Children, 2011). Historically, children and adults with disabilities in developed countries and former communist countries were more likely to be living in residential institutions. Rates of violence and abuse are often higher in residential settings. However, even in community settings, disabled children come into contact with many different adults: carers, taxi drivers, teachers, support workers, respite carers, and given that abusers are sometimes drawn to this area of work, there is likely to be a greater risk of abuse.

Since the welcome advent of community care policies, people with learning difficulties are less likely to be institutionalised, which takes them out of one situation of risk. Instead, they are likely to be living on their own or with one or two other people with learning difficulties in social housing. This housing is more likely to be located on outlying housing estates, where there are few facilities or community networks and quite possibly many disaffected young people. The outcome of this social location is that people with learning difficulties may be isolated and lonely, and they may be highly visible and vulnerable to bored youth looking for 'fun' and possibly financial gain. Keith, quoted in the *Loneliness and Cruelty* report, wanted to have friends, and mistakenly thought that his abusers were his friends. Gravell (2012: 4) concludes:

> It is the loneliness of some people with learning disabilities – their search for friendship within a selfish society and within deeply fragmented communities – that is putting them at particular risk, leading them to frequent alone hostile and permissive public spaces, and bring them to the attentions of the cruel-hearted and criminal few.

A theme of this socially created vulnerability is disempowerment. An individual may not be valued, may not be believed, and may be in a position of dependency vis-à-vis their abuser, who may be the main earner for the family. If they or their family manage to complain to the authorities, there may be no follow-up on the complaint, or they may fear repercussions (Save the Children, 2011; Sin, 2013).

One response to the perception of vulnerability is protection policies. These can infringe the choices and freedoms of individuals. Paradoxically, over-protection may put people at risk, because people do not learn the skills to analyse interactions or cope with situations. Describing the lives of two women with learning difficulties, Cindy and Jill, the researchers Welsby and Horsfall conclude: '[Cl]early the management of risk has become a restrictive barrier to live what is generally perceived to be a "normal" life' (2011: 805).

Whatever term is used – risk or vulnerability – a considered and balanced response is needed. In practice, vulnerability usually arises from the inter-action of individual and contextual factors – the characteristics of the individual, and the context in which they find themselves. The answer is not to over-protect or segregate, but to empower, support, monitor and react quickly and effectively to any signs that things are going wrong.

Understanding perpetrators

Discourse around hate crime fuels attention to the impact on victims, and creates a generalised sense of opposition to disabled people. However, a more careful attention is needed to why individuals perpetrate violence and abuse against disabled people, and what can be done to reduce this behaviour.

Despite the terrible crimes that are occasionally reported, it is necessary to note that perpetrators of violence against disabled people are essentially ordinary people. In Gravell's (2012) research with people with learning difficulties who had experienced violence, 7 per cent of acts were committed by family members, 25 per cent from known people in the neighbourhood, 17 per cent from school children, 13 per cent from predatory 'friends' and 11 per cent from strangers in the street. Unlike other hate crimes or crimes of violence, women are strongly represented among those who perpetrate violence and abuse against disabled people. It is also the case that disabled people can themselves be perpetrators.

One of the factors that may sometimes fuel violence is stress and the pressure of caring. For example, children with behavioural issues are more likely to experience physical maltreatment, which might reflect the difficulties which parents and carers have in controlling them. The behaviour does not in any sense justify the abusive treatment, but it does suggest that prevention may entail support for parents and carers, and perhaps work to identify strategies to avoid 'challenging behaviours'. More broadly, where individuals and families are struggling to cope, or are living in conditions of economic strain and stress, they are more likely to resort to violence.

Earlier it was noted that youth violence against disabled people may be more common on deprived housing estates where people with disabilities are sometimes located. The boredom and anomie of life on the margins are clearly a contributory factor. If generations of people are excluded from meaningful participation in society, they are more likely to respond with crime and violence. If disabled people are perceived as a soft touch, and to have access to welfare benefits that other people do not have, then they may become prey to resentment and possibly exploitation. Some evidence to support this speculation comes from the Emerson and Roulstone analysis of the Life Opportunities Survey, which found a strong association between poverty and exposure to violent crime and hate crime. Where poverty was low, there was no difference in exposure between disabled and non-disabled people, but as poverty increased, the chances of becoming a victim of violence also increased. If this speculation is accurate, then the long-term answer to reducing violence and abuse would require better opportunities in life for disaffected youth, not just improved policing.

There is probably some truth when Gravell (2012) claims that '[c]learly, perpetrators experience a perverse and sadistic pleasure from their acts of cruelty – from seeing others hurt, humiliated, embarrassed, demonstrated as weak and helpless. Getting a "rise", a reaction from people, is part of the fun.' As the Milgram experiments proved, human beings are capable of great cruelty. But these abusive actions are possibly much more likely on the part of people who lack power in their lives, or feel insecure or devalued. Putting other people down strengthens their own sense of self as individuals or boosts their status in their wider peer group. Particularly when disinhibited by alcohol or drugs, they make themselves feel better by victimising people who are different: elderly people, disabled people, people of foreign birth or origin.

These thoughts remain speculative, which underscores the importance of good quality research with people who commit acts of violence or abuse against disabled people. At present, very little is known about perpetrators of violence, whether this occurs within families or in the wider community. Often, sentences for hate crime are very short, and there will consequently not even be any education or rehabilitation work done with those found guilty and given custodial sentences.

Ways forward

Whether called hate crime, violence, abuse or anything else, the available evidence shows that these are common, pressing and serious human rights violations which tarnish the lives of many disabled people. Understanding violence against disabled people and the contexts in which violence occurs is key to reducing the problem. More research, of better quality, is badly needed, particularly in developing countries.

As well as research, action is needed. While the immediate need is to support the victims, the longer-term response should be to invest in prevention. Thinking more widely about what can be done to reduce violence, particularly youth and community violence, Carwyn Gravell (2012: 3) suggests three priorities:

1 Enhanced social networks for people with learning disabilities.
2 Stronger prevention and support services from mainstream organisations.
3 Creating civic mindedness and safer public spaces.

Victim support must begin with services which listen, believe and support people who have experienced violence, for example, women with learning difficulties who have suffered intimate partner violence (Walter-Brice et al., 2012). UK police and criminal justice authorities have failed to respond adequately to violence and abuse directed at disabled people (Sin, 2013). For example in the cases of Fiona Pilkington (19 complaints) and David Askey (88 complaints), multiple complaints to the police led to no solutions, with tragic final outcomes. Police stations need to be physically accessible, to be better at listening to complaints and quicker and more effective at responding. Anti-social behaviour or intimidation may not be taken seriously by police. Disabled people may often need support to give witness statements and testify in court, and this is frequently unavailable (ibid.).

As well as a better response from the police and criminal justice authorities, disabled people who have been victims of violence, harassment or bullying need support from disabled people's organisations and other voluntary groups. Support groups can help overcome the isolation of feeling a solitary victim. However, research has found that both disabled people's organisations, and Women's Aid-type organisations, failed adequately to support women who were victims of intimate partner violence (Thiara et al., 2011). The former considered the problem to be beyond their remit. The latter services were often not compliant with anti-discrimination legislation, and had low awareness of disability issues. It can be particularly difficult for people with disabilities to leave an abusive situation, because they may be dependent on their abuser, or they may find it difficult to find alternative accessible accommodation. However, there are some examples of better responses from the disability community, for example, the projects in Manchester and Tyne and Wear cited by Susie Balderston (2013), and the awareness-raising work of The Lawnmowers Theatre company of people with learning difficulties (Brandon and Keyes, 2012).

More research and better evidence are needed on what works to reduce violence against disabled people. Our team at WHO also reviewed evidence on the effectiveness of prevention and victim support measures responding to violence against disabled people (Maguire et al., forthcoming). A Korean programme raised awareness of child abuse among parents of children with disabled children. Respite care reduced stress among parents of children with developmental disabilities. Various forms of behavioural skills training or decision-making have been tried for women with mild to moderate intellectual disabilities, which have produced improvements in knowledge and skills. British trainee police officers have undergone awareness training about intellectual disability. In South Africa, a sexual assault victim empowerment programme led to victims with intellectual disability achieving the same conviction rape against their attackers as non-disabled women (25 per cent).

Thinking about violence prevention in general, WHO has found that interventions of proven effectiveness in reducing violence against non-disabled people include: developing better relationships between children and parents/caregivers; developing life skills in children and adolescents; reducing availability of alcohol, and access to guns and knives; promoting gender equality; changing cultural norms that support violence; victim identification, care and support programmes. It is likely, though it has not been tested, that these interventions would also reduce violence against disabled children and adults (WHO, 2009).

To conclude, my belief is that the debate on violence against disabled people has been derailed by arguments about hate crime, and diluted by the use of the term 'violence' as a metaphor for human rights violations in general. There is now a welcome and growing awareness that disabled people are disproportionately vulnerable to violence, due to a range of intrinsic and contextual factors. A clearer focus is required on all crimes of violence committed against children and adults with disabilities, in families, in institutions, and in communities, and the actions that the criminal justice authorities and wider society can take to reduce their incidence and recurrence, and support and protect victims. Researchers have an important role in developing understanding and evaluating prevention and victim support interventions.

13

CONCLUDING THOUGHTS

In this book, I have re-examined some of the key principles of the British disability rights movement. I have questioned the intellectual and political basis for the social model of disability and the personal assistance model of independent living. I have also questioned the rejection of cure, genetic screening, assisted suicide and charity. Throughout the book, I have suggested that academics, activists and policy-makers need to look again at cherished rhetoric and taken-for-granted assumptions. I have tried to orient my discussions in the empirical evidence – quantitative and qualitative – about the lives of disabled people. Like William of Ockham, I take an inductive approach to theory: we need explanations that are no more complex than necessary to make sense of the evidence. This seems preferable to imposing over-arching conceptual schemes, whether they originate from Marx or Foucault, and then subordinating the testimonies of research participants to those theoretical frameworks.

In writing and revising this book, I want to contribute to better understandings, better policies and better practices regarding disability and disabled people. While I challenge consensus, I want to stress three points of agreement. First, I accept that social and environmental barriers constitute major problems for many disabled people, and that removing such obstacles is the main priority for disability politics. Second, I agree that disabled people should have choices over their lives, and should be supported to live in the community. Third, I have no doubt that the medicalisation of disability and the persistent assumption that disabled people are defined by their incapacity are cultural barriers to the emancipation of disabled people which must be challenged. Seven years on from the first edition, it is very depressing to note that the current British government has attacked the living standards, withdrawn the support and threatened the independent living of disabled people.

I believe my account of disability suggests a full agenda for engaged social research. Disability studies should work to provide rich empirical studies, both quantitative and qualitative, of how disabled people experience barriers, and how they experience their impairments. In particular, the differences between disabled people are as important as the similarities, for example, examination of the role of class is paradoxically absent, even from materialist disability studies (Shakespeare, 2010). Rather than being restricted by social model orthodoxy, disability studies should be pluralist, valuing analytical rigour and open debate. Disability researchers should look outwards and engage with medical sociology, philosophy, economics and other areas of academia.

This book also highlights ways forward for emancipatory strategies. Disability movements should be cautious about assuming that either disability identity or disability rights are robust foundations for emancipation. Recognition that the majority of people with impairments have no desire to identify as disabled is overdue. So too is the appreciation that rights alone will not solve all disability problems (Young and Quibell, 2000; Barron, 2001): social justice may ultimately be the preferable goal (Sen, 1992). Disability groups should seek coalition with other parallel communities, particularly older people. It would be wrong to neglect either prevention of impairment or attention to the medical needs of disabled people (Shakespeare, 2013). Finally, neither rights nor justice renders concepts such as charity and community redundant. Supporting positive social relationships between disabled and non-disabled people and recognising the beneficial role of solidarity and mutuality are both vital to the flourishing of disabled people.

BIBLIOGRAPHY

Abberley, P. (1987) The concept of oppression and the development of a social theory of disability, *Disability, Handicap and Society*, 2(1): 5–20.
——(1992) Counting us out: a discussion of the OPCS disability surveys, *Disability, Handicap and Society*, 7(2): 139–155.
——(1996) Work, utopia and impairment, in L. Barton (ed.) *Disability and Society: Emerging Issues and Insights*, Harlow: Longman.
——(1998) The spectre at the feast: disabled people and social theory, in T. Shakespeare (ed.) *The Disability Reader: Social Science Perspectives*, London: Cassell.
——(2001) Work, disability and European social theory, in C. Barnes, M. Oliver and L. Barton (eds) *Disability Studies Today*, Cambridge: Polity.
Abraham, C. (1989) Supporting people with mental handicap in the community: a social psychological perspective, *Disability, Handicap and Society*, 4(2): 121–130.
Ahmed, S., Bryant, L.D. and Cole, P. (2012) Midwives' perceptions of their role as facilitators of informed choice in antenatal screening, *Midwifery*, 29(7): 745–750.
Ahmed, S., Hewison, J. and Bryant, L. (2008) 'Balance' is in the eye of the beholder: providing information to support informed choices in antenatal screening via Antenatal Screening Web Resource, *Health Expectations*, 10(4): 309–320.
Aitchison, C. (2003) From leisure and disability to disability leisure: developing data, definitions and discourses, *Disability and Society*, 18(7): 955–969.
Albrecht, G.L. (ed.) (1976) *The Sociology of Physical Disability and Rehabilitation*, Pittsburgh, PA: University of Pittsburgh Press.
——(1981) *Cross-National Rehabilitation Policies: A Sociological Perspective*, London: Sage.
——(1992) *The Disability Business: Rehabilitation in America*, London: Sage.
Albrecht, G.L. and Devlieger, P.J. (1999) The disability paradox: high quality of life against all odds, *Social Science and Medicine*, 48: 977–988.
Alderson, P. (1993) *Children's Consent to Surgery*, Buckingham: Open University Press.
——(2001) Down's syndrome: cost, quality and value of life, *Social Science and Medicine*, 53: 627–638.

Allison, R. (2003) Does a cleft palate justify an abortion? Curate wins right to challenge doctors, *The Guardian*, 2 December.

Amundson, R. (2010) Quality of life, disability, and hedonic psychology, *Journal for the Theory of Social Behaviour*, 40(4): 374–392.

Anderson, P. and Kitchin, R. (2000) Disability, space and sexuality: access to family planning services, *Social Science and Medicine*, 51: 1163–1173.

Andrews, J. (2005) Wheeling uphill? Reflections of practical and methodological difficulties encountered in researching the experiences of disabled volunteers, *Disability and Society*, 20(2): 201–212.

Areheart, B.A. (2011) Disability trouble, *Yale Law and Policy Review*, 29(2): 347–388.

Arias, B., Ovejero, A. and Morentin, R. (2009) Love and emotional well-being in people with intellectual disabilities, *The Spanish Journal of Psychology*, 12(1): 204–216.

Asch, A. (2000) Why I haven't changed my mind about prenatal diagnosis: reflections and refinements, in E. Parens and A. Asch (eds) *Prenatal Testing and Disability Rights*, Washington, DC: Georgetown University Press.

——(2001) Disability, bioethics and human rights, in G.L. Albrecht, K.D. Seelman and M. Bury (eds) *Handbook of Disability Studies*, Thousand Oaks, CA: Sage.

——(2003) Disability equality and prenatal testing: contradictory or compatible? *Florida State University Law Review*, 30: 315–341.

Asch, A. and Geller, G. (1996) Feminism, bioethics, and genetics, in S.M. Wolf (ed.) *Feminism and Bioethics: Beyond Reproduction*, New York: Oxford University Press.

Asch, A. and Wasserman, D. (2010) Making embryos healthy or making healthy embryos: how much of a difference between prenatal treatment and selection? in J. Nisker, F. Baylis, I. Karpin, C. McLeod and R. Mykitiuk (eds) *The 'Healthy' Embryo: Social, Biomedical, Legal and Philosophical Perspectives*, Cambridge: Cambridge University Press, pp. 201–219.

Astbury-Ward, E. (2008) Emotional and psychological impacts of abortion: a critique of the literature, *Journal of Family Planning and Reproductive Health Care*, 34(3): 181–184.

Atkin, K. and Hussain, Y. (2003) Disability and ethnicity: how young Asian disabled people make sense of their lives, in N. Watson and S. Riddell (eds) *Disability, Culture and Identity*, Harlow: Pearson Education.

Bahner, J. (2012) Legal rights or simply wishes? The struggle for sexual recognition of people with physical disabilities using personal assistance in Sweden, *Sexuality and Disability*, 30(3): 337–356.

Bailey, R. (1996) Prenatal testing and the prevention of impairment: a woman's right to choose? in J. Morris (ed.) *Encounters with Strangers: Feminism and Disability*. London: Women's Press.

Balderston, S. (2013) 'After disablist hate crime: which interventions really work to resist victimhood and build resilience with survivors?', in A. Roulstone and H. Mason-Bish (eds) *Disability, Hate Crime and Violence*, London: Routledge.

Barnes, C. (1990) *The Cabbage Syndrome: The Social Construction of Dependence*, Lewes: Falmer Press.

——(1991) *Disabled People in Britain and Discrimination*, London: Hurst and Co.

——(1992) *Disabling Imagery and the Media*, Halifax: Ryburn Publishing.

——(1995) Review of *Disability is Not Measles*, edited by Marcia Rioux, *Disability and Society*, 10(3): 380.

——(1998a) Review of *The Rejected Body*, by Susan Wendell, *Disability and Society*, 13(1): 145–147.

——(1998b) The social model of disability: a sociological phenomenon ignored by sociologists, in T. Shakespeare (ed.) *The Disability Reader*, London: Cassell.

——(1999) Disability studies: new or not-so-new directions, *Disability and Society*, 14(4): 577–580.

——(2000) A working social model? Disability, work and disability politics in the 21st century, *Critical Social Policy* 20(4): 441–457.

Barnes, C. and Mercer, G. (1996) *Exploring the Divide: Illness and Disability*, Leeds: The Disability Press.

——(2003) *Disability*, Cambridge: Polity.

——(eds) (2004) *Implementing the Social Model of Disability: Theory and Research*, Leeds: The Disability Press.

Barnes, C., Oliver, M. and Barton, L. (eds) (2002) *Disability Studies Today*, Cambridge: Polity.

——(eds) (2004) *Disability Studies Today*, 2nd edn, Cambridge: Polity.

Barnes, M. (2012) *Care in Everyday Life: An Ethic of Care in Practice*, Bristol: Policy Press.

Barr, O., McConkey, R. and McConagahie, J. (2003) Views of people with learning difficulties about current and future accommodation: the use of focus groups to promote discussion, *Disability and Society*, 18(5): 577–597.

Barrett, K.A., O'Day, B., Roche, A. and Carlson, B.L. (2009) Intimate partner violence, health status, and healthcare access among women with disabilities, *Women's Health Issues*, 19: 94–100.

Barron, K. (2001) Autonomy in everyday life, for whom? *Disability and Society*, 16 (3): 431–447.

Bartlett, P. (2010) Sex, dementia, capacity and care homes, *Liverpool Law Review*, 31: 137–154.

Batavia, A.I. (1997) Disability and physician assisted suicide, *New England Journal of Medicine*, 336: 1671–1673.

Bates, P. and Davis, F.A. (2004) Social capital, social inclusion and services for people with learning disabilities, *Disability and Society*, 19(3): 195–207.

Bauman, Z. (1993) *Postmodern Ethics*, Oxford: Blackwell.

BBC News website (2003) 'Euthanasia fears for disabled', 20 January, http://news.bbc.co.uk/1/hi/health/2668253.stm (accessed 24 January 2003).

Beardshaw, V. (1989) Conductive education: a rejoinder, *Disability, Handicap and Society*, 4(3): 297–299.

Beck-Gernsheim, E. (1990) Changing duties of parents: from education to bio-engineering? *International Social Science Journal*, 42: 451.

Bedard, C., Zhang, H.L. and Zucker, K.J. (2010) Gender identity and sexual orientation in people with developmental disabilities, *Sexuality and Disability*, 28: 165–175.

Benjamin, A. (2004) Going undercover, *The Guardian*, 14 April.

Beresford, B. (1994) *Positively Parents: Caring for a Severely Disabled Child*, London: HMSO.

Beresford, P. (2012) Psychiatric system survivors: an emerging movement, in N. Watson, A. Roulstone and C. Thomas (eds) *Routledge Handbook of Disability Studies*, London: Routledge, pp. 151–164.

Beresford, P. and Wallcraft, J. (1997) Psychiatric system survivors and emancipatory research: issues, overlaps and differences, in C. Barnes and G. Mercer (eds) *Doing Disability Research*, Leeds: The Disability Press.

Beresford, P. and Wilson, A. (2002) Genes spell danger: mental health service users/survivors, bioethics and control, *Disability and Society*, 17(5): 541–553.

Berger, P.L. and Luckmann, T. (1966) *The Social Construction of Reality: A Treatise in the Sociology of Knowledge*, Garden City, NY: Anchor Books.

Berlin, I. (1976) *Vico and Herder: Two Studies in the History of Ideas*, London: Chatto and Windus.

Bernert, D. (2011) Sexuality and disability in the lives of women with intellectual disabilities, *Sexuality and Disability*, 29(2): 129–141.

Berubé, M. (2010) Equality, freedom and/or justice for all: a response to Martha Nussbaum, in E.F. Kittay and L. Carlson (eds) *Cognitive Disability and Its Challenge to Moral Philosophy*, Chichester: Wiley-Blackwell.

Bhaskar, R. (1975) *A Realist Theory of Science*, Leeds: Leeds Books.

Bickenbach, J.E. (1993) *Physical Disability and Social Policy*, Toronto: University of Toronto Press.

——(1998) Disability and life-ending decisions, in M.P. Battin, R. Rhodes and A. Silvers (eds) *Physician Assisted Suicide: Expanding the Debate*, New York: Routledge.

——(2009) Disability, culture and the UN Convention, *Disability and Rehabilitation*, 31(14): 1111–1124.

——(2012) The International Classification of Functioning, Disability and Health and its relationship to disability studies, in N. Watson, A. Roulstone and C. Thomas (eds) *Routledge Handbook of Disability Studies*, London: Routledge, pp. 51–66.

Bickenbach, J.E., Chatterji, S., Badley, E.M. and Ustun, T.B. (1999) Models of disablement, universalism and the international classification of impairments, disabilities and handicaps, *Social Science and Medicine*, 48: 1173–1187.

Blaxter, M. (1976) *The Meaning of Disability*, London: Heinemann.

Bolt, D. (2012) Social encounters and critical avoidance, in N. Watson, A. Roulstone and C. Thomas (eds) *Routledge Handbook of Disability Studies*, London: Routledge, pp. 287–297.

Boorse, C. (1977) Health as a theoretical concept, *Philosophy of Science*, 44(4): 542–573.

Bornman, J. (2004) The World Health Organisation's terminology and classification: application to severe disability, *Disability and Rehabilitation*, 26(3): 182–188.

Bourke, S. and Burgman, I. (2010) Coping with bullying in Australian schools: how children with disabilities experience support from friends, parents and teachers, *Disability and Society*, 25(3): 359–371.

Brandon, T. and Keyes, S. (2012) Civil courage, civil societies and good Samaritans: a response to disablist hate crime, in A. Roulstone and H. Mason-Bish (eds) *Disability, Hate Crime and Violence*, London: Routledge.

Branfield, F. (1998) What are you doing here? 'Non-disabled' people and the disability movement: a response to Robert F. Drake, *Disability and Society*, 13(1): 143–144.

——(1999) The disability movement: a movement of disabled people – a response to Paul S. Duckett, *Disability and Society*, 13(3): 399–403.

Briant, E., Watson, N., Philo, G. and Inclusion London (2012) 'Bad news for disabled people: how the newspapers are reporting disability', Glasgow Media Group and Strathclyde Centre for Disability Research, Glasgow. Available at: http://www.gla.ac.uk/media/media_214917_en.pdf (accessed 20 May 2013).

Brisenden, S. (1989) Young, gifted and disabled: entering the employment market, *Disability, Handicap and Society*, 4(3): 217–220.

British Council of Disabled People (BCODP) (n.d.) 'The social model of disability and emancipatory disability research, briefing document', downloaded from www.bcodp.org.uk/about/research.shtml (accessed 23 March 2004).

Broberg, G. and Roll-Hansen, N. (eds) (1996) *Eugenics and the Welfare State: Sterilization Policies in Denmark, Sweden, Norway and Finland*, East Lansing, MI: Michigan State University Press.

Brouwer, W.B.F., Van Exel, N.J.A. and Stolk, E.A. (2005) Acceptability of less than perfect health states, *Social Science and Medicine*, 60: 237–246.

Brown, H. (1994) 'An ordinary sexual life?': a review of the normalization principle as it applies to the sexual options of people with learning disabilities, *Disability and Society*, 2: 123–144.

Brown, N. (2003) Hope against hype: accountability in biopasts, presents and futures, *Science Studies*, 16(2): 3–21.

Brown, N. and Michael, P. (2003) The sociology of expectations: retrospecting prospects and prospecting retrospects, *Technology Analysis and Strategic Management*, 15(1): 3–19.

Brown, P. (1995) Naming and framing: the social construction of diagnosis and illness, *Journal of Health and Social Behaviour*, extra issue: 34–52.

Brownridge, D.A. (2006) Partner violence against women with disabilities: prevalence, risk and explanations, *Violence Against Women*, 12: 805–822.

Brunnberg, E., Boström, M.L. and Berglund, M. (2009) Sexuality of 15/16-year-old girls and boys with and without modest disabilities, *Sexuality and Disability*, 27: 139–153.

Brunner, E. (1997) Socioeconomic determinants of health: stress and the biology of inequality, *British Medical Journal*, 314: 1472–1476.

Buchanan, A. (1996) Choosing who will be disabled: genetic intervention and the morality of inclusion, *Social Philosophy and Policy*, 13(2): 18–46.

Buchanan, A., Brock, D.W., Daniels, N. and Wikler, D. (2000) *From Chance to Choice: Genetics and Justice*, Cambridge: Cambridge University Press.

Burleigh, M. (1994) *Death and Deliverance: 'Euthanasia' in Germany, 1900–1945*, Cambridge: Cambridge University Press.

——(1998) *Ethics and Extermination: Reflections on Nazi Genocide*, Cambridge: Cambridge University Press.

Burton-Smith, R., McVilly, K.R., Yazbeck, M., Parmenter, T.R. and Tsutsui, T. (2009) Service and support needs of Australian carers supporting a family member with disability at home, *Journal of Intellectual & Developmental Disability*, 34(3): 239–247.

Bury, M. (1996) Defining and researching disability: challenges and responses, in C. Barnes and G. Mercer (eds) *Exploring the Divide: Chronic Illness and Disability*, Leeds: The Disability Press.

——(1997) *Health and Illness in a Changing Society*, London: Routledge.

——(2000) A comment on the ICIDH2, *Disability and Society*, 15(7): 1073–1077.

Butler, J. (1990) *Gender Trouble: Feminism and the Subversion of Identity*, New York: Routledge.

Cambridge, P. and Mellan, B. (2000) Reconstructing the sexuality of men with learning disabilities: empirical evidence and theoretical interpretations of need, *Disability and Society*, 15(2): 293–311.

Campbell, F.K. (2009) *Contours of Ableism: The Production of Disability and Abledness*, Basingstoke: Palgrave Macmillan.

Campbell, J. (2003) 'Don't be fooled, we don't all want to kill ourselves', available at: www.bcodp.org.uk/about/campbell.shtml (accessed 23 March 2004).

Campbell, J. and Oliver, M. (1996) *Disability Politics: Understanding Our Past, Changing Our Future*, London: Routledge.

Caplan, A.L., McGee, G. and Magnus, D. (1999) What is immoral about eugenics? *British Medical Journal*, 319: 1284.

Carmichael, A. and Brown, L. (2002) The future challenges for direct payments, *Disability and Society*, 17(7): 797–808.

Carnaby, S. and Cambridge, P. (2002) Getting personal: an exploratory study of intimate and personal care provision for people with profound and multiple intellectual disabilities, *Journal of Intellectual Disability Research*, 46(2): 120–132.

Carter, H. (2010) Police investigate death of man with learning difficulties tormented for years by gangs, *The Guardian*, 12 March.

Carvel, J. (2004) Demonstrators rattle Scope, *The Guardian*, 6 October.

——(2005) Scope for improvement: disability charity shifts its policy towards integration, *The Guardian*, 2 March.

Carver, V. and Rodda, M. (1978) *Disability and the Environment*, London: Elek Books.

Cassidy, S. (2012) Young disabled stay silent over hate crimes, *The Independent*, 22 February.

Center for Universal Design (1997) 'The Principles of Universal Design', available at: http://www.ncsu.edu/ncsu/design/cud/about_ud/udprinciplestext.htm (accessed 20 May 2013).

Chadwick, A. (1996) Knowledge, power and the Disability Discrimination Bill, *Disability and Society*, 11(1): 25–40.

Chamak, B. (2008) Autism and social movements: French parents' associations and international autistic individuals' organisations, *Sociology of Health and Illness*, 30(1): 76–96.

Chappell, A. (1998) Still out in the cold: people with learning difficulties and the social model of disability, in T. Shakespeare (ed.) *The Disability Reader*, London: Cassell.

Chappell, A.L., Goodley, D. and Lawthom, R. (2001) Making connections: the relevance of the social model of disability for people with learning difficulties, *British Journal of Learning Disabilities*, 24: 45–50.

Charlton, J. (1998) *Nothing About Us Without Us: Disability, Oppression and Empowerment*, Berkeley, CA: University of California Press.

Charmaz, K. (1995) The body, identity and self: adapting to impairment, *The Sociological Quarterly*, 36(4): 657–680.

——(2004) Premises, principles and practices in qualitative health research: revisiting the foundations, *Qualitative Health Research*, 14: 976–993.

Check, E. (2005) Screen test, *Nature*, 438, 8 December: 733.

Cherniack, E.P. (2002) Increasing use of DNR orders in the elderly worldwide: whose choice is it? *Journal of Medical Ethics*, 28: 303–307.

Chouinard, V. (2012) Pushing the boundaries of our understanding of disability and violence: voices from the Global South (Guyana), *Disability and Society*, 27(6): 777–792.

Christensen, K. (2009) In(ter)dependent lives, *Scandinavian Journal of Disability Research*, 11(2): 117–130.

——(2010) Caring about independent lives, *Disability and Society*, 25(2): 241–252.

——(2012) Towards sustainable hybrid relationships in a cash-for-care system, *Disability and Society*, 27(3): 399–412.

Clarke, C.L., Lhussier, M., Minto, C., Gibb, C.E. and Perini, T. (2005) Paradoxes, locations and the need for social coherence: a qualitative study of living with a learning difficulty, *Disability and Society*, 20(4): 405–420.

Clevnert, U. and Johansson, L. (2007) Personal assistance in Sweden, *Journal of Aging and Social Policy*, 19(3): 65–80.

Cohen, J., Van Wesemael, Y., Smets, T., Bilsen, J. and Deliens, L. (2012) Cultural differences affecting euthanasia practice in Belgium: one law but different attitudes and practices in Flanders and Wallonia, *Social Science and Medicine*, 75: 845–853.

Coleman P.K., Coyle, C.T. and Rue, V.M. (2010) Late-term elective abortions and susceptibility to posttraumatic stress syndrome, *Journal of Pregnancy*, 130: 5–19.

Coles, J. (2001) 'The social model of disability: what does it mean for practice in services for people with learning difficulties?', *Disability and Society*, 16(4): 501–510.

Connors, C. and Stalker, K. (2007) Children's experiences of disability: pointers to a social model of childhood disability, *Disability and Society*, 22(1): 19–33.

Conrad, P. and Potter, D. (2004) Human growth hormone and the temptations of biomedical enhancement, *Sociology of Health and Illness*, 26(2): 184–215.

Conroy, P. (2012) No safety net for disabled children in residential institutions in Ireland, *Disability and Society*, 27(6): 809–822.

Cooper, C. (1997) Can a fat woman call herself disabled? *Disability and Society*, 12(1): 31–42.

Cooper, M. (1999) The Australian Disability Rights Movement lives, *Disability and Society*, 14(2): 217–226.

Corker, M. (1998) *Deaf and Disabled or Deafness Disabled*, Buckingham: Open University Press.

——(1999) Conflations, differences and foundations: the limits to 'accurate' theoretical representation of disabled people's experience? *Disability and Society*, 14(5): 627–642.

Corker, M. and French, S. (eds) (1999) *Disability Discourse*, Buckingham: Open University Press.

Craib, I. (1997) Social constructionism as a social psychosis, *Sociology*, 31(1): 1–15.

Crewe, N.M. and Zola, I.K. (eds) (1978) *Independent Living for Physically Disabled People*, San Francisco: Jossey-Bass Publishers.

Cross Disorder Group of the Psychiatric Genomics Consortium (2013) Identification of risk loci with shared effects on five major psychiatric disorders: a genome-wide analysis, *The Lancet*, early online publication, 28 February.

Crow, L. (1991) 'Rippling raspberries: disabled women and sexuality', unpublished Msc dissertation, South Bank Polytechnic.

——(1992) Renewing the social model of disability, *Coalition*, July: 5–9.

——(1996) Including all our lives, in J. Morris (ed.) *Encounters with Strangers: Feminism and Disability*, London: Women's Press.

Dalley, G. (1988) *Ideologies of Caring: Rethinking Community and Collectivism*, London: Macmillan.

Danermark, B. (2001) 'Interdisciplinary research and critical realism: the example of disability research', Orebro: Swedish Institute for Disability Research, Orebro University.

Danermark, B. and Gellerstedt, L.C. (2004) Social justice: redistribution and recognition: a non-reductionist perspective on disability, *Disability and Society*, 19(4): 339–353.

Darke, P. (1998) Understanding cinematic representations of disability, in T. Shakespeare (ed.) *The Disability Reader: Social Science Perspectives*, London/New York: Cassell, pp. 181–197.

——(2004) Interview: beyond the U bend, *Disability Arts in London*, 182: 15–17.

Davis, A. (2004) 'A disabled person's perspective on euthanasia', paper presented at UK Forum on Healthcare law and ethics, University of Newcastle.

Davis, A.M., Perruccio, A.V., Ibrahim, S., Hogg-Johnson, S., Wong, R. and Badley, E.M. (2012) Understanding recovery: changes in the relationships of the International Classification of Functioning (ICF) components over time, *Social Science and Medicine*, 75: 1999–2006.

Davis, C. (1998) Caregiving, carework and professional care, in A. Brechin, J. Walmsley, J. Katz and S. Peace (eds) *Care Matters: Concepts, Practice and Research in Health and Social Care*, London: Sage.

Davis, F. (1964) Deviance disavowal and the visibly handicapped, in H. Becker (ed.) *The Other Side*, New York: Free Press.

Davis, K. (1993) On the movement, in J. Swain *et al.* (eds) *Disabling Barriers, Enabling Environments*, London: Sage, pp. 285–292.

Davis, L.J. (1995) *Enforcing Normalcy: Disability, Deafness and the Body*, London: Verso.

——(2002) *Bending over Backwards: Disability, Dismodernism and Other Difficult Positions*, New York: New York University Press.

Deal, M. (2003) Disabled people's attitudes towards other impairment groups: a hierarchy of impairment, *Disability and Society*, 18(7): 897–910.

Department of Health (2001) *Valuing People*, London: DoH.

Department of Health Community Care Statistics (2003–4) *Referrals, Assessments and Packages of Care for Adults, England: National Summary*. Available at: http://www.publications.doh.gov.uk/rap/rap-report2003–4.doc.

Desjardins, M. (2012) The sexualized body of the child, parents and the politics of 'voluntary' sterilization of people labelled intellectually disabled, in R. McRuer and A. Mollow (eds) *Sex and Disability*, Durham, NC: Duke University Press.

De Wolfe, P. (2002) Private tragedy in social context? Reflections on disability, illness and suffering, *Disability and Society*, 17(3): 255–267.

Diem, S.J., Lantos, J.D. and Tulsky, J.A. (1996) Cardiopulmonary resuscitation on television: miracles and misinformation, *New England Journal of Medicine*, 334(24):1578–1582.

Disability Awareness in Action (1997) *Disabled People and the New Genetics*, London: Disability Awareness in Action.

——(2003) UK hospital's new policy puts pressure on people to refuse treatment, *Disability Tribune*, March, p. 1.

——(n.d.) 'Social model or unsociable model', available at: www.daa.org.uk/social_model.html (accessed 26 April 2004).

Disability Rights Commission and Capability Scotland (2004) *Hate Crime against Disabled People in Scotland: A Survey Report*, Edinburgh: Capability Scotland.

DisAbility Services (n.d.) 'Community Inclusion: Enhancing Friendship Networks among People with a Cognitive Impairment', Victorian Government Department of Human Services, available at: www.dhs.vic.gov.au/disability (accessed July 2005).

Dos Santos-Zingale, M. and McColl, M.A. (2006) Disability and participation in post-conflict situations: the case of Sierra Leone, *Disability and Society*, 21(3): 243–257.

Driedger, D. (1989) *The Last Civil Rights Movement*, London: Hurst.

Duffield, V.L. (2001) Friendship and autistic spectrum disorders: a practical programme, *International Journal of Practical Approaches to Disability*, 25(1): 43.

Dunn, M.C., Clare, I.C.H. and Holland, A.J. (2008) To empower or to protect? Constructing the 'vulnerable adult' in English law and public policy, *Legal Studies*, 28(2): 234–253.

Durkin, M.S. and Gottlieb, C. (2009) Prevention versus protection: reconciling global public health and human rights perspectives on childhood disability, *Disability and Health Journal*, 2: 7–8.

Dworkin, R.M. (1984) *Life's Dominion: An Argument About Abortion, Euthanasia and Individual Freedom*, New York: Vintage Books.

Eagle, M., Baudouin, S., Chandler, C., Giddings, D., Bullock, R. and Bushby, K. (2002) Survival in Duchene Muscular Dystrophy: improvements in life expectancy since 1967 and the impact of home nocturnal ventilation, *Neuromuscular Disorders*, 12(10): 926–929.

Earle, S. (1999) Facilitated sex and the concept of sexual need: disabled students and their personal assistants, *Disability and Society*, 14(3): 309–324.

——(2001) Disability, facilitated sex and the role of the nurse, *Journal of Advanced Nursing*, 36(3): 433–440.

Edgerton, R. (1984) *The Cloak of Competence: Stigma in the Lives of the Mentally Retarded*, Berkeley, CA: University of California Press.

Editorial (1959) Kick him while he's down, *Paraplegia News*, 13(132): 2.

Edwards, J. and Boxall, K. (2010) Adults with cystic fibrosis and barriers to employment, *Disability and Society*, 25(4): 441–453.

Edwards, S.D. (2004) Disability, identity and the 'expressivist objection', *Journal of Medical Ethics*, 30: 418–420.

——(2005) *Disability: Definitions, Value and Identity*, Abingdon: Radcliffe.

Egan, J.F.X. *et al.* (2004) Down syndrome births in the United States from 1989–2001, *American Journal of Obstetrics and Gynaecology*, 191: 1044–1048.

Ehrich, K., Williams, C., Farsides, B. and Scott, R. (2012) Embryo futures and stem cell research: the management of informed uncertainty, *Sociology of Health and Illness*, 34(1): 114–129.

Elliot, C. (1999) Pursued by happiness and beaten senseless: Prozac and the American dream, *Hastings Center Report*, 30(2): 7–12.

Elstad, T.A. and Kristiansen, K. (2009) Mental health centres as 'meeting places' in the community: exploring experiences of being service users and participants, *Scandinavian Journal of Disability Research*, 11(3): 195–208.

Emens, E.F. (2009) Intimate discrimination: the state's role in the accidents of sex and love, *Harvard Law Review*, 122: 1307–1314.

Emerson, E. and McVilly, K. (2004) Friendship activities of adults with intellectual disabilities in supported accommodation in Northern England, *Journal of Applied Research in Intellectual Disabilities*, 17: 191–197.

Emerson, E. and Roulstone, A. (in press) Developing an evidence base for violent and disablist hate crime in Britain: findings from the Life Opportunities Survey, *Journal of Interpersonal Violence*.

Epstein, R. (2005) The right to die: the assisted dying for the terminally ill bill, *Legal Executive Journal*, September: 14–16.

European Network of Independent Living (n.d.) 'Policy statement'. Available at: http://www.enil.eu/policy/ (accessed 1 February 2011).

Farrugia, D. (2009) Exploring stigma: medical knowledge and the stigmatisation of parents of children diagnosed with autism spectrum disorder, *Sociology of Health and Illness*, 31(7): 1011–1027.

Ferguson, I. (2003) Challenging a 'spoiled identity': mental health service users, recognition and redistribution, in N. Watson and S. Riddell (eds) *Disability, Culture and Identity*, Harlow: Pearson Education.

Findlay, B. (1999) Disability rights and culture under attack, *Disability Arts in London*, 149: 6–7.

Finkelstein, V. (1980) *Attitudes and Disabled People*, New York, World Rehabilitation Fund.

——(1981) To deny or not to deny disability, in A. Brechin *et al.* (eds) *Handicap in a Social World*, Sevenoaks: OUP/Hodder and Stoughton.

——(2001) *A Personal Journey into Disability Politics*, Leeds: University of Leeds, Centre for Disability Studies.

Finkelstein, V., French, S. and Oliver, M. (eds) (1993) *Disabling Barriers, Enabling Environments*, London: Sage.

Finlay, I.G., Wheatley, V.J. and Izdebski, C. (2005) The House of Lords Select Committee on the Assisted Dying for the Terminally Ill Bill: implications for specialist palliative care, *Palliative Medicine*, 19: 444–453.

Finlay, M. and Lyons, E. (1998) Social identity and people with learning difficulties: implications for self-advocacy groups, *Disability and Society*, 13(1): 37–52.

Fisher, B. and Galler, R. (1988) Friendship and fairness: how disability affects friendship between women, in M. Fine and A. Asch (eds) *Women with Disabilities: Essays in Psychology, Culture and Politics*, Philadelphia, PA: Temple University Press, pp. 172–194.

Fisher, P. and Byrne, V. (2012) Identity, emotion and the internal goods of practice: a study of learning disability professionals, *Sociology of Health and Illness*, 34(1): 79–94.

Fletcher, A. (1999) *Genes Are Us? Attitudes to Genetics and Disability*, London: RADAR.

——(2006) What's in a name? *Disability Now*, January, 21.

Flory, J.H. and Kitcher, P. (2004) Global health and the scientific research agenda, *Philosophy and Public Affairs*, 32(1): 36–65.

Foucault, M. (1989) *The History of Sexuality*, vol. 1, Harmondsworth: Penguin.

——(1990) *Politics, Philosophy, Culture*, London: Routledge.

Fox, H.M. and Kim, K. (2004) Understanding emerging disabilities, *Disability and Society*, 19(4): 323–337.

Frank, E., Anderson, C. and Rubinstein, D. (1978) Frequency of sexual dysfunction in 'normal' couples, *New England Journal of Medicine*, 299: 111–115.

Franklin, S. (2003) Ethical biocapital: new strategies of cell culture, in S. Franklin and M. Lock (eds) *Rethinking Life and Death: Towards an Anthropology of the Biosciences*, Santa Fe, NM: School of American Research Press, pp. 97–128.

Fraser, N. (1989) *Unruly Practices: Power, Discourse and Gender in Contemporary Social Theory*, Minneapolis: University of Minnesota Press.

——(1995) From redistribution to recognition, *New Left Review*, 212: 68–92.

——(2000) Rethinking recognition, *New Left Review*, 3: 107–120.

Fraser, N. and Honneth, A. (2003) *Redistribution or Recognition? A Political-Philosophical Exchange*, London: Verso.

Fraser, N. and Nicholson, L. (1990) Social criticism without philosophy: an encounter between feminism and postmodernism, in L. Nicholson (ed.) *Feminism/Postmodernism*, London: Routledge.

Fraser, W.I. (1992) The professions, knowledge and practice, in S.R. Barron and J.D. Haldane (eds) *Community, Normality and Difference*, Aberdeen: Aberdeen University Press.

Freire, P. (1972) *The Pedagogy of the Oppressed*, Harmondsworth: Penguin.

French, S. (1993) Disability, impairment or something in between, in J. Swain *et al.* (eds) *Disabling Barriers, Enabling Environments*, London: Sage, pp. 17–25.

Freund, P. (2001) Bodies, disability and spaces: the social model and disabling spatial organisations, *Disability and Society*, 16(5): 689–706.

Friedman, M. (1993) Beyond caring: the de-moralization of gender, in M.J. Larrabee (ed.) *An Ethic of Care: Feminist and Interdisciplinary Perspectives*, New York: Routledge.

Fuss, D. (1989) *Essentially Speaking: Feminism, Nature and Difference*, New York: Routledge.

Gabel, S. and Peters, S. (2004) Presage of a paradigm shift? Beyond the social model of disability toward resistance theories of disability, *Disability and Society*, 19(6): 585–600.

Gallagher, H. (1995) *By Trust Betrayed: Patients, Physicians and the Licence to Kill in the Third Reich*, New York: Vandemere Press.

Galvin, R. (2003) The paradox of disability culture: the need to combine versus the imperative to let go, *Disability and Society*, 18(5): 675–690.

Ganchoff, C. (2004) Regenerating movements: embryonic stem cells and the politics of potentiality, *Sociology of Health and Illness*, 26(6): 757–774.

Garbutt, R. (2010) Exploring the barriers to sex and relationships for people with learning difficulties, in R. Shuttleworth and T. Sanders (eds) *Sex and Disability*, Leeds: The Disability Press.

Gardiner, P. (2003) A virtue ethics approach to moral dilemmas in medicine, *Journal of Medical Ethics*, 29: 297–302.

Geras, N. (1995) Language, truth and justice, *New Left Review*, 209: 110–135.

Gill, C.J. (1992) Suicide intervention for people with disabilities: a lesson in inequality, *Issues in Law & Medicine*, 8(1): 37–53.

Gillon, R. (2001) Is there a 'new ethics of abortion'? *Journal of Medical Ethics*, 27 (supplement II): ii5–ii9.

Gilman, M., Heyman, B. and Swain, J. (2000) What's in a name? The implications of diagnosis for people with learning difficulties and their family carers, *Disability and Society*, 15: 3.

Gilson, S.F., Tusler, A. and Gill, C. (1997) Ethnographic research in disability identity, self-determination and community, *Journal of Vocational Rehabilitation*, 9: 7–17.

Gleeson, B. (1999) *Geographies of Disability*, New York: Routledge.

Glendinning, C., Rummery, K., Halliwell, S., Jacobs, S. and Tyrer, J. (2000) *Buying Independence: Using Direct Payments to Purchase Integrated Health and Social Services*, Bristol: Policy Press.

Glover, J. (1977) *Causing Death and Saving Lives*, Harmondsworth: Penguin.

Goffman, E. (1968a) *Stigma: Notes on the Management of Spoiled Identity*, Harmondsworth: Penguin.

——(1968b) *Asylums: Essays on the Social Situation of Mental Patients and Other Inmates*, Harmondsworth: Penguin.

Goggin, G. and Newell, C. (2004) Uniting the nation? Disability, stem cells and the Australian media, *Disability and Society*, 19(1): 47–60.

——(2005) *Disability in Australia: Exposing a Social Apartheid*, Sydney: UNSW Press.

Gomez, M. (2011) Sexual behavior among Filipino high school students who are deaf, *Sexuality and Disability*, 29(4): 301–312.

Gooding, C. (2000) Disability Discrimination Act: from statute to practice, *Critical Social Policy*, 20(4): 533–549.

Gold, D. (1999) Friendship, leisure and support: the purposes of 'circles of friends' of young people, *Journal of Leisurability*, 26(3): 1–13.

Goodley, D. (2001) 'Learning difficulties', the social model of disability and impairment: challenging epistemologies, *Disability and Society*, 16(2): 207–231.

——(2003) Against a politics of victimisation: disability culture and self-advocates with learning difficulties, in N. Watson and S. Riddell (eds) *Disability, Culture and Identity*, Harlow: Pearson Education.

——(2011) *Disability Studies: An Interdisciplinary Introduction*, London: Sage.

Goodley, D. and Moore, M. (2000) Doing disability research: activist lives and the academy, *Disability and Society*, 15(6): 861–882.

Goodley, D. and Runswick-Cole, K. (2011) The violence of disablism, *Sociology of Health and Illness*, 33(4): 602–617.

Gordon, B.O. and Rosenblum, K.E. (2001) Bringing disability into the sociological frame: a comparison of disability with race, sex and sexual orientation statuses, *Disability and Society*, 16(1): 5–19.

Gosling, V. and Cotterill, L. (2000) An employment project as a route to social inclusion for people with learning difficulties? *Disability and Society*, 15(7): 1001–1018.

Graham, H. (1983) Caring, a labour of love, in J. Finch and D. Groves (eds) *A Labour of Love: Women, Work and Caring*, London: Routledge & Kegan Paul.

——(1991) The concept of caring in feminist research: the case of domestic service, *Sociology*, 25(1): 61–78.

Gravell, C. (2012) *Cruelty: People with Learning Disabilities and their Experience of Harassment, Abuse and Related Crime in the Community*, London: Lemos and Crane.

Grech, S. (2009) Disability, poverty and development: critical reflections on the majority world debate, *Disability and Society*, 24(6): 771–784.

Grey-Thompson, T. (2005) 'Tactile paving and other bad inventions', available at: www.bbc.co.uk/ouch/columnists/tanni/130605_index.shtml (accessed 1 August 2005).

Groce, N. (1985) *Everyone Here Spoke Sign Language: Hereditary Deafness on Martha's Vineyard*, Cambridge, MA: Harvard University Press.

Grönvik, L. (2007) The fuzzy buzz word: conceptualisation of disability in disability research classics, *Sociology of Health and Illness*, 29(5): 750–766.

Gullette, M.M. (2013) *Amour*: how can we embrace a film that is clearly an advert for euthanasia? *The Guardian*, film blog, 28 February. Available at: http://www.guardian.co.uk/film/filmblog/2013/feb/28/amour-advert-for-euthanasia?INTCMP=SRCH (accessed 13 March 2013).

Guse, T. and Harvey, C. (2010) Growing up with a sibling with dwarfism: perceptions of adult non-dwarf siblings, *Disability and Society*, 25(3): 387–401.

Gustavsson, A. (2004) The role of theory in disability research: springboard or strait-jacket, *Scandinavian Journal of Disability Research*, 6(1): 55–70.

Gustavsson, A., Sandvin, J., Traustadóttir, R. and Tøssebro, J. (2005) *Resistance, Reflection and Change: Nordic Disability Research*, Lund: Studentlitteratur.

Hacking, I. (1986) Making up people, in T.C. Helier *et al.*, *Reconstructing Individualism*, Stanford, CA: Stanford University Press.

——(1999) *The Social Construction of What?* Cambridge, MA: Harvard University Press.

Hahn, H. (1985) Towards a politics of disability: definitions, disciplines and policies, *Social Science Journal*, 22(4): 87–105.

——(1988) The politics of physical differences: disability and discrimination, *Journal of Social Issues*, 44(1): 39–47.

Hamilton, C. (2010) 'But Rachael was enjoying it too, wasn't she?' A learning disability and sexuality case study, in R. Shuttleworth and T. Sanders (eds) *Sex and Disability*, Leeds: The Disability Press.

Hampton, S.J. (2005) Family eugenics, *Disability and Society*, 20(5): 553–561.

Hanass-Hancock, J. (2009) Interweaving conceptualizations of gender and disability in the context of vulnerability to HIV/AIDS in KwaZulu-Natal, South Africa, *Sexuality and Disability*, 27: 35–47.

Happé, F. (1994) *Autism: An Introduction to Psychological Theory*, London: UCL Press.

Haraway, D. (1988) Situated knowledges: the science question in feminism and the privilege of partial perspective, *Feminist Studies*, 14(3): 575–599.

Harris, J. (1985) *The Value of Life: An Introduction to Medical Ethics*, London: Routledge & Kegan Paul.

——(1992) *Wonderwoman and Superman: The Ethics of Human Biotechnology*, Oxford: Oxford University Press.

——(1993) Is gene therapy a form of eugenics? *Bioethics*, 7: 178–187.

——(2000) The welfare of the child, *Health Care Analysis*, 8(1): 27–34.

——(2001) One principle and three fallacies of disability studies, *Journal of Medical Ethics*, 27(6): 383–388.

Harris, J. and Bamford, C. (2001) Services for Deaf and hard of hearing people, *Disability and Society*, 16(7): 969–979.

Hashiloni-Dolev, Y. and Weiner, N. (2008) New reproductive technologies, genetic counselling and the standing of the fetus: views from Germany and Israel, *Sociology of Health and Illness*, 30(7): 1055–1069.

Hasler, F. (1993) Developments in the disabled people's movement, in J. Swain *et al.* (eds) *Disabling Barriers, Enabling Environments*, London: Sage.

——(2003) 'Clarifying the evidence on direct payments into practice'. Available at: www.ncil.org.uk/evidence_paper.asp (accessed 4 March 2004).

Häyry, M. (2009) The moral contestedness of selecting 'deaf embryos', in K. Kristiansen, S. Vehmas and T. Shakespeare (eds) *Arguing about Disability: Philosophical Perspectives*, London: Routledge.

Hedlund, M. (2000) Disability as a phenomenon: a discourse of social and biological understandings, *Disability and Society*, 15(5): 765–780.

Henley, C.A. (2001) Good intentions: unpredictable consequences, *Disability and Society*, 16(7): 933–947.

Henn, W. (2000) Consumerism in prenatal diagnosis: a challenge for ethical guidelines, *Journal of Medical Ethics*, 26: 444–446.

Hevey, D. (1992) *The Creatures Time Forgot: Photography and Disability Imagery*, London: Routledge.

Hochschild, A. (1983) *The Managed Heart: The Commercialization of Human Feeling*, Berkeley, CA: The University of California Press.

Hodge, N. (2005) Reflections on diagnosing autism spectrum disorders, *Disability and Society*, 20(3): 345–349.

Holdsworth, A. (1993) Our allies within, *Coalition*, June, 4–10.

Hollomotz, A. (2011) *Learning Difficulties and Sexual Vulnerability: A Social Approach*, London: Jessica Kingsley.

Honneth, A. (1995) *The Struggle for Recognition: The Moral Grammar of Social Conflicts*, Cambridge: Polity.

Hood-Williams, J. (1996) Goodbye to sex and gender, *Sociological Review*, 44(1): 1–16.

Hughes, B. (2009) Disability activisms: social model stalwarts and biological citizens, *Disability and Society*, 24(6): 677–688.

Hughes, B., McKie, L., Hopkins, D. and Watson, N. (2005a) Love's labour's lost? Feminism, the disabled people's movement and an ethic of care, *Sociology*, 39(2): 259–275.

Hughes, B., Russell, R. and Paterson, K. (2005b) Nothing to be had 'off the peg': consumption, identity and the immobilization of young disabled people, *Disability and Society*, 20(1): 3–18.

Hughes, K., Bellis, M.A., Jones, L., Wood, L., Wood, S., Bates, G., Eckley, L., McCoy, E., Mikton, C., Shakespeare, T. and Officer, A. (2012) Prevalence and risk of violence against adults with disabilities: a systematic review and meta-analysis of observational studies, *The Lancet*, early online publication February 28 2012.

Humphrey, J.C. (1999) Disabled people and the politics of difference, *Disability and Society*, 14: 173–188.

——(2000) Researching disability politics, or, some problems with the social model in practice, *Disability and Society*, 15(1): 63–85.

Hunt, P. (ed.) (1966) *Stigma*, London: Geoffrey Chapman Publishing.

Hurst, R. (1995) Choice and empowerment: lessons from Europe, *Disability and Society*, 10(4): 529–534.

——(ed.) (1998) *Are Disabled People Included?* London: Disability Awareness in Action.

——(2000) To revise or not to revise, *Disability and Society*, 15(7): 1083–1087.

——(n.d.) 'Assisted suicide and disabled people: a briefing paper', Disability Awareness in Action website, available at: wwww.daa.org.uk/assisted_suicide. htm (accessed 26 April 2004).

Huurre, T.M. and Aro, H.M. (1998) Psychosocial development among adolescents with visual impairment, *European Child and Adolescent Psychiatry*, 7: 73–78.

Hwang, S.K. and Charnley, H. (2010) Honourable sacrifice: a visual ethnography of the family lives of Korean children with autistic siblings, *Children and Society*, 24(6): 437–448.

Imrie, R. (2004) Demystifying disability: a review of the International Classification of Functioning, Disability and Health, *Sociology of Health and Illness*, 26(3): 287–305.

JAG (n.d.) *Ten Years with Personal Assistance*. Available at: www.jag.se/kunskap.

Jamieson, L. (1998) *Intimacy: Personal Relationships in Modern Society*, Cambridge: Polity.

Jaudes, P.K. and Mackey-Bilaver, L. (2008) Do chronic conditions increase young children's risk of being maltreated? *Child Abuse and Neglect*, 32: 671–681.

Jeffreys, S. (2008) Disability and the male sexual right, *Women's Studies International Forum*, 31: 327–335.

Johnson, K., Frawley, P., Hillier, L. and Harrison, L. (2002) Living safer sexual lives: research and action, *Tizard Learning Disability Review*, 7(3): 4–9.

Johnson, K., Hillier, L., Harrison, L. and Frawley, P. (2000) *Living Safer Sexual Lives*, Melbourne: Australian Research Centre in Sex, Health and Society.

Jones, L., Bellis, M.A., Wood, S., Hughes, K., Bates, G., Eckley, L., McCoy, E., Mikton, C., Shakespeare, T. and Officer, A. (2012) Prevalence and risk of violence against children with disabilities: a systematic review and meta-analysis of observational studies, *The Lancet*, early online publication, July 12 2012.

Juengst, E.T. (1998) What does enhancement mean? in E. Parens (ed.) *Enhancing Human Traits: Social and Ethical Implications*, Washington, DC: Georgetown University Press.

Keith, L. (1996) Encounters with strangers, in J. Morris (ed.) *Encounters with Strangers: Disability and Feminism*, London: Women's Press.

Kelly, B. (2005) 'Chocolate, makes you autism': impairment, disability and childhood identities, *Disability and Society*, 20(3): 261–276.

Kelly, C. (2010) The role of mandates/philosophies in shaping interactions between disabled people and their support providers, *Disability and Society*, 25(1): 103–119.

Kelly, M.P. and Field, D. (1994) Reflections on the rejection of the bio-medical model in sociological discourse, *Medical Sociology News*, 19: 34–37.

——(1996) Medical sociology, chronic illness and the body, *Sociology of Health and Illness*, 18(2): 241–257.

Kelly, S.E. (2009) Choosing not to choose: reproductive responses of parents of children with genetic conditions or impairments, *Sociology of Health and Illness*, 31(1): 81–97.

Kermit, P. (2009) Deaf or deaf? Questioning alleged antinomies in the bioethical discourses on cochlear implantation and suggesting an alternative approach to d/Deafness, *Scandinavian Journal of Disability Research*, 11(2): 159–174.

Kerr, A. and Shakespeare, T. (2002) *Genetic Politics: From Eugenics to Genome*, Cheltenham: New Clarion Press.

Kevles, D.J. (1985) *In the Name of Eugenics: Genetics and the Uses of Human Heredity*, New York: Knopf.

King, D.S. (1999) Preimplantation genetic diagnosis and the 'new' eugenics, *Journal of Medical Ethics*, 25(2): 176–182.

Kitcher, P. (1997) *Lives to Come: The Genetic Revolution and Human Possibilities*, New York: Simon & Schuster.

Kittay, E.F. (1999) *Love's Labour: Essays on Women, Equality and Dependency*, New York: Routledge.

Kittay, E.F. and Carlson, L. (eds) (2010) *Cognitive Disability and Its Challenge to Moral Philosophy*, Chichester: Wiley-Blackwell.

Kreuter, M., Siosteen, A. and Biering-Sorensen, F. (2008) Sexuality and sexual life in women with spinal cord injury: a controlled study, *Journal of Rehabilitative Medicine*, 40: 61–69.

Kripke, S. (1980) *Naming and Necessity*, Oxford: Blackwell.

Kröger, T. (2009) Care research and disability studies: nothing in common? *Critical Social Policy*, 29: 398–420.

Kuhse, H. and Singer, P. (1985) *Should the Baby Live? The Problem of Handicapped Infants*, Oxford: Oxford University Press.

Kulick, D. and Rydström, J. (forthcoming) *Excessibility Guidelines: Sex, Disability, and the Ethics of Engagement*, Duke University Press.

Laura, R.S. (ed.) (1980) *Problems of Handicap*, Melbourne: Macmillan.

Lee, P. (2002) Shooting for the moon: politics and disability at the beginning of the twenty-first century, in C. Barnes, M. Oliver and L. Barton (eds) *Disability Studies Today*, Cambridge: Polity.

Leece, D. and Leece, J. (2006) Direct payments: creating a two-tiered system in social care? *British Journal of Social Work*, 36: 1379–1393.

Leece, J. (2004) Money talks, but what does it say? Direct payments and the commodification of care, *Practice: Social Work in Action*, 16(3): 211–221.

Leece, J. and Peace, S. (2010) Developing new understandings of independence and autonomy in the personalized relationship, *British Journal of Social Work*, 40: 1847–1865.

Leff, J. (2001) *The Unbalanced Mind*, London: Phoenix.

Leipoldt, E. (2005) 'Embryonic stem cell research: a sob story', Online Opinion. Available at: www.onlineopinion.com.au/print.asp?article=172 posted September 14 2005 (accessed 10 October 2005).

Lenney, M. and Sercombe, H. (2002) 'Did you see that guy in the wheelchair down the pub?' Interactions across difference in a public place, *Disability and Society*, 17(1): 5–18.

Lester, H. and Tritter, J.Q. (2005) 'Listen to my madness': understanding the experiences of people with serious mental illness, *Sociology of Health and Illness*, 27(5): 649–669.

Levy, N. (2002) Reconsidering cochlear implants: the lesson of Martha's Vineyard, *Bioethics*, 16(2): 134–153.

Lifton, R.J. (1986) *The Nazi Doctors: Medical Killing and the Psychology of Genocide*, London: Macmillan.

Liggett, H. (1988) Stars are not born: an interpretative approach to the politics of disability, *Disability, Handicap & Society*, 3(3):263–276.

Linton, S. (1998) *Claiming Disability: Knowledge and Identity*, New York: New York University Press.

Lippman, A. (1994) Prenatal genetic testing and screening: constructing needs and reinforcing inequalities, in A. Clarke (ed.) *Genetic Counselling: Practice and Principles*, London: Routledge.

Littlewood, J. (2004) 'Looking back over 40 years and what the future holds', Joseph Levy Memorial Lecture and the Ettore Rossi Medal Lecture, 27th European Cystic Fibrosis Conference, Birmingham.

Llewellyn, A. and Hogan, K. (2000) The use and abuse of models of disability, *Disability and Society*, 15(1): 157–165.

Lock, S., Jordan, L., Bryan, K. and Maxim, J. (2005) Work after stroke: focusing on barriers and enablers, *Disability and Society*, 20(1): 33–47.

Locker, D. (1983) *Disability and Disadvantage*, London: Tavistock.

Longmore, P.K. (1997) Conspicuous contribution and American cultural dilemmas: telethon rituals of cleansing and renewal, in D.T. Mitchell and S.L. Snyder (eds) *The Body and Physical Difference: Discourses of Disability*, Ann Arbor, MI: University of Michigan.

——(2003) *Why I Burned My Book and Other Essays on Disability*, Philadelphia, PA: Temple University Press.

Lynch, K., Baker, J. and Lyons, M. (2009) *Affective Equality: Love, Care and Injustice*, Basingstoke: Palgrave Macmillan.

Macdonald, S.J. (2009) Windows of reflection: conceptualizing dyslexia using the social model of disability, *Dyslexia*, 15(4): 347–362.

MacIntyre, A. (1999) *Dependent Rational Animals: Why Human Beings Need the Virtues*, London: Duckworth.

Mackenzie, C. and Scully, J.L. (2008) Moral imagination, disability and embodiment, *Journal of Applied Philosophy*, 24(4): 335–351.

Maclean, A. (1993) *The Elimination of Morality: Reflections on Utilitarianism and Bioethics*, London: Routledge.

Madigan, R. and Milner, J (1999) Access for all: housing design and the Disability Discrimination Act 1995, *Critical Social Policy*, 19(3): 396–409.

Maguire, H., Mikton, C. and Shakespeare, T. (forthcoming) Responding to violence against persons with disabilities: a review of prevention and victim support measures, *Journal of Interpersonal Violence*.

Magnusson, R.S. (2002) *Angels of Death: Exploring the Euthanasia Underground*, New Haven, CT: Yale University Press.

Manthorpe, J., Moriarty, J. and Cornes, M. (2011) Keeping it in the family? People with learning disabilities and families employing their own care and support workers: findings from a scoping review of the literature, *Journal of Intellectual Disabilities*, 15: 195–207.

Mao, X. (1998) Chinese geneticists' views on ethical issues in genetic testing and screening: evidence for eugenics in China, *American Journal of Human Genetics*, 63(3): 688–695.

Marfisi, C. (2002) Personally speaking: a critical reflection of factors which blur the original vision of personal assistance services, *Disability Studies Quarterly*, 22(1): 25–30.

Marinelli, R.P. and Dell Orto, A.E. (1984) *The Psychological and Social Impact of Physical Disability*, New York: Springer.

Marshall, T.H. (1950) *Citizenship and Social Class*, Cambridge: Cambridge University Press.

Martin, P. (1999) Genes and drugs: the social shaping of gene therapy and the reconstruction of genetic disease, in P. Conrad and J. Gabe (eds) *Sociological Perspectives on the New Genetics*, Oxford: Blackwell.

Martz, E. (2001) Acceptance of imperfection, *Disability Studies Quarterly*, 21(3): 160–165.

Mauldin, L. (2012) Parents of deaf children with cochlear implants: a study of technology and community, *Sociology of Health and Illness*, 34(4): 529–543.

Mayo-Wilson, E., Montgomery, P. and Dennis, J.A. (2008) 'Personal assistance for adults (19–64) with physical impairments', Cochrane Database of Systematic Reviews (Online). Available at: 2008 3CD006856, PMID: 18646171.

McCarthy, M. (2008) Prescribing contraception to women with intellectual disabilities: general practitioners' attitudes and practices, *Sexuality and Disability*, 29(4): 339–349.

McColl, M.A., Jarzynowska, A. and Shortt, S.E.D. (2010) Unmet health needs of people with disabilities: population level evidence, *Disability and Society*, 25(2): 205–218.

McConkey, R. and Ryan, D. (2001) Experiences of staff in dealing with client sexuality in services for teenagers and adults with intellectual disability, *Journal of Intellectual Disability Research*, 45(1): 83–87.

McDermott, S. (2012) Crime risk associated with disability, *Disability and Health Journal*, 5: 211–212.

McLaughlin, J. (2003) Screening networks: shared agendas in feminist and disability movement challenges to antenatal screening and abortion, *Disability and Society*, 18(3): 297–310.

McMaugh, A. (2011) En/countering disablement in school life in Australia: children talk about peer relations and living with illness and disability, *Disability and Society*, 26(7): 853–866.

McRuer, R. (2006) *Crip Theory: Cultural Signs of Queerness and Disability*, New York: New York University Press.

McRuer, R. and Mollow, A. (eds) (2012) *Sex and Disability*, Durham, NC: Duke University Press.

McVilly, K.R., Stancliffe, R.J., Parmenter, T.R. and Burton-Smith, R.M. (2006) Self-advocates have the last say on friendship, *Disability and Society*, 21(7): 693–708.

Meekosha, H. (2004) Drifting down the Gulf Stream: navigating the cultures of disability, *Disability and Society*, 19(7): 721–734.

——(2011) Decolonising disability: thinking and acting globally, *Disability and Society*, 26(6): 667–682.

Meekosha, H. and Shuttleworth, R. (2009) What's so critical about critical disability studies? *Australian Journal of Human Rights*, 15(1): 47–75.

Meltzer, N., Singleton, A., Bebbington, P., Brugha, T. and Jenkins, R. (2002) *The Social and Economic Circumstances of Adults with Mental Disorders*, London: The Stationery Office.

Mencap (2000) *Living in Fear*, London: Mencap.

Mercer, G. (2002) Emancipatory research, in C. Barnes, M. Oliver and L. Barton (eds) *Disability Studies Today*, Cambridge: Polity.

Miller, L.L., Harvath, T.A., Ganzini, L., Goy, E.R., Delorit, M.A. and Jackson, A. (2004) Attitudes and experiences of Oregon hospice nurses and social workers regarding assisted suicide, *Palliative Medicine*, 18: 685–691.

Milner, P. and Kelly, B. (2009) Community participation and inclusion: people with disabilities defining their place, *Disability and Society*, 24(1): 47–62.

Mirfin-Veitch, B. (2003) *Relationships and Adults with an Intellectual Disability: Review of the Literature Prepared for the National Advisory Committee on Health and Disability to Inform Its Project on Services for Adults with an Intellectual Disability*, Wellington: National Health Committee.

Mitchell, D. and Snyder, S. (2012) Minority model: from liberal to neoliberal futures of disability, in N. Watson, A. Roulstone and C. Thomas (eds) *Routledge Handbook of Disability Studies*, London: Routledge, pp. 42–50.

Mitra, M., Manning, S.E. and Lu, E. (2012) Physical abuse around the time of pregnancy among women with disabilities, *Maternal and Child Health Journal*, 16: 802–806.

Mitra, M. and Mouradian, M. (in press) Intimate partner violence in the relationships of men with disabilities in the US, *Journal of Interpersonal Violence*.

Mladenov, T. (2012) Personal assistance for disabled people and the understanding of human being, *Critical Social Policy*, 32: 242–261.

Mohammed, M.A., Mant, J., Bentham, J., Stevens, A. and Hussain, S. (2005) Process of care and mortality of stroke patients with and without a do not resuscitate order in the West Midlands, UK, *International Journal for Quality in Health Care*, October 7, 1–5.

Mohapatra, S. and Mohanty, M. (2005) *Abuse and Activity Limitation: A Study on Domestic Violence Against Disabled Women in Orissa, India*, Orissa: Swabhiman.

Mohr, M. and Kettler, D. (1997) Ethical aspects of resuscitation, *British Journal of Anaesthesia*, 79: 253–259.

Moloney, P. (2010) 'How can a chord be weird if it expresses your soul?' Some critical reflections on the diagnosis of Asperger's syndrome, *Disability and Society*, 25(2): 135–148.

Morales, G.E., Lopez, E.O. and Mullet, E. (2011) Acceptability of sexual relationship among people with learning disabilities: family and professional caregivers' views in Mexico, *Sexuality and Disability*, 29: 165–174.

Morris, J. (1991) *Pride Against Prejudice*, London: Women's Press.

——(1992) Personal and political: a feminist perspective on researching physical disability, *Disability, Handicap and Society*, 7(2):157–166.

——(1993a) *Independent Lives? Community Care and Disabled People*, London: Macmillan.

——(1993b) Gender and disability, in J. Swain, V. Finkelstein, S. French and M. Oliver (eds) *Disabling Barriers, Enabling Environments*, London: Sage, pp. 85–92.

——(1995) Creating a space for absent voices: disabled women's experience of receiving assistance with daily living activities, *Feminist Review*, 51: 68–93.

——(ed.) (1996) *Encounters with Strangers: Feminism and Disability*, London: Women's Press.

——(2004) Independent living and community care: a disempowering framework, *Disability and Society*, 19(5); 427–442.

Muenchberger, H., Ehrlich, C., Kendall, E. and Vit, M. (2012) Experience of place for young adults under 65 years with complex disabilities moving into purpose-built residential care, *Social Science and Medicine*, 75: 2151–2159.

Murray, P. (2002) *Hello! Are You Listening? Disabled Teenagers' Experience of Access to Inclusive Leisure*, York: Joseph Rowntree Foundation.

Naraine, M. and Lindsay, P. (2011) Social inclusion of employees who are blind or low vision, *Disability and Society*, 26(4): 389–403.

Noonan, A. and Taylor Gomez, M. (2011) Who's missing? Awareness of lesbian, gay, bisexual and transgender people with intellectual disability, *Sexuality and Disability*, 29: 175–180.

Noreau, L. and Boschen, K. (2010) Intersection of participation and environmental factors: a complex interactive process, *Archives of Physical Medicine and Rehabilitation*, 91(suppl.), 10: 44–53.

Novas, C. (2006) The political economy of hope: patients' organizations, science and biovalue, *Biosocieties*, 1: 289–305.

Nozick, R. (1975) *Anarchy, State and Utopia*, Oxford: Basil Blackwell.

Nussbaum, M. (2006) *Frontiers of Justice: Disability, Nationality, Species Membership*, Cambridge, MA: Harvard University Press.

Oakley, A. (1972) *Sex, Gender and Society*, London: Gower.

O'Brien, J. (1987) A guide to lifestyle planning: using the activities catalogue to integrate services and natural support systems, in B. Wilcox and G.T. Bellamy (eds) *The Activities Catalogue: An Alternative Curriculum for Youth and Adults with Severe Disabilities*, Baltimore, MD: Brookes.

O'Brien, R. (2001) *Crippled Justice: The History of Modern Disability Policy in the Workplace*, Chicago: University of Chicago Press.

Office of Disability Issues (2012) *Facts and Figures*. Available at: http://odi.dwp.gov.uk/disability-statistics-and-research/disability-facts-and-figures.php#imp (consulted March 13, 2013).

Oliver, M. (1978) Medicine and disability: steps in the wrong direction, *International Journal of Medical Engineering and Technology*, 2(3): 136–138.

——(1983) *Social Work with Disabled People*, Basingstoke: Macmillan.

——(1989) Conductive education: if it wasn't so sad it would be funny, *Disability, Handicap and Society*, 4(2): 197–2000.

——(1990) *The Politics of Disablement*, London: Macmillan.

——(1992a) Changing the social relations of research production? *Disability, Handicap and Society*, 7(2): 101–114.

——(1992b) Intellectual masturbation: a rejoinder to Söder and Booth, *European Journal of Special Needs Education*, 7(1): 20–28.

——(1993) *Disability, Citizenship and Empowerment*, Milton Keynes: Open University Press.

——(1996) *Understanding Disability: From Theory to Practice*, Basingstoke: Macmillan.

——(2004) The social model in action: if I had a hammer, in C. Barnes and G. Mercer (eds) *Implementing the Social Model of Disability: Theory and Research*, Leeds: The Disability Press, pp. 18–47.

Oliver, M. and Barnes, C. (2012) *The New Politics of Disablement*, Basingstoke: Macmillan.

Oliver, M. and Hasler, F. (1987) Disability and self-help: a case study of the Spinal Injuries Association, *Disability, Handicap and Society*, 2(2): 113–125.

Oliver, M. and Sapey, B. (1999) *Social Work with Disabled People*, 2nd edn, Basingstoke: Palgrave Macmillan.

Orkin, S.H. and Motulsky, A.G. (1995) 'Report and recommendations of the panel to assess the NIH investment in research on gene therapy', National Institutes of Health. Available at: www.nih.gov/news/panelrep.html (accessed 19 January 2006).

Othman, A.S. and Engkasan, J.P. (2011) Sexual dysfunction following spinal cord injury: the experiences of Malaysian women, *Sexuality and Disability*, 29: 329–337.

Pagan, R. (2012) Transitions to part-time work at older ages: the case of people with disabilities in Europe, *Disability and Society*, 27(1): 95–115.

Pahl, R. (2000) *On Friendship*, Cambridge: Polity.

Parens, E. (ed.) (2006) *Surgically Shaping Children*, Washington, DC: Georgetown University Press.

Parens, E. and Asch, A. (eds) (2000) *Prenatal Testing and Disability Rights*, Washington, DC: Georgetown University Press.

Parfit, D. (1984) *Reasons and Persons*, Oxford: Clarendon Press.

Paterson, K. and Hughes, B. (1999) Disability studies and phenomenology: the carnal politics of everyday life, *Disability and Society*, 14(5): 597–610.

Paul, D.B. (1992) Eugenic anxieties, social realities, and political choices, *Social Research*, 59(3); 663–683.

Pearson, C. (2012) Independent living, in N. Watson, A. Roulstone and C. Thomas (eds) *Routledge Handbook of Disability Studies*, London: Routledge, pp. 240–252.

Perske, T. (1988) *Circles of Friends*, Nashville, TN: Abingdon Press.

Pescosolido, B.A. (2001) The role of social networks in the lives of persons with disabilities, in G.L. Albrecht, K.D. Seelman and M. Bury (eds) *Handbook of Disability Studies*, Thousand Oaks, CA: Sage.

Peters, S. (2000) Is there a disability culture? A syncretisation of three possible world views, *Disability and Society*, 15(4): 583–601.

Peters, S., Gabel, S. and Symeonidou, S. (2009) Resistance, transformation and the politics of hope: imagining a way forward for the disabled people's movement, *Disability and Society*, 24(5): 543–556.

Pfeiffer, D. (1998) The ICIDH and the need for its revision, *Disability and Society*, 3(4): 503–523.

——(2000) The devil is in the details: the ICIDH2 and the disability movement, *Disability and Society*, 15(7): 1079–1082.

——(2001) The conceptualization of disability, in S. Barnart and B.M. Altman (eds) *Exploring Theories and Expanding Methodologies: Where Are We and Where Do We Need to Go? Research in Social Science and Disability*, vol. 2, Amsterdam: JAI.

Pilnick, A. (2008) 'It's something for you both to think about': choice and decision making in nuchal translucency screening for Down's syndrome, *Sociology of Health and Illness*, 30(4): 511–530.

Pinfold, V. (2004) *Social Participation*, report prepared for the Social Exclusion Unit, Rethink Mental Illness.

Plummer, K. (1995) *Telling Sexual Stories: Power, Change, and Social Worlds*, London: Routledge.

Press, N. and Brown, C. (1997) Why women say yes to prenatal diagnosis, *Social Science and Medicine*, 45: 979–989.

Price, D. and Barron, L. (1999) Developing independence: the experience of the Lawnmowers Theatre Company, *Disability and Society*, 14: 819–830.

Price, J. and Shildrick, M. (1998) Uncertain thoughts on the dis/abled body, in M. Shildrick and J. Price (eds) *Vital Signs: Feminist Reconfigurations of the Biological Body*, Edinburgh: Edinburgh University Press, pp. 224–249.

Prideaux, S., Roulstone, A., Harris, J. and Barnes, C. (2009) Disabled people and self-directed support schemes: reconceptualising work and welfare in the 21st century, *Disability and Society*, 24(5): 557–569.

Priestley, M. (1998) Constructions and creations: idealism, materialism and disability theory, *Disability and Society*, 13(1): 75–94.

——(2004) *Disability: A Life Course Approach*, Cambridge: Polity.

Priestley, M., Corker, M. and Watson, N. (1999) Unfinished business: disabled children and disability identity, *Disability Studies Quarterly*, 19(2): 87–98.

Priestley, M., Waddington, L. and Bessozi, C. (2010) Towards an agenda for disability research in Europe: learning from disabled people's organizations, *Disability and Society*, 25(6): 731–746.

Quarmby, K. (2011) *Scapegoat: Why We Are Failing Disabled People*, London: Portobello Books.

Radcliffe Richards, J. (2002) How not to end disability, *San Diego Law Journal*, 39: 693.

Rae, A. (2012) Time to talk: assisted suicide – the last taboo, *Coalition*, December: 9–12.

Rainey, S.S. (2011) *Love, Sex, and Disability: The Pleasures of Care*, Boulder, CO: Lynne Reinner.

Rapp, R. (1997) *Testing Women, Testing the Fetus*, London: Routledge.

Rawles, S. (2004) Fringe benefits, *The Guardian*, March 31.

Read, J. (1998) Conductive education and the politics of disablement, *Disability and Society*, 13(2): 279–293.

Redley, M., Banks, C., Foody, K. and Holland, A. (2012) Healthcare for men and women with learning disabilities: understanding inequalities in access, *Disability and Society*, 27(6): 747–759.

Reeve, D. (2003) 'Encounters with Strangers': psycho-emotional dimensions of disability in everyday life, paper presented at the UK Disability Studies Conference, Lancaster, available at: http://www.lancs.ac.uk/depts/apsocsci/events/dsa-conf2003/papers.htm.

——(2012) 'Psycho-emotional disablism: the missing link?', in N. Watson, A. Roulstone and C. Thomas (eds) *Routledge Handbook of Disability Studies*, London: Routledge, pp. 78–92.

Reid, B., Sinclear, M., Barr, O., Dobbs, F. and Crealey, G. (2009) A meta-synthesis of pregnant women's decision-making processes with regard to antenatal screening for Down's syndrome, *Social Science and Medicine*, 69: 1561–1573.

Reinders, H.S. (2008) *Receiving the Gift of Friendship: Profound Disability, Theological Anthropology, and Ethics*, Grand Rapids, MI: William B. Erdmans Publishing Company.

Resuscitation Council (2001) 'Decisions relating to cardiopulmonary resuscitation: a joint statement by the British Medical Association, the Resuscitation Council (UK) and the Royal College of Nursing'. Available at: www.resus.org.uk/pages/dnar.htm (accessed 12 January 2006).

Reynolds, J. and Walmsley, J. (1998) Care, support or something else, in A. Brechin, J. Walmsley, J. Katz and S. Peace (eds) *Care Matters: Concepts, Practice and Research in Health and Social Care*, London: Sage.

Reynolds, T.M. (2003) Downs syndrome screening is unethical: views of today's research ethics committees, *Journal of Clinical Pathology*, 56: 268–270.

Rickell, A. (2003) Our disability is political, *The Guardian*, 1 October.

——(2006) Key notes, *Disability Now*, January: 20.

Riddick, B. (2000) An examination of the relationship between labelling and stigmatisation with special reference to dyslexia, *Disability and Society*, 15(4): 653–668.

Riley, D. (1988) *Am I That Name?* Basingstoke: Macmillan.

Rioux, M. (1994) New research directions and paradigms: disability is not measles, in M. Rioux and M. Bach (eds) *Disability Is Not Measles: New Research Paradigms in Disability*, North York: L'Institut Roeher Institute.

Roberts, J. (2012) 'Wakey wakey baby': narrating four-dimensional (4D) bonding scans, *Sociology of Health and Illness*, 34(2): 299–314.

Robertson, P. *et al.* (2001) Social networks of people with intellectual disabilities in residential settings, *Mental Retardation*, 39: 201–214.

Rock, P.J. (1996) Eugenics and euthanasia: a cause for concern for disabled people, particularly disabled women, *Disability and Society*, 11(1): 121–128.

Roets, G. (2009) Unravelling Mr President's nomad lands: travelling to interdisciplinary frontiers of knowledge in disability studies, *Disability and Society*, 24(6): 689–701.

Rogers, L (1999) Having disabled baby will be 'sin' says scientist, *Sunday Times*, 4 July.

Rose, N. (2001) The politics of life itself, *Theory, Culture & Society*, 18(6): 1–30.

Rose, P. and Kiger, G. (1995) Intergroup relations: political action and identity in the deaf community, *Disability & Society*, 10(4): 521–528.

Roulstone, A. (2012) Disabled people, work and employment: a global perspective, in N. Watson, A. Roulstone and C. Thomas (eds) *Routledge Handbook of Disability Studies*, London: Routledge, pp. 211–224.

Roulstone, A. and Mason-Bish, H. (eds) (2013) *Disability, Hate Crime and Violence*, London: Routledge.

Roulstone, A., Thomas, P. and Balderston, S. (2011) Between hate and vulnerability: unpacking the British criminal justice system's construction of disablist hate crime, *Disability and Society*, 26(3): 351–364.

Russell, G., Kelly, S.E., Ford, T. and Steer, C. (2012) Diagnosis as social determinant: the development of prosocial behaviour before and after an autistic spectrum disorder, *Social Science and Medicine*, 75: 1642–1649.

Russell, M. (2002) What disability civil rights cannot do: employment and political economy, *Disability and Society*, 17(2): 117–135.

Safilios-Rothschild, C. (1970) The sociology and social psychology of disability and rehabilitation, *Australian Occupational Therapy Journal*, 19: 147.

——(1976) Disabled persons' self-definitions and their implications for rehabilitation, in G.L. Albrecht (ed.) *The Sociology of Physical Disability and Rehabilitation*, Pittsburgh, PA: University of Pittsburgh Press.

Samaha, A.M. (2007) 'What good is the social model of disability?' Chicago Public Law and Legal Theory Working Paper no 166, The Law School, University of Chicago. Available at: www.law.uchicago.edu/academics/public-law/index.html.

Sample, I. (2005) Human stem cells allow paralysed mice to walk again, *The Guardian*, 20 September.

Sapey, B., Stuart, J. and Donaldson, G. (2005) Increases in wheelchair use and perceptions of disablement, *Disability and Society*, 20(5): 489–505.

Save the Children (2011) *Out From the Shadows: Sexual Violence Against Children with Disabilities*, London: Save the Children UK.

Savulescu, J. (2001) Is current practice around late termination of pregnancy eugenic and discriminatory? Maternal interests and abortion, *Journal of Medical Ethics*, 27: 165–171.

——(2002) Abortion, embryo destruction and the future of value argument, *Journal of Medical Ethics*, 28: 133–135.

Saxton, M. (2000) Why members of the disability community oppose prenatal diagnosis and selective abortion, in E. Parens and A. Asch (eds) *Prenatal Testing and Disability Rights*, Washington, DC: Georgetown University Press.

Sayer, A. (2011) *Why Things Matter to People: Social Science, Values and Ethical Life*, Cambridge: Cambridge University Press.

Sayers, G., Schofield, I. and Aziz, M. (1997) An analysis of CPR decision-making by elderly patients, *Journal of Medical Ethics*, 23: 207–212.

Schur, L. (2002) Dead-end jobs or a path to economic well-being? The consequences of non-standard work among people with disabilities, *Behavioral Sciences and the Law*, 20: 601–620.

Schweik, S.M. (2009) *The Ugly Laws: Disability in Public*, New York: New York University Press.

Schwennesen, N. and Koch, L. (2012) Representing and intervening: 'doing' good care in first trimester prenatal knowledge production and decision-making, *Sociology of Health and Illness*, 34(2): 283–298.

Scourfield, P. (2005) Implementing the Community Care (Direct Payments) Act: will the supply of personal assistants meet the demand and at what price? *Journal of Social Policy*, 34(3): 469–488.

Scully, J.L. (2008) *Disability Bioethics: Moral Bodies, Moral Difference*, Lanham, MD: Rowman and Littlefield.

——(2012) Deaf identities in disability studies: with us or without us? in N. Watson, A. Roulstone and C. Thomas (eds) *Routledge Handbook of Disability Studies*, London: Routledge, pp. 109–121.

Scully, J.L. and Rehmann-Sutter, C. (2001) When norms normalize: the case of genetic 'enhancement', *Human Gene Therapy*, 12: 87–95.

Seale, C. (2006) National survey of end-of-life decisions made by UK medical practitioners, *Palliative Medicine*, 20(1): 3–10.

Sen, A. (1992) *Inequality Reexamined*, Oxford: Clarendon Press.

Sevenhuijsen, S. (1998) *Citizenship and the Ethics of Care: Feminist Considerations on Justice, Morality and Politics*, London: Routledge.

Seymour, W. and Lupton, D. (2004) Holding the line online: exploring wired relationships for people with disabilities, *Disability and Society*, 19(4): 291–305.

Shakespeare, T. (1992) A response to Liz Crow, *Coalition*, Sept.: 40–42.

——(1993) Disabled people's self-organisation: a new social movement? *Disability, Handicap and Society*, 8(3): 249–264.

——1994) Cultural representations of disabled people: dustbins for disavowal? *Disability and Society*, 9(3): 283–299.

——(1995a) Back to the future? New genetics and disabled people, *Critical Social Policy*, 44/45: 22–35.

——(1995b) Disability, identity, difference, in C. Barnes and G. Mercer (eds) *Chronic Illness and Disability: Bridging the Divide*, Leeds: Disability Press.

——(1998a) Choices and rights: eugenics, genetics and disability equality, *Disability and Society*, 13(5): 665–682.

——(1998b) Social constructionism as a political strategy, in I. Velody and R. Williams (eds) *The Politics of Constructionism*, London: Sage, pp. 168–181.

——(1999a) Losing the plot? Discourses on genetics and disability, *Sociology of Health and Illness*, 21(5): 669–688.

——(1999b) What is a disabled person? in M. Jones and L.B. Marks (eds) *Disability, Diversability and Legal Change*, The Hague: Martinus Nijhoff Publishers.

——(2000) *Help*, Birmingham: Venture Press.

——(2004) Social models of disability and other life strategies, *Scandinavian Journal of Disability Research*, 6(1): 8–21.

——(2005a) The social context of reproductive choice, in D. Wasserman, J. Bickenbach and R. Wachbroit (eds) *Quality of Life and Human Difference: Genetic Testing, Health Care, and Disability*, Cambridge: Cambridge University Press.

——(2005b) Disability, genetics and global justice, *Social Policy and Society*, 4(1): 87–95.

——(2010) It's the economy, stupid! The ironic absence of class analysis in British disability studies, in A. Matsui *et al.* (eds) *Creating a Society for All: Disability and Economy*, Leeds: Disability Press.

——(2013) Nasty, brutish and short, in J. Bickenbach, F. Feder, and B. Schmitz (eds) *Disability and the Good Human Life*, Cambridge: Cambridge University Press.

Shakespeare, T. and Corker, M. (eds) (2002) *Disability/Postmodernity: Embodying Disability Theory*, London: Continuum.

Shakespeare, T.W. and Erickson, M. (2000) Different strokes: beyond biological essentialism and social constructionism, in S. Rose and H. Rose (eds) *Coming to Life*, New York: Little, Brown.

Shakespeare, T., Gillespie-Sells, K. and Davies, D. (1996) *The Sexual Politics of Disability*, London: Cassell.

Shakespeare, T., Thompson, S. and Wright, M.J. (2009) No laughing matter: medical and social factors in restricted growth, *Scandinavian Journal of Disability Research*, 12(1): 19–31.

Shakespeare, T.W. and Watson, N. (1995) 'Habeamus corpus? Disability studies and the issue of impairment', paper presented at Quincentennial Conference, University of Aberdeen.

——(1997) Defending the social model, *Disability and Society*, 12(2): 293–300.

——(2001a) The social model of disability: an outdated ideology? In S. Barnart and B.M. Altman (eds) *Exploring Theories and Expanding Methodologies: Where Are We And Where Do We Need To Go? Research in Social Science and Disability*, vol. 2, Amsterdam: JAI.

——(2001b) Making the difference: disability, politics and recognition, in G. Albrecht *et al.* (eds) *Handbook of Disability Studies*, Thousand Oaks, CA: Sage.

Shantha, N., Granger, K., Arora, A. and Polson, D. (2009) Women's choice for Down's screening: a comparative experience in three district general hospitals, *European Journal of Obstetrics and Gynaecology and Reproductive Biology*, 146: 61–64.

Sharp, K. and Earle, S. (2002) Feminism, abortion and disability: irreconcilable differences, *Disability and Society*, 17(2): 137–146.

Sheldon, S. and Wilkinson, S. (2001) Termination of pregnancy for reason of foetal disability: are there grounds for a special exception in law? *Medical Law Review*, 9: 85–109.

Sherry, M. (2002) 'If I only had a brain': examining the effects of brain injury in terms of disability, impairment, identity and embodiment, unpublished PhD dissertation, University of Queensland.

——(2010) *Disability Hate Crimes: Does Anyone Really Hate Disabled People?* Avebury: Ashgate.

Shier, M., Graham, J.R. and Jones, M.E. (2009) Barriers to employment as experienced by disabled people: a qualitative analysis in Calgary and Regina, Canada, *Disability and Society*, 24(1): 63–76.

Shildrick, M. (1997) *Leaky Bodies and Boundaries: Feminism, Postmodernism and (Bio) ethics*, London: Routledge.

——(2012) Critical disability studies; rethinking the conventions for the age of postmodernity, in N. Watson, A. Roulstone and C. Thomas (eds) *Routledge Handbook of Disability Studies*, London: Routledge, pp. 30–41.

Sim, A.J., Milner, J., Love, J. and Lishman, J. (1998) Definitions of need: can disabled people and care professionals agree? *Disability and Society*, 13(1): 53–74.

Sin, C.H. (2013) Making disablist hate crime visible: addressing the challenges of improving reporting, in A. Roulstone and H. Mason-Bish (eds) *Disability, Hate Crime and Violence*, London: Routledge.

Sin, C.H., Hedges, A., Cook, C., Mguni, N. and Comber, N. (2009) *Disabled People's Experiences of Targeted Violence and Hostility*, London: Equalities and Human Rights Commission.

Singer, J. (1999) 'Why can't you be normal for once in your life?' From a 'problem with no name' to the emergence of a new category of difference, in M. Corker and S. French (eds) *Disability Discourse*, Buckingham: Open University Press.

Singer, P. (1993) *Practical Ethics*, New York: Cambridge University Press.

Skär, L. and Tam, M. (2001) My assistant and I: disabled children's and adolescents' roles and relationships to their assistants, *Disability and Society*, 16(7): 917–932.

Skär, R.N.L. (2003) Peer and adult relationships of adolescents with disabilities, *Journal of Adolescence*, 26: 635–649.

Skirton, H. and Barr, O. (2007) Influences on the uptake of antenatal screening for Down syndrome: a review of the literature, *Evidence Based Midwifery*, 5(1): 4–9.

——(2010) Antenatal screening and informed choice: a cross-sectional survey of parents and professionals, *Midwifery*, 26: 596–602.

Smart, A. (2003) Reporting the dawn of the post-genomic era: who wants to live forever? *Sociology of Health and Illness*, 25(1): 24–49.

Smith, A. and Twomey, B. (2002) Labour market experience of people with disabilities, *Labour Market Trends*, August: 415–427.

Smith, B. and Sparkes, A.C. (2004) Men, sport and spinal cord injury: an analysis of metaphors and narrative types, *Disability and Society*, 19(6): 613–626.

Smith, N., Middleton, S., Ashton-Brooks, K., Cox, L. and Dobson, B. with Reith, L. (2005) *Disabled People's Costs of Living: 'More Than You Would Think'*, York: Joseph Rowntree Foundation.

Smittkamp, J. (1964) NPF Director's Report, *Paraplegia News*, 17(185): 6.

Snyder, S. and Mitchell, D. (2006) *Cultural Locations of Disability*, Chicago: University of Chicago Press.

Söder, M. (2009) Tensions, perspectives and themes in disability studies, *Scandinavian Journal of Disability Research*, 11(2): 67–81.

Spandler, H. (2004) Friend or foe? Towards a critical assessment of direct payments, *Critical Social Policy*, 79(2): 187–209.

Spriggs, M. and Savulescu, J. (2002) The Perruche judgement and the 'right not to be born', *Journal of Medical Ethics*, 28: 63–64.

Stainton, T. and Boyce, S. (2004) 'I have got my life back': users' experiences of direct payments, *Disability and Society*, 19(5): 443–454.

Stalker, K. (2012) Theorizing the position of people with learning difficulties within disability studies, in N. Watson, A. Roulstone and C. Thomas (eds) *Routledge Handbook of Disability Studies*, London: Routledge.

Stalker, K., Baron, S., Riddell, S. and Wilkinson, H. (1999) Models of disability: the relationship between theory and practice in non-statutory organisations, *Critical Social Policy*, 19(1): 5–29.

Stalker, K. and McArthur, K. (2012) Child abuse, child protection and disabled children: a review of recent research, *Child Abuse Review*, 21: 24–40.

Statham, H., Solomou, W. and Green, J.M. (2001) *When a Baby Has an Abnormality: A Study of Parents' Experiences*, Cambridge: Centre for Family Research.

Stark, S. (2001) Creating disability in the home: the role of environmental barriers in the United States, *Disability and Society*, 16(1): 37–50.

Stockdale, A. (1999) Waiting for the cure: mapping the social relations of human gene therapy research, in P. Conrad and J. Gabe (eds) *Sociological Perspectives on the New Genetics*, Oxford: Blackwell.

Stone, D.A. (1984) *The Disabled State*, Basingstoke: Macmillan.

Stone, E. (1997) From the research notes of a foreign devil: disability research in China, in C. Barnes and G. Mercer (eds) *Doing Disability Research*, Leeds: The Disability Press.

——(1999) Modern slogan, ancient script: impairment and disability in the Chinese language, in M. Corker and S. French (eds) *Disability Discourse*, London: Sage.

Strathclyde Centre for Disability Research and Glasgow Media Unit (2012) *Bad News for Disabled People: How the Newspapers Are Reporting Disability*, Glasgow: Inclusion London and University of Glasgow.

Sunderland, N., Catalano, T. and Kendall, E. (2009) Missing discourses: concepts of joy and happiness in disability, *Disability and Society*, 24(6): 703–714.

Sutherland, A. (1981) *Disabled We Stand*, London: Souvenir Press.

Swain, J. and French, S. (2000) Towards an affirmation model of disability, *Disability and Society*, 15(4): 569–582.

Swain, J., French, S., Barnes, C. and Thomas, C. (eds) (2004) *Disabling Barriers, Enabling Environments*, London: Sage.

Swain, J., French, S. and Cameron, C. (eds) (2003) *Controversial Issues in a Disabling Society*, Buckingham: Open University Press.

Swango-Wilson, A. (2011) Meaningful sex education programs for individuals with intellectual/developmental disabilities, *Sexuality and Disability*, 29: 113–118.

Tajfel, H. (1978) *The Social Psychology of Minorities*, London: Minority Rights Group.

Takala, T. (2009) Gender, disability and personal identity: moral and political problems in community thinking, in K. Kristiansen, S. Vehmas and T. Shakespeare (eds) *Arguing about Disability: Philosophical Perspectives*, London: Routledge.

Taylor, M. (1997) *The Best of Both Worlds: The Voluntary Sector and Local Government*, York: Joseph Rowntree Foundation.

Taylor, S.J. and Bogdan, R. (1989) On accepting relationships between people with mental retardation and non-disabled people: towards an understanding of acceptance, *Disability, Handicap and Society*, 4(1): 21–36.

Thiara, R.K., Hague, G. and Mullender, A. (2011) Losing out on both counts: disabled women and domestic violence, *Disability and Society*, 26(6): 757–771.

Thomas, C. (1998) 'The body and society: impairment and disability', paper presented at BSA Annual Conference: Making Sense of the Body, Edinburgh.

——(1999) *Female Forms: Experiencing and Understanding Disability*, Buckingham: Open University Press.

——(2004a) How is disability understood? *Disability and Society*, 19(6): 563–568.

——(2004b) Rescuing a social relational understanding of disability, *Scandinavian Journal of Disability Research*, 6(1): 22–36.

——(2007) *Sociologies of Disability and Illness: Contested Ideas in Disability Studies and Medical Sociology*, Basingstoke: Palgrave Macmillan.

——(2012) Theorising disability and chronic illness: where next for perspectives in medical sociology? *Social Theory and Health*, 10: 209–228.

Thompson, S., Shakespeare, T. and Wright, M. (2010) Disability and identity across the life course: the restricted growth experience, *Medische Anthropologie*, 22(2): 237–251.

Thomson, R.G.T. (1996) *Extraordinary Bodies: Figuring Physical Disability in American Culture and Literature*, New York: Columbia University Press.

——(2009) *Staring: How We Look*, Oxford: Oxford University Press.

Tiefer, L. (1995) *Sex Is Not a Natural Act*, Boulder, CO: Westview Press.

Tierney, S. (2001) A reluctance to be defined 'disabled': how can the social model of disability enhance understanding of anorexia? *Disability and Society*, 16(5): 749–764.

Timpanaro, S. (1975) *On Materialism*, London: New Left Books.

Trani, J. *et al.* (2010) *Disability In and Around Urban Areas of Sierra Leone*, London: Leonard Cheshire International.

Traustadóttir, R. (1993) The gendered context of friendships, in A.N. Amado (ed.) *Friendship and Community Connections between People with and without Developmental Disabilities*, Baltimore, MD: Paul Brookes Publishing.

——(2000) Friendship: love or work? In R. Traustadóttir and K. Johnson (eds) *Women with Intellectual Disabilities: Finding a Place in the World*, London: Jessica Kingsley Publishers.

——(2001) Research with others: reflections on representation, difference and othering, *Scandinavian Journal of Disability Research*, 3(2): 9–28.

Tregaskis, C. (2004a) *Constructions of Disability: Researching the Interface Between Disabled and Non-Disabled People*, London: Routledge.

——(2004b) Applying the social model in practice: some lessons from countryside recreation, *Disability and Society*, 19(6): 601–612.

Tremain, S. (1998) 'Feminist approaches to naturalizing disabled bodies or, does the social model of disablement rest upon a mistake?', paper presented at Annual Meeting of the Society for Disability Studies, Oakland, CA.

——(2002) On the subject of impairment, in M. Corker and T. Shakespeare (eds) *Disability/Postmodernity: Embodying Disability Theory*, London: Continuum.

——(ed.) (2005) *Foucault and the Government of Disability*, Ann Arbor, MI: University of Michigan Press.

Tremblay, M., Campbell, A. and Hudson, G.L. (2005) When elevators were for pianos: an oral history account of the civilian experience of using wheelchairs in Canadian society. The first twenty-five years: 1945–1970, *Disability and Society*, 20, 2: 103–116.

Tringham, G.M., Nawaz, T.S., Holding, S., Mcfarlane, J. and Lindow, S.W. (2011) Introduction of first trimester combined TET increases uptake of Down's syndrome screening, *European Journal of Obstetrics and Gynecology and Reproductive Biology*, 159: 95–98.

Tronto, J.C. (1993) *Moral Boundaries: A Political Argument for an Ethic of Care*, London: Routledge.

Tsouroufli, M. (2011) Routinisation and constraints on informed choice in a one-stop clinic offering first trimester chromosomal antenatal screening for Down's syndrome, *Midwifery*, 27: 431–436.

Tucker, B.P. (1998) Deaf culture, cochlear implants, and elective disability, *Hastings Center Report*, 28(4): 6–14.

Ungerson, C. (1987) *Policy is Personal: Sex, Gender and Informal Care*, London: Tavistock.

——(1999) Personal assistants and disabled people: an examination of a hybrid form of work and care, *Work, Employment and Society*, 13(4): 583–600.

——(2004) Whose empowerment and independence? A cross-national perspective on 'cash for care' schemes, *Ageing and Society*, 24: 189–212.

——(2005) Care, work and feeling, *Sociological Review*, 53(2): 188–203.

United Nations (1993) *Standard Rules on Equalisation of Opportunities for Disabled Persons*, New York: United Nations.

——(2006) *Convention on the Rights of Persons with Disabilities*, New York: United Nations.

United States Department of Justice (2012) *Crime against Persons with Disabilities 2009–2011: Statistical Tables*, Office of Justice Programmes, Bureau of Justice Statistics, December 2012, NCJ 240299.

UPIAS (1976) *Fundamental Principles of Disability*, London: UPIAS.

Ursic, C. (1996) Social (and disability) policy in the new democracies of Europe (Slovenia by way of example), *Disability and Society*, 11(1): 91–105.

Van den Ven, L., Post, M., de Witte, L. and van den Heuvel, W. (2005) It takes two to tango: the integration of people with disabilities into society, *Disability and Society*, 20(3): 311–329.

Van der Klift, E. and Kunc, N. (1994) 'Hell-bent on helping: benevolence, friendship and the politics of help', available at: www.noormemma.com/arhellbe.htm (accessed 2 September 2004).

Vanier, J. (1999) *Becoming Human*, London: Darton, Longman and Todd.

Vehmas, S. (2002) Parental responsibility and the morality of selective abortion, *Ethical Theory and Moral Practice*, 5: 463–484.

——(2003a) Live and let die? Disability in bioethics, *New Review of Bioethics*, 1(1): 145–157.

——(2003b) The grounds for preventing impairments: a critique, in M. Häyry and T. Takala (eds) *Scratching the Surface of Bioethics*, Amsterdam: Rodopi.

——(2004) Ethical analysis of the concept of disability, *Mental Retardation*, 42(3): 209–222.

——(2010) The who or what of Steve: severe cognitive impairment and its implications, in M. Häyry, T. Takala, P. Herrissone-Kelly and G.Árnason (eds) *Arguments and Analysis in Bioethics*, Amsterdam: Rodopi.

——(2012) What can philosophy tell us about disability? In N. Watson, A. Roulstone and C. Thomas (eds) *Routledge Handbook of Disability Studies*, London: Routledge, pp. 298–309.

Vehmas, S. and Mäkelä, P. (2008) A realist account on the ontology of impairment, *Journal of Medical Ethics*, 34: 93–95.

Vernon, A. (1996) A stranger in many camps: the experience of disabled black and ethnic minority women, in J. Morris (ed.) *Encounters with Strangers: Feminism and Disability*, London: Women's Press.

——(1999) The dialectics of multiple identities and the disabled people's movement, *Disability and Society*, 14(3): 385–398.

Vernon, A. and Qureshi, H. (2000) Community care and independence: self-sufficiency or empowerment? *Critical Social Policy*, 63(2): 255–276.

Wagg, A., Kinrions, M. and Stewart, K. (1995) Cardiopulmonary resuscitation: doctors and nurses expect too much, *Journal of the Royal College of Physicians of London*, 29: 20–4.

Wall, P. (1999) *Pain: The Science of Suffering*, London: Weidenfeld and Nicolson.

Walter-Brice, A., Cox, R., Priest, H. and Thompson, F. (2012) What do women with learning disabilities say about their experiences of domestic abuse within the context of their intimate partner relationships? *Disability and Society*, 27(4): 503–517.

Warren, M.A. (1993) Abortion, in P. Singer (ed.) *A Companion to Ethics*, Oxford: Blackwell.

——(1997) *Moral Status: Obligations to Persons and Other Living Things*, Oxford: Clarendon Press.

Wasserman, D. (2001) Philosophical issues in the definition and social response to disability, in G. Albrecht, K. Seelman and M. Bury (eds) *The Handbook of Disability Studies*, Thousand Oaks, CA: Sage.

Watermeyer, B. (2009) Claiming loss in disability, *Disability & Society*, 24(1): 91–102.

——(2012) Is it possible to create a politically engaged, contextual psychology of disability? *Disability and Society*, 27(2): 161–174.

Watson, N. (2002) Well, I know this is going to sound very strange to you, but I don't see myself as a disabled person: identity and disability, *Disability and Society*, 17(5): 509–523.

——(2003) Daily denials: the routinisation of oppression and resistance, in N. Watson and S. Riddell (eds) *Disability, Culture and Identity*, Harlow: Pearson Education.

——(2012) Researching disablement, in N. Watson, A. Roulstone and C. Thomas (eds) *Routledge Handbook of Disability Studies*, London: Routledge, pp. 93–105.

Watson, N., McKie, L., Hughes, B., Hopkins, D. and Gregory, S. (2004) (Inter)dependence, needs and care: the potential for disability and feminist theorists to develop an emancipatory model, *Sociology*, 38(2): 331–350.

We Are Spartacus (2012) *Responsible Reform*. Available at: www.wearespartacus.org.uk (accessed 13 March 2013).

Weeks, J., Heaphy, B. and Donovan, C. (2001) *Same Sex Intimacies: Families of Choice and Other Life Experiments*, London: Routledge.

Welsby, J. and Horsfall, D. (2011) Everyday practices of exclusion/inclusion: women who have an intellectual disability speaking for themselves? *Disability and Society*, 26(7): 795–808.

Wendell, S. (1996) *The Rejected Body: Feminist Philosophical Reflections on Disability*, New York: Routledge.

Wertz, D. (1998) Eugenics is alive and well, *Science in Context*, 11(3 and 4): 493–510.

Wheeler, M. (2011) Syndrome or difference: a critical review of medical conceptualisations of Asperger's syndrome, *Disability and Society*, 26(7): 839–851.

White-Van Mourik, M. (1994) Termination of a second-trimester pregnancy for fetal abnormality: psychosocial aspects, in A. Clarke (ed.) *Genetic Counselling: Practice and Principles*, London: Routledge.

Wikler, D. (1999) Can we learn from eugenics? *Journal of Medical Ethics*, 25(2): 183–194.

Williams, C., Alderson, P. and Farsides, B. (2002) What constitutes 'balanced' information in the practitioners' portrayals of Down's syndrome? *Midwifery*, 18: 230–237.

Williams, C., Kitzinger, J. and Henderson, L. (2003) Envisaging the embryo in stem cell research: rhetorical strategies and media reporting of the ethical debates, *Sociology of Health and Illness*, 25(7): 793–814.

Williams, C., Sandall, J., Lewando-Hundt, G., Heyman, B., Spencer, K. and Grellier, R. (2005) Women as moral pioneers? Experiences of first trimester antenatal screening, *Social Science and Medicine*, 61: 1983–1992.

Williams, F. (2001) In and beyond New Labour: towards a new political ethics of care, *Critical Social Policy*, 21(4): 467–493.

Williams, G. (1983) The movement for independent living: an evaluation and a critique, *Social Science and Medicine*, 17(15): 1003–1010.

Williams, I. (1989) *The Alms Trade: Charities, Past, Present and Future*, London: Unwin Hyman.

Williams, S.J. (1999) Is anybody there? Critical realism, chronic illness and the disability debate, *Sociology of Health and Illness*, 21(6): 797–819.

Williams, V., Ponting, L. and Ford, K. (2009) 'I do like the subtle touch': interactions between people with learning difficulties and their personal assistants, *Disability and Society*, 24(7): 815–828.

Wilson, A., Riddell, S. and Baron, S. (2000) Welfare for those who can? The impact of the quasi-market on the lives of people with learning difficulties, *Critical Social Policy*, 20(4): 479–502.

Wilson-Kovacs, D., Ryan, M.K., Haslam, A. and Rabinovich, A. (2008) 'Just because you can get a wheelchair in the building doesn't necessarily mean that you can still participate': barriers to the career advancement of disabled professionals, *Disability and Society*, 23(7): 705–717.

Wood Mak, Y.Y. and Elwyn, G. (2005) Voices of the terminally ill: uncovering the meaning of desire for euthanasia, *Palliative Medicine*, 19: 343–350.

Woodin, S. (2006) 'Social relationships and disabled people: the impact of direct payments', unpublished PhD dissertation, University of Leeds.

Woods, S. (2002) Respect for autonomy and palliative care, in H. Ten Have and D. Clark (eds) *The Ethics of Palliative Care*, Buckingham: Open University Press.

——(2005) Respect for persons: autonomy and palliative care, *Medicine Health Care and Philosophy*, 8: 243–253.

Woolf, J. (2010) Cognitive disability in a society of equals, in E.F. Kittay and L. Carlson (eds) *Cognitive Disability and Its Challenge to Moral Philosophy*, Chichester: Wiley-Blackwell.

World Health Organization (1980) *International Classification of Impairments, Disabilities and Handicaps*, Geneva: World Health Organization.

——(2001) *International Classification of Functioning, Disability and Health*, Geneva: World Health Organization.

——(2009) *Violence Prevention: The Evidence*, Geneva: World Health Organization.

——(2011) *World Report on Disability*, Geneva: World Health Organization.

Wotton, R. and Isbister, S. (2010) Sex workers, in R. Shuttleworth and T. Sanders eds) *Sex and Disability: Politics, Identity and Access*, Leeds: The Disability Press.

Wright, B.A. (1960) *Physical Disability: A Psychological Approach*, New York: Harper and Row.

Wright, D. (2011) *Downs: The History of a Disability*, Oxford: Oxford University Press.

Wright, D. and Digby, A. (1996) *From Idiocy to Mental Deficiency: Medical Perspectives on People with Learning Disabilities*, London: Routledge.

Wuthnow, R. (1991) *Acts of Compassion: Caring for Others and Helping Ourselves*, Princeton, NJ: Princeton University Press.

Yamaki, C.K. and Yamazaki, Y. (2004) 'Instruments', 'employees', 'companions', 'social assets': understanding relationships between persons with disabilities and their assistants in Japan, *Disability and Society*, 19(1): 31–46.

Young, D.A. and Quibell, R. (2000) Why rights are never enough: rights, intellectual disability and understanding, *Disability and Society*, 15(5): 747–764.

Young, I.M. (1990) *Justice and the Politics of Difference*, Princeton, NJ: Princeton University Press.

——(1997) Asymmetrical reciprocity: on moral respect, wonder, and enlarged thought, *Constellations*, 3(3): 340–363.

Young, L.L. (2012) Validating difference and counting the cost of exclusion in the lives of people who identify as on the autistic spectrum, *Disability and Society*, 27(2): 291–294.

Zeiler, K. (2005) *Chosen Children? An Empirical Study and a Philosophical Analysis of Moral Aspects of Pre-Implantation Genetic Diagnosis and Germ-Line Gene Therapy*, Linköping: Linköping University Studies in Art and Science.

Zola, I.K. (1989) Towards the necessary universalizing of a disability policy, *The Milbank Quarterly*, 67(suppl. 2, Pt. 2): 401–428.

INDEX